METHODS IN MOLECULAR BIOLOGY

Series Editor
John M. Walker
School of Life and Medical Sciences
University of Hertfordshire
Hatfield, Hertfordshire, UK

For further volumes:
http://www.springer.com/series/7651

For over 35 years, biological scientists have come to rely on the research protocols and methodologies in the critically acclaimed *Methods in Molecular Biology* series. The series was the first to introduce the step-by-step protocols approach that has become the standard in all biomedical protocol publishing. Each protocol is provided in readily-reproducible step-by-step fashion, opening with an introductory overview, a list of the materials and reagents needed to complete the experiment, and followed by a detailed procedure that is supported with a helpful notes section offering tips and tricks of the trade as well as troubleshooting advice. These hallmark features were introduced by series editor Dr. John Walker and constitute the key ingredient in each and every volume of the *Methods in Molecular Biology* series. Tested and trusted, comprehensive and reliable, all protocols from the series are indexed in PubMed.

Antibody-Drug Conjugates

Methods and Protocols

Edited by

L. Nathan Tumey

Department of Pharmacy and Pharmaceutical Sciences, Binghamton University, Binghamton, NY, USA

Humana Press

Editor
L. Nathan Tumey
Department of Pharmacy
and Pharmaceutical Sciences
Binghamton University
Binghamton, NY, USA

ISSN 1064-3745 ISSN 1940-6029 (electronic)
Methods in Molecular Biology
ISBN 978-1-4939-9928-6 ISBN 978-1-4939-9929-3 (eBook)
https://doi.org/10.1007/978-1-4939-9929-3

This Humana imprint is published by the registered company Springer Science+Business Media, LLC, part of Springer Nature.
The registered company address is: 233 Spring Street, New York, NY 10013, U.S.A.

Preface

The design, preparation, and bioanalysis of antibody drug conjugates (ADCs) have become progressively more sophisticated over the past decade. Thanks to the persistence of a handful of research groups, ADCs are now viewed as a proven therapeutic modality for the targeted delivery of chemotherapeutic agents. From the outside, the technology is deceptively simple. A targeting antibody delivers a covalently attached payload to a cell type of interest, wherein the molecule is internalized and lysosomally processed and the payload is released. However, a quick look "under the hood" reveals that the failure rate of ADC discovery programs is not so different than small molecule discovery efforts and that there remain a tremendous number of unknown variables when designing these therapeutic agents. As such, the diversity of ADC technology has exploded over the past 10 years in trying and addressing the shortcomings in first-generation ADCs. ADCs in clinical and preclinical development now employ a dizzying array of technology that spans multiple types of antibody backbones, over a dozen varieties of payload classes, various cleavable and non-cleavable linker chemistries, and numerous conjugation technologies. For the bench-top scientists charged with evaluating and advancing these research programs, the technical hurdles can seem overwhelming. This book has been designed keeping these scientists in mind. We have pulled together a team of authors who are lab-based scientists who have performed many of the key conjugations, bioanalyses, and in vitro assays for the ADCs that are now in advanced preclinical and clinical evaluation. The goal of this book is not to provide an exhaustive list of procedures, but rather to highlight some of the key methodologies that are commonly employed across multiple ADC programs. It is our hope that this book will help to lower the "activation barrier" that is often present when entering a new discipline and will provide a "toolbox" of sorts for the next generation of aspiring ADC scientists who will, no doubt, advance the field into new and exciting therapeutic arenas.

Binghamton, NY, USA *L. Nathan Tumey*

Contents

Contributors

Yilma T. Adem • *Pharmaceutical Development Department, Genentech (A Member of the Roche Group), South San Francisco, CA, USA*
Pragya Adhikari • *Department of Protein Chemistry, Genentech, Inc., South San Francisco, CA, USA*
Yasuaki Anami • *Texas Therapeutics Institute, The Brown Foundation Institute of Molecular Medicine, The University of Texas Health Science Center at Houston, Houston, TX, USA*
Susan L. Bane • *Department of Chemistry, Binghamton University, State University of New York, Binghamton, NY, USA*
Alain Beck • *Pierre Fabre Laboratories, IRPF—Centre d'Immunologie Pierre-Fabre (CIPF), Saint-Julien-en-Genevois, France*
Calvin L. Becker • *Abbvie Inc., North Chicago, IL, USA*
Andrew J. Bessire • *Medicine Design, Pfizer Worldwide R&D, Groton, CT, USA*
Matthew Bird • *Abzena Ltd., Cambridge, UK*
Jeffrey Casavant • *Pfizer, Inc., Groton, CT, USA*
Hsuan-Ping Chang • *Department of Pharmaceutical Sciences, School of Pharmacy and Pharmaceutical Sciences, The State University of New York, University at Buffalo, Buffalo, NY, USA*
Soraya Chapel • *Institut des Sciences Analytiques, CNRS, UMR 5280, Université de Lyon, Villeurbanne, France*
Tak Ian Chio • *Department of Chemistry, Binghamton University, State University of New York, Binghamton, NY, USA*
Sarah Cianférani • *Laboratoire de Spectrométrie de Masse Bio-Organique (LSMBO), IPHC, UMR 7178, Université de Strasbourg, CNRS, Strasbourg, France*
Olivier Colas • *Pierre Fabre Laboratories, IRPF—Centre d'Immunologie Pierre-Fabre (CIPF), Saint-Julien-en-Genevois, France*
Robert J. Duffy • *Abbvie Inc., Redwood City, CA, USA*
Anthony Ehkirch • *Laboratoire de Spectrométrie de Masse Bio-Organique (LSMBO), IPHC, UMR 7178, Université de Strasbourg, CNRS, Strasbourg, France*
Ryan Fleming • *Antibody Discovery and Protein Engineering, Biologic Therapeutics, AstraZeneca, Gaithersburg, MD, USA*
Yannis-Nicolas François • *Laboratoire de Spectrométrie de Masse des Interactions et des Systèmes (LSMIS), UMR 7140 (Unistra-CNRS), Université de Strasbourg, Strasbourg, France*
Mark Frigerio • *Abzena Ltd., Cambridge, UK*
Rabah Gahoual • *Laboratoire Vecteurs Pour l'Imagerie Moléculaire et le Ciblage Thérapeutique (VICT), Faculté de Pharmacie, Université Paris Descartes, Paris, France*
Jorge Gandarilla • *Abbvie Inc., North Chicago, IL, USA*
Davy Guillarme • *School of Pharmaceutical Sciences, University of Geneva, Geneva, Switzerland; University of Lausanne, Lausanne, Switzerland*
Jianxin Guo • *Pharmaceutical R&D, Pfizer, Inc., Chesterfield, MO, USA*
Linjie Han • *Process Analytical Chemistry, AbbVie Inc., North Chicago, IL, USA*
Jintang He • *Genentech Inc., South San Francisco, CA, USA*

SABINE HEINISCH • *Institut des Sciences Analytiques, CNRS, UMR 5280, Université de Lyon, Villeurbanne, France*

OSCAR HERNANDEZ-ALBA • *Laboratoire de Spectrométrie de Masse Bio-Organique (LSMBO), IPHC, UMR 7178, Université de Strasbourg, CNRS, Strasbourg, France*

ADRIAN D. HOBSON • *Abbvie Global Biologics, AbbVie Bioresearch Center, Worcester, MA, USA*

SURINDER KAUR • *Genentech Inc., South San Francisco, CA, USA*

EMMANUELLE LEIZE-WAGNER • *Laboratoire de Spectrométrie de Masse des Interactions et des Systèmes (LSMIS), UMR 7140 (Unistra-CNRS), Université de Strasbourg, Strasbourg, France*

GAOYUAN LU • *School of Pharmacy, China Pharmaceutical University, Nanjing, Jiangsu, People's Republic of China*

MICHAEL J. MCPHERSON • *Abbvie Global Biologics, AbbVie Bioresearch Center, Worcester, MA, USA*

VAMSI KRISHNA MUDHIVARTHI • *Pharmaceutical R&D, Pfizer, Inc., Chesterfield, MO, USA*

DURGESH V. NADKARNI • *Pfizer Inc., Chesterfield, MO, USA*

WENJING NING • *Process Analytical Chemistry, AbbVie Inc., North Chicago, IL, USA*

JOAO NUNES • *Abzena Ltd., Cambridge, UK*

HELÉN NYHLÉN • *Genovis AB, Lund, Sweden*

RACHANA OHRI • *Department of Protein Chemistry, Genentech, Inc., South San Francisco, CA, USA*

FREDRIK OLSSON • *Genovis AB, Lund, Sweden*

SUJIET PUTHENVEETIL • *AbbVie Bioresearch Center, R&D, Worcester, MA, USA; Pfizer, Inc., Groton, CT, USA*

ANOKHA S. RATNAYAKE • *Pfizer, Inc., Groton, CT, USA*

STEVEN M. RICHTER • *Abbvie Inc., North Chicago, IL, USA*

FLORENT ROUVIÈRE • *Institut des Sciences Analytiques, Université de Lyon, Villeurbanne, France*

JOSIANE SAADÉ • *Laboratoire de Spectrométrie de Masse des Interactions et des Systèmes (LSMIS), UMR 7140 (Unistra-CNRS), Université de Strasbourg, Strasbourg, France*

JACK SADOWSKY • *Department of Protein Chemistry, Genentech, Inc., South San Francisco, CA, USA*

HUA SANG • *Department of Pharmacy, Affiliated Hospital of Nantong University, Nantong, Jiangsu, People's Republic of China; Key Laboratory of Drug Metabolism and Pharmacokinetics, State Key Laboratory of Natural Medicines, China Pharmaceutical University, Nanjing, Jiangsu, People's Republic of China*

MORGAN SARRUT • *Institut des Sciences Analytiques, Université de Lyon, Villeurbanne, France*

DHAVAL K. SHAH • *Department of Pharmaceutical Sciences, School of Pharmacy and Pharmaceutical Sciences, The State University of New York, University at Buffalo, Buffalo, NY, USA*

JONATHAN SJÖGREN • *Genovis AB, Lund, Sweden*

CHAKRAPANI SUBRAMANYAM • *Medicine Design, Pfizer Worldwide R&D, Groton, CT, USA*

YANG TIAN • *School of Pharmacy, China Pharmaceutical University, Nanjing, Jiangsu, People's Republic of China*

HANNA TOFTEVALL • *Genovis AB, Lund, Sweden*

KYOJI TSUCHIKAMA • *Texas Therapeutics Institute, The Brown Foundation Institute of Molecular Medicine, The University of Texas Health Science Center at Houston, Houston, TX, USA*
L. NATHAN TUMEY • *Department of Pharmacy and Pharmaceutical Sciences, Binghamton University, Binghamton, NY, USA; Pfizer Inc., Groton, CT, USA*
ELSA WAGNER-ROUSSET • *Pierre Fabre Laboratories, IRPF—Centre d'Immunologie Pierre-Fabre (CIPF), Saint-Julien-en-Genevois, France*
NING WAN • *Key Laboratory of Drug Metabolism and Pharmacokinetics, State Key Laboratory of Natural Medicines, China Pharmaceutical University, Nanjing, Jiangsu, People's Republic of China*
GUANGJI WANG • *Key Laboratory of Drug Metabolism and Pharmacokinetics, State Key Laboratory of Natural Medicines, China Pharmaceutical University, Nanjing, Jiangsu, People's Republic of China*
CONG WEI • *Drug Metabolism and Pharmacokinetics, Biogen Inc., Cambridge, MA, USA*
SHENGJIA WU • *Department of Pharmaceutical Sciences, School of Pharmacy and Pharmaceutical Sciences, The State University of New York, University at Buffalo, Buffalo, NY, USA*
KEYANG XU • *Genentech Inc., South San Francisco, CA, USA*
HUI YE • *Key Laboratory of Drug Metabolism and Pharmacokinetics, State Key Laboratory of Natural Medicines, China Pharmaceutical University, Nanjing, Jiangsu, People's Republic of China*
NEELIE ZACHARIAS • *Department of Protein Chemistry, Genentech, Inc., South San Francisco, CA, USA*
QUNYING ZHANG • *Process Analytical Chemistry, AbbVie Inc., North Chicago, IL, USA*
YANQUN ZHAO • *Process Analytical Chemistry, AbbVie Inc., North Chicago, IL, USA*

Chapter 1

An Overview of the Current ADC Discovery Landscape

L. Nathan Tumey

Abstract

The prototypical ADC mechanism involving antigen-mediated uptake and lysosomal release is both elegantly simple and scientifically compelling. However, recent clinical-stage failures have prompted a reevaluation of this delivery paradigm and have resulted in an array of new technologies that have the potential to improve the safety and efficacy of up and coming programs. These innovations can generally be categorized into seven areas that will be elaborated on in this chapter: (1) Exploiting new payload mechanisms; (2) Increasing the drug–antibody ratio (DAR); (3) Increasing the antibody penetration; (4) Overcoming ADC resistance mechanisms; (5) Increasing the efficiency of ADC uptake and processing; (6) Mitigating off-target payload exposure; and (7) Employment of noncytotoxic payloads. It is our belief that these seven areas capture the current "landscape" of innovations that are taking place in the design of next-generation ADCs. Together, these advancements are reshaping the ADC field and providing a path forward in the face of the recent clinical setbacks.

Key words ADC, Resistance, Toxicity, Conjugation, DAR, Tumor penetration, Payload

1 Introduction

Drug discovery is not for the faint of heart. As anyone who has spent time in the field knows, promising therapeutic agents in late-stage trials can essentially disappear at a moment's notice after a disastrous clinical report; and drugs that seemed destined for obscurity can suddenly become major blockbusters. For good or for bad, the field of antibody–drug conjugates (ADCs) has proven to be a microcosm of the broader drug-discovery engine. The past 10 years of ADC discovery has seen incredible scientific innovation coupled with massive clinical failures and unexpected successes. The goal of this chapter is to highlight some of the changes in the field in recent years and to offer a "snapshot" of the most promising innovations that are currently being explored.

Typical ADCs consist of three key components: An antibody targeting vehicle, a cytotoxic drug, and a covalent linker that connects the system together. Upon binding to the receptor on the target cell, the ADC is internalized via a clathrin-mediated

L. Nathan Tumey (ed.), *Antibody-Drug Conjugates: Methods and Protocols*, Methods in Molecular Biology, vol. 2078, https://doi.org/10.1007/978-1-4939-9929-3_1,

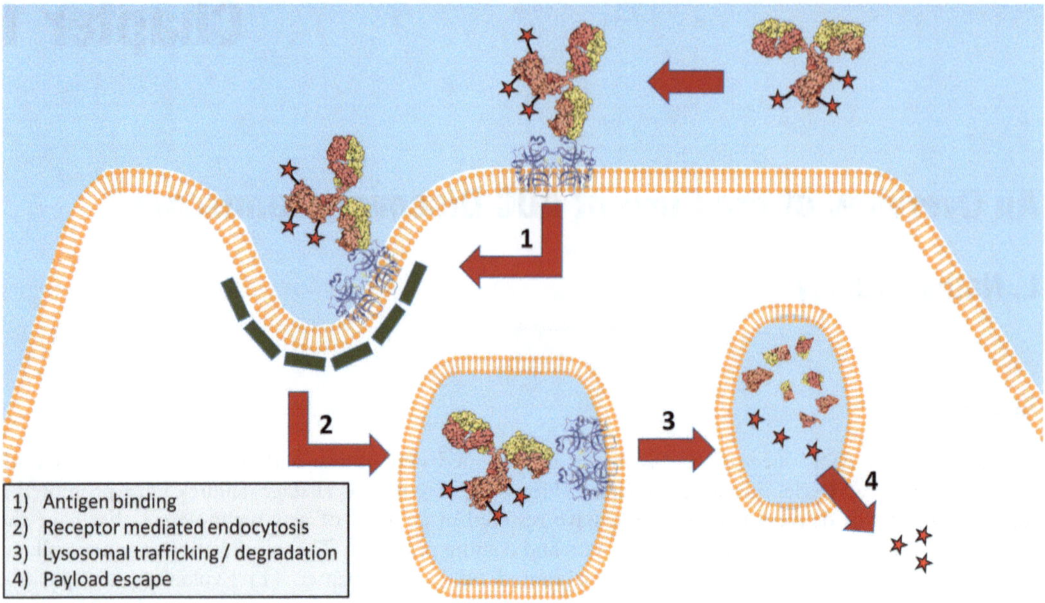

Fig. 1 Prototypical ADC uptake mechanism

endocytosis and trafficked to the lysosome. Lysosomal proteolysis cleaves the covalent linkage between the antibody and payload, thus allowing the payload to escape the lysosome and bind to its intracellular target (Fig. 1). The antibody is designed to target antigens that are uniquely expressed on the tissue of interest, typically cancer cells. Great effort is typically employed to ensure that the selected antigen has minimal expression in normal tissue, especially in highly perfused tissue. The linker is carefully selected to be rapidly cleaved in the lysosome while having minimal cleavage during its extended time in circulation (often 2 weeks or more) [1]. Linker design is also critically important in determining propensity for aggregation and the rate of premature linker cleavage in plasma [1, 2]. The ADC payload must be exquisitely potent due to the limited number of receptor interactions that are possible at a given time. Note that unlike passive diffusion, the rate of drug entry into the cell is easily saturated once all receptors have been engaged with an antibody partner. Thus, it is typically believed that only low-nM intracellular concentrations of active drug can be realized using ADC technology. Once the payload is released from the antibody (depending on its physical properties) it has the potential to freely diffuse through the cell membrane and affect nearby non-antigen expressing cells thus inducing the so-called bystander activity.

The above description represents the idealized scenario and deliberately neglects to mention many of the key "unknowns" in the field where innovation is most ripe. For the sake of organizing our discussion, we will categorize recent technological innovations into seven areas: (1) Exploiting new payload mechanisms;

(2) Increasing the drug–antibody ratio (DAR); (3) Increasing the antibody penetration; (4) Overcoming ADC resistance mechanisms; (5) Increasing the efficiency of ADC uptake and processing; (6) Mitigating off-target payload exposure; and (7) Employment of noncytotoxic payloads. These areas of innovations are by no means exhaustive and certainly we will not address every technologically interesting advancement that has been reported in recent years. However, it is our belief that these seven areas capture the current "landscape" of innovations that are taking place in the design of next-generation ADCs.

2 Exploiting New Payload Mechanisms

A full discussion of the breadth of cytotoxic payloads employed in ADCs is beyond the scope of this chapter and has been reviewed elsewhere [3]. However, it is worth noting that many of these new classes of payloads are mechanistically related to the present cohort of clinically validated payloads. For example, the clinical success of auristatin and maytansinoid payloads (tubulin-binding agents) has prompted enormous efforts to identify alternative structural classes of molecules that exploit this mechanism. This has resulted in the advancement of tubulysin [4–6], eribulin [7], cryptophycin [8], and cemadotin [9] ADCs, in addition to new structural variants of auristatin [10–12] and maytansinoid payloads [13, 14]. Likewise, the clinical success of calicheamycin ADCs has inspired a new generation of DNA-damaging payloads including uncialamycin [15], pyrrolo[2,1-c] [1, 4] benzodiazepines (PBDs) [16–18], and duocarmycins [19, 20]. While these payloads continue to advance through preclinical and clinical development, recent high-profile failures of multiple ultra-potent DNA damaging ADCs [21, 22] have prompted considerable interest in alternative anti-proliferative mechanisms.

Building on the success of tubulin-binding agents, a team from Beyer reported a series of ADCs that block the activity of kinesin spindle protein (KSP), an ATP-dependent microtubule motor that is involved in the separation of centrosomes during mitosis [23]. Interestingly, in spite of the presence of an obvious amine handle for linker conjugation, these payloads were initially attached by a noncleavable linker to a maleimide conjugation handle. (*ADC1*) Conjugation via endogenous cysteine residues resulted in DAR3-4 ADCs that exhibited sub-nM potency against antigen expressing cell lines. While not explicitly stated, a design theme for this series of ADCs seems to be the delivery of an impermeable payload that minimizes bystander activity while maximizing intracellular payload concentration. As such, a cleavable ADC (*ADC2*) was designed to release a highly polar zwiterionic lysine-adduct, as shown in Fig. 2. Indeed, the released species for these ADCs were

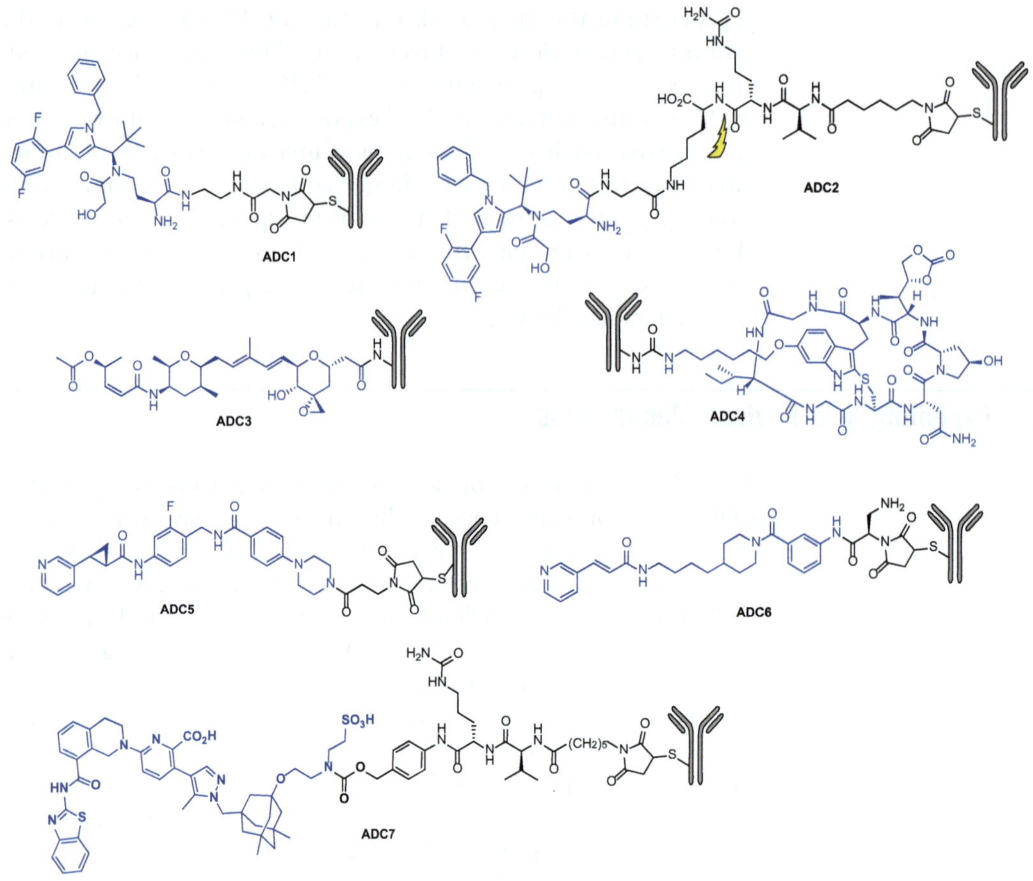

Fig. 2 Recently disclosed payload classes for use in ADCs

shown to be minimally effective in a cytotoxicity assay in spite of their impressive efficacy as conjugates. Interestingly, both ADCs appear to be designed to release an amino-acid linked payload that is perhaps a substrate of an amino acid transporter that has been speculated to be an important mechanism of lysosomal escape [24].

In 2016, a team from Pfizer reported generating ADCs that deliver a potent RNA splicing inhibitor known as thialanstatin A (also known as spliceostatin) [25]. Unlike auristatins and maytansinoids, these compounds do not have a readily available amine or thiol handle that is suitable for conjugation. Instead, a carboxylic acid on the payload was directly attached to lysine residues of the antibody by a "linker-less" NHS-ester-mediated conjugation. (*ADC3*) Similar to early-generation auristatin ADCs, the loading was found to significantly impact the efficacy. The optimal efficacy was observed with an ADC with a DAR of 3.2. Both high-loaded (DAR 4.2) and low-loaded (DAR 2.2) ADCs were less efficacious. Interestingly, a later report showed that the hinge-cysteine conjugated thialanstatin A resulted in quite weak in vivo efficacy. Thus, in order to retain the lysine-based conjugation method, a site-specific method that employed multivalent peptidic linkers was reported [26]. In short, a small lysine-containing peptide was allowed to react with the NHS-activated thialanstatin and subsequently "clicked" into place using a site-specific azide handle. The resulting homogeneous DAR4 thialanstatin conjugates exhibited efficacy in a Her2 model at doses as low as 1.5 mg/kg. Interestingly, while prior reports of site-specific conjugation methods typically focus on stability and metabolism issues [27], this report shows that site of conjugation can play a significant role in in vitro cytotoxicity. Presumably this is due to site-dependent lysosomal catabolism, similar to the mechanism reported by Bessire [28].

Continuing with the theme of blocking RNA processing, a number of reports have emerged describing inhibitors of RNA polymerase, the key enzyme responsible for the formation of mRNA. The centrality of this mechanism for all biological processes suggests that RNA polymerase inhibitors will have toxicity across both proliferating and quiescent cells. The most well-studied of the RNA polymerase inhibitors are toxins derived from the *Amanita* genus of mushrooms, known collectively as amatoxins. An early amatoxin linked to an anti-EpCAM antibody exhibited efficacy in a pancreatic cancer line following a 2 mg/kg dose, but exhibited severe toxicity at doses of 6 mg/kg and higher [29]. Building on this work, a number of patents have now been filed on amanatin-based ADCs, such as the one shown in Fig. 2 [30–32] (*ADC4*). While amanatin ADCs (like their small-molecule payloads) have been known to exhibit severe toxicity, a serendipitous observation reported in 2015 may render a path forward for this class of molecules. A well-known tumor suppressor gene known as TP53 is frequently found to be deleted in human tumors, thus leading to uncontrolled cell growth. A key subunit of RNA polymerase, known as POLR2A, is a genetic neighbor of TP53, and is frequently downregulated in hemizygous TP53 deletions, thus rendering the cells hypersensitive to RNA polymerase inhibitors [33]. Thus, amatoxin-ADCs may be particularly useful in TP53-downregulated tumors.

In a move away from mitotic and transcriptional inhibitors, teams from Novartis and Seattle Genetics simultaneously disclosed ADCs designed to block cellular metabolism by inhibiting the formation of nicotinamide adenine dinucleotide (NAD^+) [34, 35]. The ADCs, shown in Fig. 2 (*ADC4* and *ADC5*), deliver potent inhibitors of nicotinamide phosphoribosyltransferase (NAMPT), a critical enzyme involved in the biosynthesis of NAD^+. Unlike some of the aforementioned mechanisms, inhibitors of NAMPT were demonstrated to be cytotoxic irrespective of the mitotic state of the cells. Perhaps most importantly, a null-targeted version of *ADC5* was shown to be well tolerated in rats at doses of up to 100 mg/kg—well above the dose that is typically tolerated by

DNA-damaging and tubulin-binding ADCs. Efficacy was reported in a variety of tumor xenograft models at doses of 10–20 mg/kg.

Rather than directly blocking an essential metabolic pathway, a recent report demonstrates an interesting approach to sensitize cells to apoptosis by inhibiting an anti-apoptotic protein known as Bcl-x_L. While the specific details have not yet been published, the team from AbbVie has reported a series of ADCs, exemplified by *ADC7*, which enhance the activity of docetaxel at doses of 3–10 mg/kg [36, 37]. Importantly, these ADCs do not appear to result in thrombocytopenia, a common side effect of Bcl-x_L inhibitors that have been evaluated in the clinic. Given the immense progress in our understanding of cell signaling in recent years, agents that induce apoptosis and autophagy are certain to become more widely explored as ADC payloads.

2.1 Increasing the Drug–Antibody Ratio (DAR)

Based on the classical ADC mechanism outlined in Fig. 1, it is clear that the intracellular drug concentration will be related to the number of receptors that are able to engage with an ADC. Low numbers of receptors will naturally result in low cellular uptake. In order to compensate for this, a classical approach has been to increase the drug–antibody ratio (DAR) in order to maximize the number of drugs that are delivered per binding event. This can naturally lead to examples of the so-called super-stoichiometric activity, wherein a modest increase in drug loading can lead to a dramatic increase in biological activity. One example of this can be seen in the 2011 report from Zhao in which an increase in the loading of a maytansinoid conjugate by 2.5-fold led to an increase in the in vitro ADC activity by approximately 50-fold [38]. An even more dramatic example can be seen in the aforementioned thailanstatin ADCs in which increasing the loading of an anti-Her2 conjugate from ~1.6 to 4.5 increased the in vitro cytotoxicity against a moderate-expresser (MDA-MB-361-DYT2) by approximately 2500-fold. These examples illustrate the benefits of increasing the drug loading [25].

However, based on the seminal work of Hamblett [39], it has long been known that increasing the drug loading often has an adverse effect on pharmacokinetic exposure. For this reason, the vast majority of clinical-stage ADCs has employed ADCs with DAR values of ~2-4. However, the past 5 years has seen a dramatic shift in this paradigm due to advances in our understanding about how biophysical properties of ADCs impact their PK. Hydrophobicity has been found to be a key driver of these findings. A fascinating example of this was reported in 2015 by Lyon. In this study, the authors incorporated a glycolytic-release chemistry and a PEG chain within the linker (*ADC8*) in order to "mask" the hydrophobicity of the MMAE payload (Fig. 3) [10]. In doing so, they were able to develop a DAR8 ADC that had equivalent pharmacokinetics to the naked antibody. This has now become a common strategy

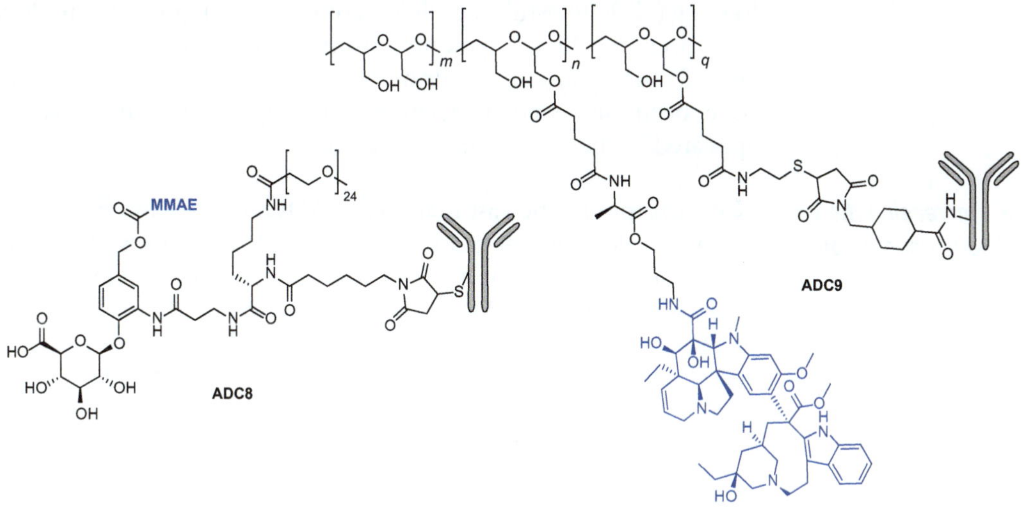

Fig. 3 Strategies for increasing the DAR of ADCs by maximizing the polarity of the linker (*ADC8*) and by incorporating polymeric linkers (*ADC9*)

and DAR8 intra-chain cysteine ADCs are now routinely used provided that the linker-payload is sufficiently polar to prevent accelerated clearance [35, 40, 41]. Additionally, a variety of chemical strategies have been used to incorporate polar functional groups into the linker with the explicit goal of decreasing the hydrophobicity of the ADC. This includes the incorporation of phosphates [42, 43], sulfates [38], tertiary amines [44], and quaternary amines [6].

While it is now commonly known that polar functionality in the linker can "mask" the hydrophobicity of a payload, it is less commonly known that the site of conjugation can have a dramatic impact on ADC hydrophobicity. Several recent studies have recently demonstrated that carefully chosen sites of conjugation can allow for the attachment of very hydrophobic payloads with minimal impact on hydrophobicity, as measured by HIC [27, 45, 46]. Using these sites, conjugates with DAR as high as eight has been achieved with a minimal impact on PK [46]. It should be noted that these sites have the potential to be useful locations for the attachment of dendrimeric or polymeric linkers, as described below.

Using the polar linker technology described above, a maximal DAR of 8 can be achieved using endogenous cysteine residues. However, an alternative strategy has been developed in which a dendrimeric or polymeric linker is used in order to increase the loading far beyond eight. Interestingly, this strategy was first reported back in 1991—long before the current cohort of clinical ADCs had been developed [47]. More recently, a team from Mersana has developed a poly-1-hydroxylmethylethylene hyrdoxymethylformal (PHF) linker that can be tuned for various levels of loading (*ADC9*). Multiple clinical conjugates using this technology have been developed, typically loading ~20 payloads per antibody (Fig. 3) [48]. Related dendrimeric and polymeric linker strategies have been discussed at scientific meetings, but none have yet appeared in the peer-reviewed literature.

2.2 Increasing the Antibody Penetration

Not surprisingly, the vast majority of ADCs in the clinic are targeting hematological malignancies. Without doubt, this is due to the easy tissue access that ADCs have to the circulatory system upon IV dosing. However, as ADC technology has matured, it is becoming increasingly common to target solid tumors. In order for ADCs to access the solid tumor, they must diffuse into the appropriate tissue prior to engaging with the cell-surface antigen—not a small task considering that many tumors are poorly vascularized. Thus, the recent failures of many ADCs for solid tumors indications is frequently attributed to poor tumor penetration. For this reason, there has been significant effort in recent years to move away from full-size antibodies (150 kd) to smaller antibody-like fragments (10–50 kd) that may offer improved tissue penetration.

While the impetus for this move to smaller antibody fragments is logical, a recent report provides quantitative support for this strategy by showing evidence that tissue distribution of antibody fragments is inversely proportional to molecular weight [49]. Thus, there have been several recent reports of Fab (50 kd), scFv (25 kd), and nanobody (15 kd) conjugates designed to improve tumor penetration [50–54]. While the decreased size of the protein certainly improves tissue exposure, the plasma half-life and the overall exposure is typically reduced considerably due to two factors: (1) Loss of FcRN-recycling and (2) Increased renal filtration. There have been a variety of approaches for overcoming these issues, including fusion with serum albumen, conjugation to dextran, and attachment of large PEG modifiers [55]. However, these approaches all result in a significantly increased size thus negating much of the diffusion advantage that initiated the use of antibody fragments in the first place.

Thus, various "hybrid" approaches have been recently developed that may address this limitation. For example, Schneider describes the generation of ScFvs that are dosed in a biodegradable hydrogel. The increased size of the hydrogel prevents renal filtration, thus increasing the half-life from 4 h (scFv) to 2 days (scFv-hydrogel). As the hydrogel degrades, the ScFv is released into circulation and enabling tissue penetration—as demonstrated by the high volume of distribution compared to a typical mAb [56]. As an alternative approach, even smaller single-chain antibody fragments known as "nanobodies" (~15 kd) have been linked to albumin-binding domains in order to prolong the half-life [54]. While these approaches have generally only been described for unmodified scFvs and nanobodies, they no doubt will be useful approaches for drug-conjugated scFvs and nanobodies as well.

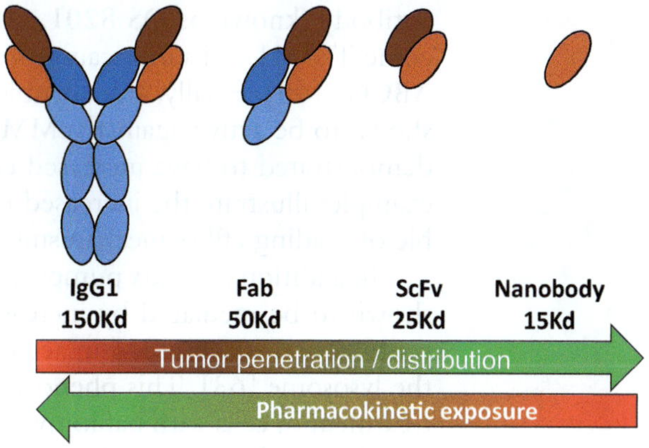

Fig. 4 Relationship between protein size and PK/distribution

2.3 Overcoming ADC Resistance Mechanisms

Resistance to ADC therapy is mediated by a number of factors including downregulation of antigen expression, changes in ADC trafficking pathways, impaired lysosomal processing, increased expression of efflux pumps, and altered apoptotic signaling pathways. These mechanisms have been reviewed elsewhere and a full discussion of them is beyond the scope of this chapter [24, 57]. Rather, we wish to highlight a few examples of ADC-design strategies that have been reported for overcoming these resistance mechanisms (Fig. 4).

Many chemotherapeutic agents are actively effluxed from cells by a variety of pumps such as MDR1 (PGP), BCRP, and MRP1. As such, it is hardly surprising that ADC efficacy has been shown to be impacted by these same efflux mechanisms. For example, Loganzo demonstrated that a MDA-MB-361-DYT2 cell line continuously exposed to low levels of T-DM1 (trastuzumab DM1) developed resistance via increased expression of MRP1 [58]. Similar experiments employing brentuximab vedotin (anti-CD30 vcMMAE) resulted in a resistant cell line with increased expression of MDR1 [59]. The authors went on to show that several tumor samples isolated from patients who had become resistant to brentuximab vedotin exhibited measurable levels of MDR1, MRP1, and MRP3. Based on these (and related) studies, there have been significant efforts to design ADCs that are less susceptible to resistance induced by efflux mechanisms. One of the earliest strategies to address this issue involved attachment of a sulfate or PEG chain to the linker of a maytansinoid payload thus rendering the ADC more potent against MDR1-expressing cell lines [38, 60]. Alternatively, there have been significant efforts to design ADC payloads that are inherently resistant to efflux. For example, there is growing interest in tubulysin ADCs in spite of its mechanistic and physiochemical similarity to existing tubulin-binding payloads, thanks to its well-known resistance to PGP efflux [4, 5, 61] (*ADC10*). Likewise, an exatecan topoisomerase I inhibitor attached to a Her2 antibody (known as DS-8201, *ADC11*) has been shown to overcome T-DM1 resistance caused by overexpression of ABCC2 and ABCG2 [40]. Finally, a doxorubicin conjugate (*ADC12*) has been shown to be active against vcMMAE-resistant cells lines that were demonstrated to have increased expression of MDR1 [62]. These examples illustrate the increased interest in payloads that are capable of evading efflux mechanisms.

In addition to efflux pumps, resistance to T-DM1 has also been shown to be mediated by increased lysosomal pH and decreased protease activity resulting in accumulation of unprocessed ADC in the lysosome [63]. This phenotype could be recapitulated by pretreatment of cells with bafilomycin, a well-studied V-ATPase inhibitor that results in neutralization of lysosomal pH. The mechanism of T-DM1 catabolism has been studied in depth and is known to require total antibody proteolysis in order to release the active lysine-linked DM1. In contrast, the widely utilized mcValCitPABC-MMAE ("vcMMAE") system only requires a single proteolysis event (cleavage of ValCit-PAB) in order to release the active MMAE payload. Therefore, it follows that vcMMAE ADCs may be less susceptible to resistance mechanisms that involve defects in lysosomal processing. Indeed, a recent report demonstrates that T-DM1 resistance can be overcome through the use of an analogous ADC with a proteolytically cleavable linker [64]. In this light, it is interesting to note recent study showing that cathepsin is not required for the lysosomal cleavage of the ever-popular ValCit linker, suggesting that multiple lysosomal proteases can cleave peptidic linkers and therefore resistance to ADCs is unlikely to be mediated by a single mutant protease [65]. While not demonstrated yet in the literature, it is also conceivable that cell lines with decreased lysosomal protease activity may still be susceptible to ADCs that employ peptidic linkers attached at highly exposed sites or ADCs that employ linkers with alternative cleavage mechanisms, such as glucuronidase or phosphatase-mediated cleavage [27, 42, 66].

Finally, a significant factor in ADC resistance is decreased antigen expression and/or decreased lysosomal trafficking. Decreased antigen expression certainly arises from the fact that antigen expression in tumor tissue is notoriously heterogeneous. Cells with low antigen expression can evade ADC-mediated toxicity and over time can become the predominant cell type. In order to prevent the outgrowth of low-antigen expressing cells, a permeable payload can be employed that diffuses from high-antigen tissues into adjacent low-antigen tissues. This so-called bystander effect has been effectively employed to target heterogeneous cell populations [67]. Rather than reducing antigen expression, some cell types have developed resistance by decreased efficiency of lysosomal trafficking. This can potentially be overcome by co-targeting antigens (using a bispecific antibody) that are known to be rapidly internalized and trafficked to the lysosome, such as APLP2 [68]. This strategy is also useful for generally increasing the potency and efficacy of ADCs, and will therefore be discussed in Subheading 2.4.

2.4 Increasing the Efficiency of ADC Uptake and Processing

While the canonical ADC internalization mechanism elegantly shuttles the antigen-antibody complex from the cell surface directly to the lysosome, the reality is far more complex. For example, in 2004 Austin demonstrated that Her2 is constitutively endocytosed and recycled—and only a fraction of antibody-bound Her2 makes its way to the lysosome [69]. Interestingly, the authors of this study showed that geldanamycin increased the proportion of Her2 trafficked to the lysosome—ultimately resulting in lower surface expression of Her2. This result demonstrates that intracellular ADC trafficking can have a significant impact on lysosomal uptake and payload release.

Building on this result, there have been a number of strategies reported over the past 5 years that aim to increase lysosomal uptake. For example, a team from AstraZeneca reported a biparatropic-ADC that targets two different domains of Her2 [5]. The authors claim that the dual-targeting mechanism results in "clustering" of Her2 receptors and improved internalization. Rather than cross-linking receptors, several other teams have employed bispecific antibodies (or other dual-targeting approaches) that bind both to a tumor-specific antigen and to an antigen that is known to be efficiently internalized or lysosomally trafficked. For example, Strop reports a bispecific antibody in which one arm targets Her2, an antigen known to be highly expressed on various breast cancers, and one arm targets APLP2, a low-expressing antigen that is efficiently trafficked to the lysosome [68]. In a related approach, Goeij reported a bispecific antibody in which one arm bound Her2 and a second arm bound CD63, a membrane-bound protein (also known as LAMP1) that is typically found in endosomes and lysosomes [70]. The authors showed that the bispecific ADC was more potent than either monospecific ADC in a moderate-expressing SK-OV-3 cell line. Likewise, Adreev reports a bispecific antibody in which one arm binds Her2 and one arm binds prolactin receptor (PRLR), a protein expressed in breast tissue and known to be efficiently internalized and trafficked to the lysosome [71]. Once again, the authors found that the activity of the bispecific conjugate was greatly enhanced as compared with the monospecific Her2 conjugate. Together, these studies illustrate the importance of understanding lysosomal trafficking and paint a path forward for increasing the potency and payload-delivery efficiency of ADCs (Fig. 5) (Table 1).

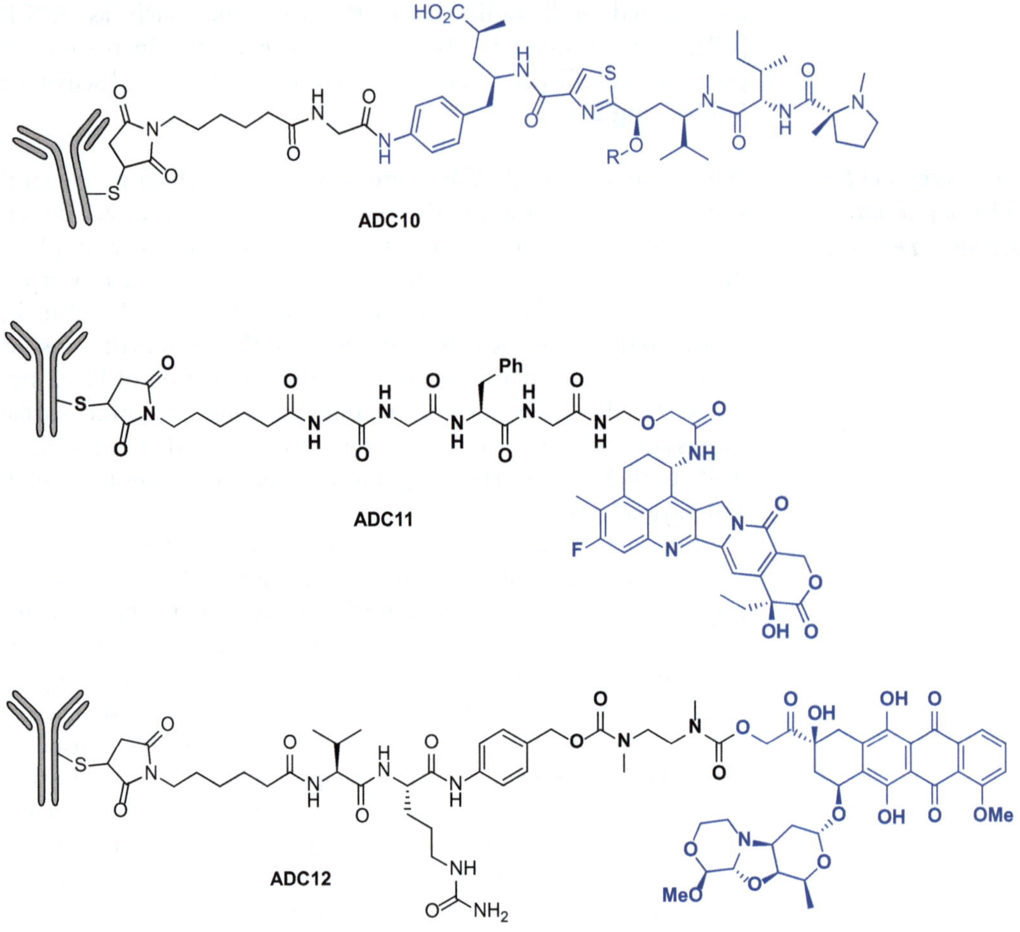

Fig. 5 ADCs employing payloads known to be resistant to efflux pumps

Table 1
Overview of ADC resistance mechanisms and possible strategies for overcoming them

ADC resistance mechanism	Possible pathways for overcoming
PGP efflux	Use of payloads that are inherently resistant to efflux [4, 5, 40, 61] Use of noncleavable linkers that incorporate highly polar features [38, 60]
Decreased lysosomal function	Use of payloads employing easily cleaved proteolytic linkers [64] Attachment at exposed sites that are easily cleaved [27]
Altered antigen uptake	Employment of bispecific antibodies or biparatropic antibodies that are more efficiently internalized and routed to the lysosome [68]
Reduced antigen expression	Use of cell-permeable payloads that can diffuse into adjacent (low expressing) cells [67]

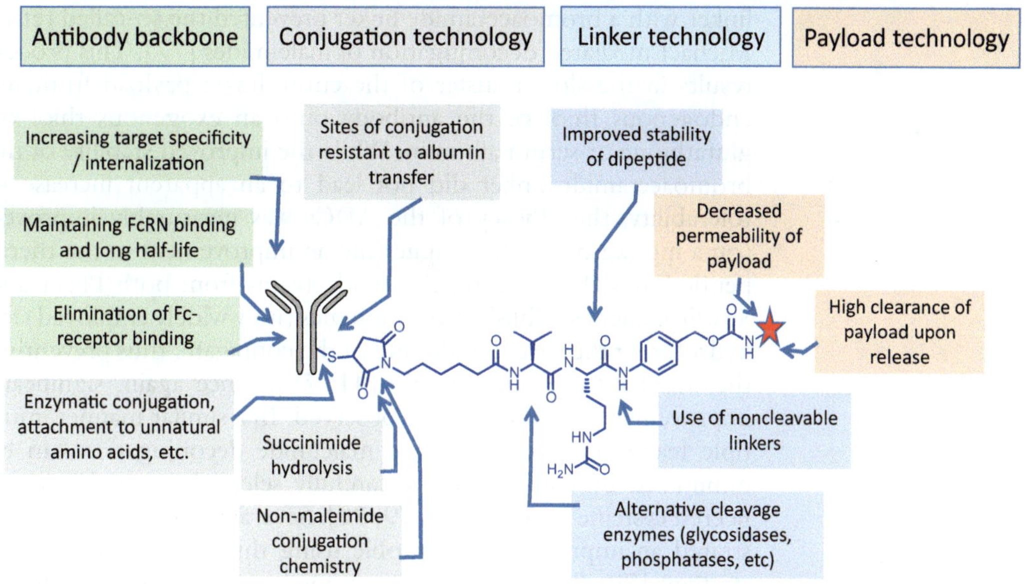

Fig. 6 Overview of methods employed for minimizing toxicity due to premature payload cleavage in circulation

2.5 Mitigating Off-Target Payload Exposure

Certainly the most attractive feature of the ADC mechanism is the ability to restrict the exposure of the cytotoxic payloads to only antigen-expressing tissues. However, as two recent late-stage clinical failures have demonstrated [22, 72], toxicity continues to be a significant hurdle in spite of the targeted delivery mechanism. In some cases, the toxicity appears to be "on-target", that is, mediated by internalization into antigen-expressing cells. For example the skin toxicity observed in a Trop2 ADC from Pfizer is speculated to be due to antigen expression in epithelial tissue [73, 74]. However, for most ADCs, including the two aforementioned late-stage clinical failures, significant toxicity was observed that appeared to be unrelated to the antigen expression. Indeed, several authors have noted that the clinically observed toxicity profile for most ADCs tends to be far more dependent upon the identity of the payload employed rather than on the identity of the antigen target [75, 76]. This strongly suggests that free (untargeted) payload exposure is somehow leading to ADC toxicity in spite of the elegance of the mechanism outlined in Fig. 1. For this reason, a variety of strategies have been introduced in recent years to mitigate nontargeted payload release. While a full discussion of these strategies is beyond the scope of this review, an overview of the methods employed for minimizing and mitigating the effects of premature payload release is outlined in Fig. 6 and the highlights will be discussed below.

Early attempts to minimize free payload exposure focused on improving the stability of the conjugation technology. A seminal study by Alley in 2008 demonstrated that replacing the maleimide linker with a bromoacetamide linker prevented the so-called retro-Michael-mediated deconjugation of maleimides [77]. This process results in the slow transfer of the entire linker-payload from the endogenous thiol of the antibody onto an exogenous thiol on glutathione or serum albumin. While the improved stability of the bromoacetamide linker did not lead to an apparent increase in tolerability, the efficacy of the ADCs was measurably improved (on a mg/kg basis) thus suggesting an improvement in the therapeutic index. Building on this work, teams from both Pfizer and Seattle Genetics published technologies (now widely employed) for hydrolyzing the succinimide ring of the conjugate, thus preventing the transfer to serum albumin [41, 78]. Once again, significant improvements in efficacy were observed. In a similar manner, multiple teams have reported that maleimide deconjugation can be minimized by conjugating to carefully selected genetically engineered cysteine residues [27, 79, 80]. Several reports have demonstrated an improved safety profile using this engineered cysteine strategy [79, 81]. The aforementioned technologies all rely on maleimide chemistry, which is well precedented, kinetically favorable, and versatile. However, the problems associated with deconjugation have prompted a variety of groups to develop cysteine-reactive functional groups that are inherently resistant to deconjugation. These electrophiles include 2-bromomaleimides [82], cyanoethynyl benzenes [83], masked acrylates [84], and heteroaryl sulfones [85].

Taking this strategy a step further, numerous bioconjugation technologies have now been identified that completely move away from cysteine chemistry altogether. For example, Strop and Schibli nearly simultaneously reported an elegant approach for using microbial transglutaminase to attach amine-containing payloads to endogenous or genetically introduced glutamine residues in the antibody backbone, thus linking the payload to the antibody via a highly stable amide linkage [86, 87]. Using related chemistry, a C-terminal LPETGGGGG tag on the antibody serves as a substrate for sortase A, resulting in a transamidation of a payload that is tagged with a poly-glycine peptide linker [88, 89]. Additionally, there have been tremendous strides made in the genetic introduction of unnatural amino acids into antibodies via the amber stop codon (TAG). The most prominent examples of this chemistry use para-azidomethyl-L-phenylalanine (pAMF) and para-acetyl-L-phenylalanine (pAcPhe) [90, 91]. These methods typically rely on a so-called click reaction, which is simply a bio-orthogonal coupling that is kinetically favorable under dilute aqueous conditions [92, 93]. A variety of other related site-specific conjugation approaches have also been described, including conjugation to the glycosyl group [94] and to engineered and endogenous tyrosine residues [95]. The reader is encouraged to consult one of several excellent reviews that have recently provided an overview of site-specific conjugation technology [96, 97].

While the initial goal in developing site-specific conjugation technology was to improve the stability of the maleimide linkage and to improve the homogeneity of the samples, an interesting and unexpected consequence of this new chemistry was the observation that peptide linkers attached at particular sites were subject to cleavage by plasma esterases and/or proteases [87]. This is a significant concern given the ultrapotent toxicity that typically characterizes ADC payloads. Due to the rapid movement of the field towards site-specific conjugation technologies, it is of critical importance to identify the factors that may render a given conjugation site to be prone towards premature linker cleavage and to identify strategies that improve the stability of the linker. Three strategies have emerged to address this premature cleavage: (1) Conjugation at antibody sites that sterically prevent access of the protease or esterase [27, 87]; (2) Optimization of the peptide cleavage element (in particular the P3 pocket) in order to slow down the plasma cleavage rate [98–100]; and (3) the use of non-protease cleavage technologies such as phosphatase and glucuronidase cleavage [42, 101]. Each of these strategies has seen significant preclinical success and many of these technologies have advanced into clinical development.

In spite of the fact that the aforementioned strategies have been applied to multiple clinical-stage programs, payload-mediated toxicity continues to be a significant problem. The two previously mentioned clinical setbacks (SGN-CD33A and Rova-T) both employed some of the strategies outlined above in order to minimize premature payload loss in circulation [22, 72]. In spite of this, significant ADC toxicity prevented the administration of dose levels needed for significant efficacy. Thus, the general consensus in the ADC field is that some of the observed clinical toxicity must be driven by nonspecific (or nonintended) cell-mediated effects—and not purely by prematurely released payload. One possible culprit is receptors that specifically recognize the Fc-domain of the antibody. There are numerous such receptors, the most well-studied of which is the FcγR. Recently, a team from Seattle Genetics showed that the FcγR-binding affinity of an anti-CD30 ADC was partially responsible for the observed efficacy in a solid tumor model [102]. While the focus of the discussion was on the role that FcγR may play in efficacy, it must also be considered as a possible source for premature payload release in macrophages and a possible mechanism of ADC toxicity. With this in mind, it is interesting to note that multiple recent ADC programs have employed antibodies with ablated FcγR binding [5]. Additionally, it should be noted that aglycosyl and deglycosyl IgG1 ADCs (of which several have entered the clinic) have significantly attenuated (or completely attenuated) FcγR binding [103].

One often overlooked, but vitally important, aspect to payload disposition is the fact that antibody clearance takes place via a lysosomal catabolism pathway. Thus, no matter how specific the expression profile is, the ADC will eventually get cleared through nonspecific pinocytosis pathways in endothelial cells. Most ADCs bind to the neonatal Fc receptor (FcRn) at low pH and are effectively recycled upon pinocytosis. This is the mechanism providing the extended half-life for plasma proteins such as IgG1 and serum albumin. Thus, ADCs that have impaired FcRn recycling exhibit a short half-life and, as a consequence, increased toxicity due to more rapid payload release in endothelial tissue [104]. Consequently, one strategy for minimizing ADC toxicity due to nonspecific payload release is to maximize the circulating half-life. Consistent with this data, Lyon and colleagues have shown that hydrophobic ADCs are cleared significantly faster than matched hydrophilic counterparts, thus resulting in increased toxicity [10]. While the mechanism of the clearance for hydrophobic ADCs remains unclear, it is interesting to note that a related study demonstrated that hydrophobicity is inversely correlated with FcRn binding at pH 6. This suggests that the increased clearance observed for hydrophobic ADCs is not due to attenuated FcRn binding [105]. Taken together, these stories strongly indicate that increased ADC clearance is associated with increased off-target toxicity.

Finally, it should be noted that there have been increased efforts to employ payloads with poor permeability in order to minimizing off-target toxicity. Classical small molecule drugs require passive permeability to gain access to the intracellular protein target. In contrast, ADCs gain access via endocytosis and lysosomal uptake. Thus, assuming lysosomal escape, the payload can gain access to the cytoplasm. At this point, permeable payloads may escape from the cell and permeate into nearby tissue (the so-called bystander effect). However, some ADC design efforts have specifically employed impermeable payloads in order to prevent payload escape thus allowing intracellular concentrations to build up [106]. This strategy also has the potential to impact ADC safety—as the payload that is released during normal clearance processes is unable to escape from endothelial cell and may therefore have reduced toxicity in liver and other organs. Additionally, impermeable payloads will not be subject to uptake following extracellular cleavage processes. This is particularly relevant given the recent finding that a secreted protease, neutrophil elastase, may be implicated in ADC-induced neutropenia [107]. Time will tell whether this interesting emerging strategy will have an impact on the therapeutic index of cytotoxic ADCs.

2.6 Employment of Noncytotoxic Payloads

As ADC technology has become increasingly sophisticated and as a variety of in vitro assays are now available for triaging ADCs in development, it should come as no surprise that this technology is now beginning to be explored for a wide variety of therapeutic applications outside of oncology. Rather than elaborating on this concept, the reader is encouraged to move on to Chapter 2 of this book for a complete discussion of these recent developments.

3 Conclusions

The ADC mechanism outlined in Fig. 1 remains both elegantly simple and scientifically compelling in spite of some of the failures and difficulties of recent years, prodded along by a number of recent developments in the field. New payload mechanisms are now being employed that may provide an additional safety margin over existing cytotoxic DNA-damaging payloads. In contrast to just a few years ago, there is now significant interest in administration of high-DAR ADCs that may offer improved efficacy as compared to earlier-generation ADCs. Antibody fragments are being explored to increase the tumor penetration and tissue distribution. Payloads and linkers are being specifically designed to overcome resistance mechanisms. Bispecific ADCs are being employed to increase the efficiency of internalization and lysosomal trafficking. Various strategies have been designed to minimize payload-mediated toxicity in nontargeted cells. Finally, the technology itself (in all these permutations) is being applied towards a wider variety of therapeutic applications than ever could have been envisioned just 5 years ago. Together, we firmly believe that these innovations will have a profound impact on patients and that ADCs will have an increasingly important role to play in the pharmaceutical marketplace.

References

1. Tumey LN, Han S (2018) ADME considerations for the development of biopharmaceutical conjugates using cleavable linkers. Curr Top Med Chem 17:3444–3462. https://doi.org/10.2174/1568026618666180118154017
2. Rago B, Clark T, King L et al (2016) Calculated conjugated payload from immunoassay and LC-MS intact protein analysis measurements of antibody-drug conjugate. Bioanalysis 8:2205–2217. https://doi.org/10.4155/bio-2016-0160
3. Tumey LN (2018) Next generation payloads for ADCs. Humana Press, Cham, pp 187–214
4. Tumey LN, Leverett CA, Vetelino B et al (2016) Optimization of tubulysin antibody-drug conjugates: a case study in addressing ADC metabolism. ACS Med Chem Lett 7:977–982. https://doi.org/10.1021/acsmedchemlett.6b00195
5. Li JY, Perry SR, Muniz-Medina V et al (2016) A biparatopic HER2-targeting antibody-drug conjugate induces tumor regression in primary models refractory to or ineligible for HER2-targeted therapy. Cancer Cell 29:117–129. https://doi.org/10.1016/j.ccell.2015.12.008
6. Burke PJ, Hamilton JZ, Pires TA et al (2016) Development of novel quaternary ammonium linkers for antibody-drug conjugates. Mol Cancer Ther 15:938–945. https://doi.org/10.1158/1535-7163.MCT-16-0038
7. Albone Earl F, Cheng X, Custar Daniel W, et al (2017) Eribulin-based antibody-drug conjugates and methods of use. International patent WO2017151979A1
8. Steinkuhler M. C, Gallinari M. P, Osswald B, et al (2016) Cryptophycin-based antibody-drug conjugates with novel self-immolative

linkers. International Patent WO2016146638A1

9. Bernardes GJL, Casi G, Truessel S et al (2012) A traceless vascular-targeting antibody-drug conjugate for Cancer therapy. Angew Chemie, Int Ed 51:941–944. https://doi.org/10.1002/anie.201106527
10. Lyon RP, Bovee TD, Doronina SO et al (2015) Reducing hydrophobicity of homogeneous antibody-drug conjugates improves pharmacokinetics and therapeutic index. Nat Biotechnol 33:733–736. https://doi.org/10.1038/nbt.3212
11. Maderna A, Doroski M, Subramanyam C et al (2014) Discovery of cytotoxic Dolastatin 10 analogues with N-terminal modifications. J Med Chem 57:10527–10543. https://doi.org/10.1021/jm501649k
12. Geierstanger J, Grunewald B, Yunho OW, et al (2015) Cytotoxic peptides and conjugates thereof. US patent US20160311853
13. Kovtun YV, Audette CA, Mayo MF et al (2010) Antibody-maytansinoid conjugates designed to bypass multidrug resistance. Cancer Res 70:2528–2537. https://doi.org/10.1158/0008-5472.CAN-09-3546
14. Pillow TH, Tien J, Parsons-Reponte KL et al (2014) Site-specific trastuzumab maytansinoid antibody-drug conjugates with improved therapeutic activity through linker and antibody engineering. J Med Chem 57:7890–7899. https://doi.org/10.1021/jm500552c
15. Chowdari NS, Gangwar S, Sufi B (2013) Enediyne compounds, conjugates thereof, and uses and methods thereof. International Patent WO2013122823
16. Jeffrey SC, Burke PJ, Lyon RP et al (2013) A potent anti-CD70 antibody-drug conjugate combining a dimeric pyrrolobenzodiazepine drug with site-specific conjugation technology. Bioconjug Chem 24:1256–1263. https://doi.org/10.1021/bc400217g
17. Saunders LR, Bankovich AJ, Anderson WC et al (2015) A DLL3-targeted antibody-drug conjugate eradicates high-grade pulmonary neuroendocrine tumor-initiating cells in vivo HHS public access. Sci Transl Med 7:302–136. https://doi.org/10.1126/scitranslmed.aac9459
18. Thevanayagam L, Bell A, Chakraborty I et al (2013) Novel detection of DNA-alkylated adducts of antibody-drug conjugates with potentially unique preclinical and biomarker applications. Bioanalysis 5:1073–1081. https://doi.org/10.4155/bio.13.57
19. Carter CA, Waud WR, Li LH et al (1996) Preclinical antitumor activity of bizelesin in mice. Clin Cancer Res 2:1143–1149
20. Chari RVJ, Jackel KA, Bourret LA et al (1995) Enhancement of the selectivity and antitumor efficacy of a CC-1065 analog through immunoconjugate formation. Cancer Res 55:4079–4084
21. Walter RB (2018) Investigational CD33-targeted therapeutics for acute myeloid leukemia. Expert Opin Investig Drugs 27:339–348. https://doi.org/10.1080/13543784.2018.1452911
22. Adams B (2019) AbbVie takes $4B hit on Rova-T failures. https://www.fiercebiotech.com/biotech/abbvie-takes-4b-hit-rova-t-failures. Accessed 18 Feb 2019
23. Lerchen H-G, Wittrock S, Stelte-Ludwig B et al (2018) Antibody-drug conjugates with Pyrrole-based KSP inhibitors as the payload class. Angew Chemie Int Ed 57:15243–15247. https://doi.org/10.1002/anie.201807619
24. Loganzo F, Sung M, Gerber H-P (2016) Mechanisms of resistance to antibody–drug conjugates. Mol Cancer Ther 15:2825–2834. https://doi.org/10.1158/1535-7163.MCT-16-0408
25. Puthenveetil S, Loganzo F, He H et al (2016) Natural product splicing inhibitors: a new class of antibody-drug conjugate (ADC) payloads. Bioconjug Chem 27. https://doi.org/10.1021/acs.bioconjchem.6b00291
26. Puthenveetil S, He H, Loganzo F et al (2017) Multivalent peptidic linker enables identification of preferred sites of conjugation for a potent thialanstatin antibody drug conjugate. PLoS One 12. https://doi.org/10.1371/journal.pone.0178452
27. Tumey LN, Li F, Rago B et al (2017) Site selection: a case study in the identification of optimal cysteine engineered antibody drug conjugates. AAPS J 19. https://doi.org/10.1208/s12248-017-0083-7
28. Bessire AJ, Ballard TE, Charati M et al (2016) Determination of antibody-drug conjugate released payload species using directed in vitro assays and mass spectrometric interrogation. Bioconjug Chem 27:1645–1654. https://doi.org/10.1021/acs.bioconjchem.6b00192
29. Moldenhauer G, Salnikov AV, Lüttgau S et al (2012) Therapeutic potential of amanitin-conjugated anti-epithelial cell adhesion molecule monoclonal antibody against pancreatic carcinoma. J Natl Cancer Inst 104:622–634. https://doi.org/10.1093/jnci/djs140

30. Grunewald J, Jin Y, Ou W, Uno T (2016) Preparation of amatoxin derivatives and their immunoconjugates as inhibitors of RNA polymerase for treating cell proliferative disorders. International patent WO2016071856 A1
31. Mendelsohn BA, Moon SJ (2013) Amatoxin derivatives and cell-permeable conjugates thereof as inhibitors of RNA polymerase. International patent WO2014043403 A1
32. Muller C, Anderl J, Simon W, et al (2014) Amatoxin derivatives. International patent WO2014/135282
33. Liu Y, Zhang X, Han C et al (2015) TP53 loss creates therapeutic vulnerability in colorectal cancer. Nature 520(7549):697–701. https://doi.org/10.1038/nature14418
34. Karpov AS, Abrams T, Clark S et al (2018) Nicotinamide phosphoribosyltransferase inhibitor as a novel payload for antibody-drug conjugates. ACS Med Chem Lett 9:838–842. https://doi.org/10.1021/acsmedchemlett.8b00254
35. Neumann CS, Olivas KC, Anderson ME et al (2018) Targeted delivery of cytotoxic NAMPT inhibitors using antibody-drug conjugates. Mol Cancer Ther 17 (12):2633–2642. https://doi.org/10.1158/1535-7163.MCT-18-0643
36. Tao Z-F, Doherty G, Wang X, et al (2016) Preparation of Bcl-xL inhibitory compounds having low cell permeability and antibody drug conjugates containing them. International patent WO2016094509 A1
37. Ackler SL, Bennett NB, Boghaert ER, et al (2016) Bcl-xl inhibitory compounds and antibody drug conjugates including the same. United States patent US20160158377A1
38. Zhao RY, Wilhelm SD, Audette C et al (2011) Synthesis and evaluation of hydrophilic linkers for antibody maytansinoid conjugates. J Med Chem 54:3606–3623. https://doi.org/10.1021/jm2002958
39. Hamblett KJ, Senter PD, Chace DF et al (2004) Effects of drug loading on the antitumor activity of a monoclonal antibody drug conjugate. Clin Cancer Res 10:7063–7070. https://doi.org/10.1158/1078-0432.CCR-04-0789
40. Ogitani Y, Aida T, Hagihara K et al (2016) DS-8201a, a novel HER2-targeting ADC with a novel DNA topoisomerase I inhibitor, demonstrates a promising antitumor efficacy with differentiation from T-DM1. Clin Cancer Res 22:5097–5108. https://doi.org/10.1158/1078-0432.CCR-15-2822
41. Lyon RP, Setter JR, Bovee TD et al (2014) Self-hydrolyzing maleimides improve the stability and pharmacological properties of antibody-drug conjugates. Nat Biotechnol 32:1059–1062. https://doi.org/10.1038/nbt.2968
42. Kern JC, Cancilla M, Dooney D et al (2016) Discovery of pyrophosphate diesters as tunable, soluble, and bioorthogonal linkers for site-specific antibody-drug conjugates. J Am Chem Soc 138:1430–1445. https://doi.org/10.1021/jacs.5b12547
43. Kern JC, Dooney D, Zhang R et al (2016) Novel phosphate modified cathepsin B linkers: improving aqueous solubility and enhancing payload scope of ADCs. Bioconjug Chem 27:2081–2088. https://doi.org/10.1021/acs.bioconjchem.6b00337
44. Lin R-H, Lin S-Y, Hsieh Y-C, Huang C-C (2014) Hydrophilic self-immolative linkers and conjugates thereof. United States patent US9089614B2
45. Benjamin SR, Jackson CP, Fang S et al (2019) Thiolation of Q295: site-specific conjugation of hydrophobic payloads without the need for genetic engineering. Mol Pharm 16 (6):2795–2807. acs.molpharmaceut.9b00323. https://doi.org/10.1021/acs.molpharmaceut.9b00323
46. Strop P, Delaria K, Foletti D et al (2015) Site-specific conjugation improves therapeutic index of antibody drug conjugates with high drug loading. Nat Biotechnol 33:694–696. https://doi.org/10.1038/nbt.3274
47. Shih LB, Goldenberg DM, Xuan H et al (1991) Anthracycline immunoconjugates prepared by a site-specific linkage via an amino-dextran intermediate carrier. Cancer Res 51:4192–4198
48. Yurkovetskiy AV, Yin M, Bodyak N et al (2015) A polymer-based antibody-vinca drug conjugate platform: characterization and preclinical efficacy. Cancer Res 75:3365–3372. https://doi.org/10.1158/0008-5472.CAN-15-0129
49. Li Z, Krippendorff B-F, Sharma S et al (2016) Influence of molecular size on tissue distribution of antibody fragments. MAbs 8:113–119. https://doi.org/10.1080/19420862.2015.1111497
50. Puthenveetil S, Musto S, Loganzo F et al (2016) Development of solid-phase site-specific conjugation and its application toward generation of dual labeled antibody and fab drug conjugates. Bioconjug Chem 27 (4):1030–1039. https://doi.org/10.1021/acs.bioconjchem.6b00054

51. Woitok M, Klose D, Di Fiore S et al (2017) OncoTargets and therapy Dovepress comparison of a mouse and a novel human scFv-snaP-auristatin F drug conjugate with potent activity against egFr-overexpressing human solid tumor cells. Onco Targets Ther:10–3313. https://doi.org/10.2147/OTT.S140492
52. Pola R, Král V, Filippov SK et al (2019) Polymer cancerostatics targeted by recombinant antibody fragments to GD2-positive tumor cells. Biomacromolecules 20:412–421. https://doi.org/10.1021/acs.biomac.8b01616
53. Deonarain MP, Yahioglu G, Stamati I, Marklew J (2015) Emerging formats for next-generation antibody drug conjugates. Expert Opin Drug Discov 10:463–481. https://doi.org/10.1517/17460441.2015.1025049
54. Bannas P, Hambach J, Koch-Nolte F (2017) Nanobodies and nanobody-based human heavy chain antibodies as antitumor therapeutics. Front Immunol 8:1603. https://doi.org/10.3389/fimmu.2017.01603
55. Patricia Herrington-Symes A, Farys M, Khalili H, Brocchini S (2013) Antibody fragments: prolonging circulation half-life special issue-antibody research. Adv Biosci Biotechnol 4:689–698. https://doi.org/10.4236/abb.2013.45090
56. Schneider EL, Hearn BR, Pfaff SJ et al (2016) Approach for half-life extension of small antibody fragments that does not affect tissue uptake. Bioconjug Chem 27:2534–2539. https://doi.org/10.1021/acs.bioconjchem.6b00469
57. García-Alonso S, Ocaña A, Pandiella A (2018) Resistance to antibody–drug conjugates. Cancer Res 78:2159–2165. https://doi.org/10.1158/0008-5472.CAN-17-3671
58. Loganzo F, Tan X, Sung M et al (2015) Tumor cells chronically treated with a trastuzumab-maytansinoid antibody-drug conjugate develop varied resistance mechanisms but respond to alternate treatments. Mol Cancer Ther 14:952–963. https://doi.org/10.1158/1535-7163.MCT-14-0862
59. Chen R, Hou J, Newman E et al (2015) CD30 Downregulation, MMAE resistance, and MDR1 upregulation are all associated with resistance to brentuximab vedotin. Mol Cancer Ther 14:1376–1384. https://doi.org/10.1158/1535-7163.MCT-15-0036
60. Erickson HK, Lewis Phillips GD, Leipold DD et al (2012) The effect of different linkers on target cell catabolism and pharmacokinetics/pharmacodynamics of trastuzumab maytansinoid conjugates. Mol Cancer Ther 11:1133–1142. https://doi.org/10.1158/1535-7163.mct-11-0727
61. Flygare JA, Pillow T, Staben L (2016) Quaternary amine compounds and antibody-drug conjugates thereof. United States patent US20170232113A1
62. Yu SF, Zheng B, Go M et al (2015) A novel anti-CD22 anthracycline-based antibody-drug conjugate (ADC) that overcomes resistance to auristatin-based ADCs. Clin Cancer Res 21:3298–3306. https://doi.org/10.1158/1078-0432.CCR-14-2035
63. Ríos-Luci C, García-Alonso S, Díaz-Rodríguez E et al (2017) Resistance to the antibody–drug conjugate T-DM1 is based in a reduction in lysosomal proteolytic activity. Cancer Res 77:4639–4651. https://doi.org/10.1158/0008-5472.CAN-16-3127
64. Wang H, Wang W, Xu Y et al (2017) Aberrant intracellular metabolism of T-DM1 confers T-DM1 resistance in HER2-positive gastric cancer cells. Cancer Sci 8(7):1458–1468. https://doi.org/10.1111/cas.13253
65. Pillow TH, Lee B-C, Ma Y et al (2017) Cathepsin B is dispensable for cellular processing of cathepsin B-cleavable antibody–drug conjugates. Cancer Res 77:7027–7037. https://doi.org/10.1158/0008-5472.can-17-2391
66. Kolakowski RV, Haelsig KT, Emmerton KK et al (2016) The methylene Alkoxy carbamate self-immolative unit: utilization for the targeted delivery of alcohol-containing payloads with antibody???Drug conjugates. Angew Chemie - Int Ed 55:7948–7951. https://doi.org/10.1002/anie.201601506
67. Kovtun YV, Audette CA, Ye Y et al (2006) Antibody-drug conjugates designed to eradicate tumors with homogeneous and heterogeneous expression of the target antigen. Cancer Res 66:3214–3221. https://doi.org/10.1158/0008-5472.CAN-05-3973
68. DeVay RM, Delaria K, Zhu G et al (2017) Improved lysosomal trafficking can modulate the potency of antibody drug conjugates. Bioconjug Chem 28(4):1102–1114. acs.bioconjchem.7b00013. https://doi.org/10.1021/acs.bioconjchem.7b00013
69. Austin CD, De Maziè AM, Pisacane PI et al (2004) Endocytosis and sorting of ErbB2 and the site of action of Cancer therapeutics trastuzumab and geldanamycin. Mol Biol Cell 15:5268–5282. https://doi.org/10.1091/mbc.E04
70. de Goeij BE, Vink T, Ten Napel H et al (2016) Efficient payload delivery by a bispecific antibody-drug conjugate targeting

HER2 and CD63. Mol Cancer Ther 15 (11):2688–2697
71. Andreev J, Thambi N, Perez Bay AE et al (2017) Bispecific antibodies and antibody--drug conjugates (ADCs) bridging HER2 and prolactin receptor improve efficacy of HER2 ADCs. Mol Cancer Ther 16:681–693. https://doi.org/10.1158/1535-7163.MCT-16-0658
72. Press release, Seattle Genetics, Inc.; "Seattle genetics discontinues phase 3 CASCADE trial of vadastuximab talirine (SGN-CD33A) in frontline acute myeloid leukemia. http://investor.seattlegenetics.com/news-releases/news-release-details/seattle-genetics-discontinues-phase-3-cascade-trial-vadastuximab. Accessed 7 May 2019
73. King GT, Eaton KD, Beagle BR et al (2018) A phase 1, dose-escalation study of PF-06664178, an anti-Trop-2/Aur0101 antibody-drug conjugate in patients with advanced or metastatic solid tumors. Investig New Drugs 36:836–847. https://doi.org/10.1007/s10637-018-0560-6
74. Strop P, Tran T-T, Dorywalska M et al (2016) RN927C, a site-specific Trop-2 antibody-drug conjugate (ADC) with enhanced stability, is highly efficacious in preclinical solid tumor models. Mol Cancer Ther 15:2698–2708. https://doi.org/10.1158/1535-7163.MCT-16-0431
75. Lyon R (2018) Drawing lessons from the clinical development of antibody-drug conjugates. Drug Discov Today Technol 30:105–109. https://doi.org/10.1016/J.DDTEC.2018.10.001
76. Masters JC, Nickens DJ, Xuan D et al (2018) Clinical toxicity of antibody drug conjugates: a meta-analysis of payloads. Investig New Drugs 36(1):121–135
77. Alley SC, Benjamin DR, Jeffrey SC et al (2008) Contribution of linker stability to the activities of anticancer immunoconjugates. Bioconjug Chem 19:759–765. https://doi.org/10.1021/bc7004329
78. Tumey LNN, Charati M, He T et al (2014) Mild method for succinimide hydrolysis on ADCs: impact on ADC potency, stability, exposure, and efficacy. Bioconjug Chem 25:1871–1880. https://doi.org/10.1021/bc500357n
79. Shen B-Q, Xu K, Liu L et al (2012) Conjugation site modulates the in vivo stability and therapeutic activity of antibody-drug conjugates. Nat Biotechnol 30:184–189. https://doi.org/10.1038/nbt.2108
80. Ohri R, Bhakta S, Fourie-O'Donohue A et al (2018) High-throughput cysteine scanning to identify stable antibody conjugation sites for maleimide- and disulfide-based linkers. Bioconjug Chem 29(2):473–485. https://doi.org/10.1021/acs.bioconjchem.7b00791
81. Junutula JR, Flagella KM, Graham RA et al (2010) Engineered thio-trastuzumab-DM1 conjugate with an improved therapeutic index to target human epidermal growth factor receptor 2-positive breast cancer. Clin Cancer Res 16:4769–4778. https://doi.org/10.1158/1078-0432.CCR-10-0987
82. Nunes JPM, Vassileva V, Robinson E et al (2017) Use of a next generation maleimide in combination with THIOMAB™ antibody technology delivers a highly stable, potent and near homogeneous THIOMAB™ antibody-drug conjugate (TDC). RSC Adv 7:24828–24832. https://doi.org/10.1039/C7RA04606E
83. Kolodych S, Koniev O, Baatarkhuu Z et al (2015) CBTF: new amine-to-Thiol coupling reagent for preparation of antibody conjugates with increased plasma stability. Bioconjug Chem 26:197–200. https://doi.org/10.1021/bc500610g
84. Badescu G, Bryant P, Swierkosz J et al (2014) A new reagent for stable Thiol-specific conjugation. Bioconjug Chem 25:460–469. https://doi.org/10.1021/bc400245v
85. Patterson JT, Asano S, Li X, et al (2015) Improving the serum stability of site-Specific antibody conjugates with Sulfone linkers. Bioconj Chem 25(8):1402–1407
86. Dennler P, Chiotellis A, Fischer E et al (2014) Transglutaminase-based chemo-enzymatic conjugation approach yields homogeneous antibody-drug conjugates. Bioconjug Chem 25:569–578. https://doi.org/10.1021/bc400574z
87. Strop P, Liu S-HH, Dorywalska M et al (2013) Location matters: site of conjugation modulates stability and pharmacokinetics of antibody drug conjugates. Chem Biol 20:161–167. https://doi.org/10.1016/j.chembiol.2013.01.010
88. Stefan N, Gébleux R, Waldmeier L et al (2017) Highly potent, anthracycline-based antibody-drug conjugates generated by enzymatic, site-specific conjugation. Mol Cancer Ther 16:879–892. https://doi.org/10.1158/1535-7163.MCT-16-0688
89. Beerli RR, Hell T, Merkel AS, Grawunder U (2015) Sortase enzyme-mediated generation of site-specifically conjugated antibody drug conjugates with high in vitro and in vivo potency. PLoS One 10(7):e0131177. https://doi.org/10.1371/journal.pone.0131177
90. Zimmerman ES, Heibeck TH, Gill A et al (2014) Production of site-specific antibody-

drug conjugates using optimized non-natural amino acids in a cell-free expression system. Bioconjug Chem 25:351–361. https://doi.org/10.1021/bc400490z

91. Axup Jun Y, Bajjuri Krishna M, Ritland M et al (2012) Synthesis of site-specific antibody-drug conjugates using unnatural amino acids. Proc Natl Acad Sci U S A 109:16101–16106

92. Chio TI, Gu H, Mukherjee K et al (2019) Site-specific bioconjugation and multi-bioorthogonal labeling via rapid formation of a boron–nitrogen heterocycle. Bioconjug Chem 30(5):1554–1564. acs.bioconjchem.9b00246. https://doi.org/10.1021/acs.bioconjchem.9b00246

93. Patterson DM, Prescher JA (2015) Orthogonal bioorthogonal chemistries. Curr Opin Chem Biol 28:141–149. https://doi.org/10.1016/J.CBPA.2015.07.006

94. Qasba PK (2015) Glycans of antibodies as a specific site for drug conjugation using glycosyltransferases. Bioconjug Chem 26:2170–2175. https://doi.org/10.1021/acs.bioconjchem.5b00173

95. Bruins JJ, Westphal AH, Albada B et al (2017) Inducible, site-specific protein Labeling by tyrosine oxidation-strain-promoted (4 + 2) cycloaddition. Bioconjug Chem 28:1189–1193. https://doi.org/10.1021/acs.bioconjchem.7b00046

96. Tsuchikama K, An Z (2018) Antibody-drug conjugates: recent advances in conjugation and linker chemistries. Protein Cell 9:33–46. https://doi.org/10.1007/s13238-016-0323-0

97. Gao W, Zhang J, Xiang J et al (2016) Recent advances in site specific conjugations of antibody drug conjugates (ADCs). Curr Cancer Drug Targets 16:469–479

98. Dorywalska M, Dushin R, Moine L et al (2016) Molecular basis of valine-citrulline-PABC linker instability in site-specific ADCs and its mitigation by linker design. Mol Cancer Ther 15(5):958–970. https://doi.org/10.1158/1535-7163.MCT-15-1004

99. Singh R, Setiady YY, Ponte J et al (2016) A new triglycyl peptide linker for antibody-drug conjugates (ADCs) with improved targeted killing of cancer cells. Mol Cancer Ther 15:1311–1320. https://doi.org/10.1158/1535-7163.MCT-16-0021

100. Anami Y, Yamazaki CM, Xiong W et al (2018) Glutamic acid-valine-citrulline linkers ensure stability and efficacy of antibody-drug conjugates in mice. Nat Commun 9:2512. https://doi.org/10.1038/s41467-018-04982-3

101. Jeffrey SC, Andreyka JB, Bernhardt SX et al (2006) Development and properties of β-Glucuronide linkers for monoclonal antibody-drug conjugates. Bioconjug Chem 17:831–840. https://doi.org/10.1021/bc0600214

102. Li F, Ulrich M, Jonas M et al (2017) Tumor-associated macrophages can contribute to antitumor activity through FcγR-mediated processing of antibody–drug conjugates. Mol Cancer Ther 16(7):1347–1354. https://doi.org/10.1158/1535-7163.mct-17-0019

103. Pawlowski JW, Bajardi-Taccioli A, Houde D et al (2018) Influence of glycan modification on IgG1 biochemical and biophysical properties. J Pharm Biomed Anal 151:133–144. https://doi.org/10.1016/j.jpba.2017.12.061

104. Hamblett KJ, Le T, Rock BM et al (2016) Altering antibody-drug conjugate binding to the neonatal fc receptor impacts efficacy and tolerability. Mol Pharm 13:2387–2396. https://doi.org/10.1021/acs.molpharmaceut.6b00153

105. Brachet G, Respaud R, Arnoult C et al (2016) Increment in drug loading on an antibody--drug conjugate increases its binding to the human neonatal fc receptor in vitro. Mol Pharm 13:1405–1412. https://doi.org/10.1021/acs.molpharmaceut.6b00082

106. Brandish PE, Palmieri A, Antonenko S et al (2018) Development of anti-CD74 antibody–drug conjugates to target glucocorticoids to immune cells. Bioconjug Chem 29:2357–2369. https://doi.org/10.1021/acs.bioconjchem.8b00312

107. Zhao H, Gulesserian S, Malinao MC et al (2017) A potential mechanism for ADC-induced neutropenia: role of neutrophils in their own demise. Mol Cancer Ther 16:1866–1876. https://doi.org/10.1158/1535-7163.MCT-17-0133

Chapter 2

Pushing the Envelope: Advancement of ADCs Outside of Oncology

Michael J. McPherson and Adrian D. Hobson

Abstract

The majority of ADCs in preclinical and clinical development are for oncology indications where cytotoxic payloads are targeted to antigen-expressing cancer cells. However, the modulation of pathogenic cellular activity via ADC-mediated delivery of bioactive small molecules is also an attractive concept for non-oncology indications leading to an expanded application of the technology. Here we summarize those ADCs that have been described so far for non-oncology applications and which cover a variety of payload mechanisms beyond cell killing, from early in vitro proof-of-concept experiments to clinical trials. As our understanding of ADC technology continues to grow, it is anticipated that the development of ADCs as therapeutics for disease areas outside of oncology will also increase.

Key words Non-oncology ADC, Anti-inflammatory, Glucocorticoid, Antibiotic, Payload, Antibody drug conjugate, Inflammatory disease

1 Introduction

There has been significant effort within oncology research to harness the potential of antibody drug conjugates (ADCs) as targeted therapeutics. Guided delivery of cytotoxic payloads to widen their therapeutic index has resulted in the successful FDA approval of five ADCs to date to treat various forms of cancer. However, the principles of the ADC platform could be applied to any disease area where site-specific release of pharmacologically active small molecules could have an efficacious response and minimize off-target effects [1]. Multiple factors can decide the successful development of an ADC including target selection, payload potency/mode-of-action, linker design, and attachment chemistry to name a few. We begin this section by highlighting several examples where ADC technology has been applied to modulate aberrant cellular activity within non-oncology settings.

L. Nathan Tumey (ed.), *Antibody-Drug Conjugates: Methods and Protocols*, Methods in Molecular Biology, vol. 2078, https://doi.org/10.1007/978-1-4939-9929-3_2, © Springer Science+Business Media, LLC, part of Springer Nature 2020

2 Antibody Drug Conjugates Described for Non-Oncology Applications

2.1 Payload Class: Glucocorticoid Receptor Modulator (GRM)

2.1.1 Anti-E Selectin Dexamethasone Conjugate

Synthetic glucocorticoid receptor modulators such as dexamethasone, prednisolone, and budesonide are a potent class of small molecules used in the treatment of inflammatory disorders but their utility in the chronic treatment of disease is limited by their severe side effects such as hypertension, weight gain, diabetes, skin thinning, and osteoporosis [2]. Several approaches to retain the anti-inflammatory efficacy of synthetic glucocorticoids while sparing the unwanted toxicities have been described [3]. However these methodologies have been met with little success primarily due to the lack of tissue-specific selectivity. Therefore, new approaches to target the delivery of steroids to pathogenic cells within sites of inflammation and thus limiting systemic exposure are highly desired.

Inflamed endothelium plays an important role in leukocyte adhesion and recruitment in chronic inflammatory disease where cells can extravasate into tissue and perpetuate further damage. Thus targeting glucocorticoids to activated endothelial cells and limiting leukocyte infiltration presents an attractive approach. In one of the first examples to test this hypothesis, the authors [4] generated an anti-E-selection dexamethasone conjugate through reaction of dexamethasone-21-hemisuccinate to free lysines on an anti-E-selectin antibody (Fig. 1). E-selectin (CD62E) is an adhesion molecule uniquely expressed on activated but not on resting endothelial cells. Although selective binding and internalization of the ADC on TNFα-stimulated endothelial cells was demonstrated with a resulting decrease in the pro-inflammatory cytokine IL-8 mRNA, the lack of a nontargeted dexamethasone conjugate control in these early in vitro studies makes it difficult to interpret a targeted glucocorticoid effect through E-selectin-mediated uptake or loss of payload due to linker instability in the culture media.

2.1.2 Anti-CD163 Dexamethasone Conjugate

An ADC approach has also been described to target glucocorticoid to the endocytic receptor CD163. CD163 is a scavenger receptor for hemoglobin and is highly expressed on activated macrophages in chronic inflammatory diseases such as atherosclerosis, rheumatoid arthritis, and inflammatory bowel disease [5–7]. Using similar chemistry to the anti-E-selectin ADC, an anti-CD163 dexamethasone conjugate was synthesized [8] through coupling of primary amines on an anti-rat CD163 mAb to dexamethasone-hemisuccinate *N*-hydroxysuccinide (NHS) ester in a controlled reaction to limit the drug:antibody ratio (DAR) to four dexamethasone molecules per antibody (Fig. 2). In an LPS-induced acute rat model of inflammation, the anti-CD163 ADC was able to demonstrate the inhibition of elevated serum levels of the pro-inflammatory cytokines, TNFα and IL-1, in a similar level to

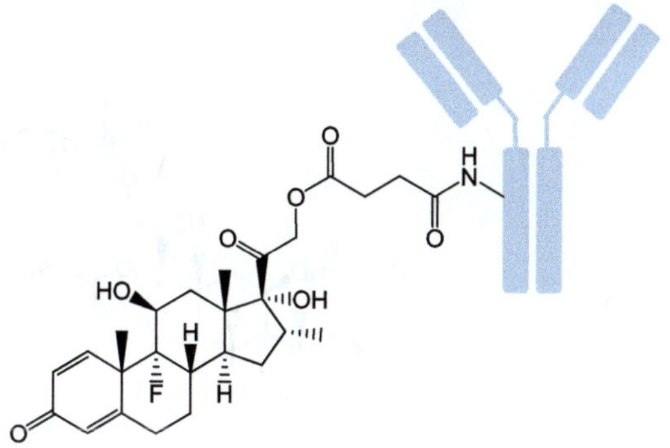

Fig. 1 Anti-E selectin dexamethasone conjugate

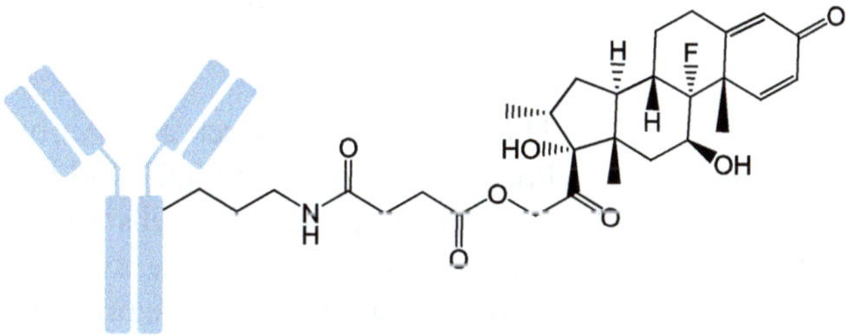

Fig. 2 Anti-CD163 dexamethasone conjugate

small molecule dexamethasone. However in healthy rats, the same efficacious dose of anti-CD163 ADC spared the unwanted side effects of systemic dexamethasone treatment including cortisol suppression, thymic atrophy, and body weight loss thus suggesting that a therapeutic window through ADC targeting was attainable.

2.1.3 Anti-CD70-Budesonide Conjugate

Perhaps sensing limitations in the stability of ester conjugates in vivo [9], scientists at Merck and Ambrx embarked on a new approach to conjugate glucocorticoids to a targeted antibody [10]. Using a novel, phosphate-based, cathepsin B-sensitive linker (CatPhos) that allows for budesonide attachment through its primary hydroxyl, they generated site-specific conjugates onto an anti-CD70 antibody incorporating unnatural amino acids (Fig. 3). The linker strategy, designed to rapidly release free budesonide in the lysosome, resulted in robust stability in human blood and favorable physicochemical properties.

Using a human renal cell carcinoma cell line expressing CD70, anti-CD70 budesonide ADCs were evaluated for steroid-dependent activity by monitoring expression of the glucocorticoid-induced leucine zipper mRNA by Real -Time–Polymerase Chain Reaction (RT-PCR). Both phosphate- and pyrophosphate-based anti-CD70 ADCs demonstrated potent induction of GILZ mRNA transcript compared to nontargeted

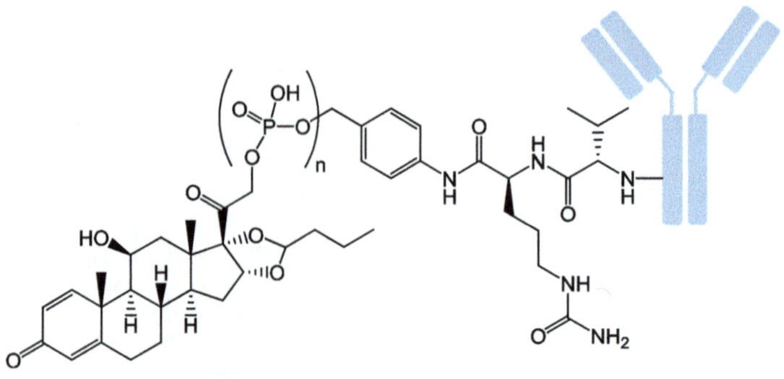

Fig. 3 Anti-CD70 budesonide conjugate

ADCs demonstrating a viable linker strategy for conjugating other bioactive small molecules containing an aliphatic alcohol.

2.1.4 Anti-CD74 Fluticasone Propionate Conjugate

The scientists at Merck and Ambrx extended their work on Cat-Phos linkers to target CD74 [11], a MHC class II protein expressed on antigen presenting cells that may play a pathogenic role in autoimmune diseases like systemic lupus erythematosus (SLE). Conjugation of fluticasone propionate via the 11-hydroxyl position through a pyrophosphate bridge afforded an anti-CD74 antibody conjugate (Fig. 4a) that demonstrated upregulation of GILZ mRNA in CD74-expressing Hut-78 cells. However, lack of in vivo activity in huCD74-Tg mice led to concerns regarding payload permeability and so the team focused on identifying a glucocorticoid designed to accumulate in cells upon ADC catabolism (Fig. 4b). B cell-dependent activity was observed with anti-CD74-AXC496 ADC (Fig. 4c) in a human peripheral blood mononuclear cell (PBMC) mixed cell culture system compared to the more permeable payload ADC, anti-CD74-flu449.

2.1.5 Anti-PRLR Glucocorticoid Conjugate

Scientists at Regeneron Pharmaceuticals have described an antibody glucocorticoid conjugate targeting the Prolactin Receptor (PRLR) [12]. PRLR is a cytokine receptor that is expressed in a subset of breast cancers and is implicated in its pathogenesis [13]. To generate the ADC, first, an azido-containing PEG linker was transferred onto Q295 and Q297 of the antibody enzymatically using microbial transglutaminase. Next, a protease-sensitive glucocorticoid linker was coupled to the azido-functionalized antibody through click chemistry to give a DAR of four (Fig. 5). The PRLR ADC was tested in a cell reporter assay expressing human PRLR where luciferase expression is controlled by glucocorticoid activity. The PRLR ADC demonstrated nanomolar activity in this bioassay compared to a nontargeted control ADC. However, it is not known if this ADC has progressed into in vivo studies.

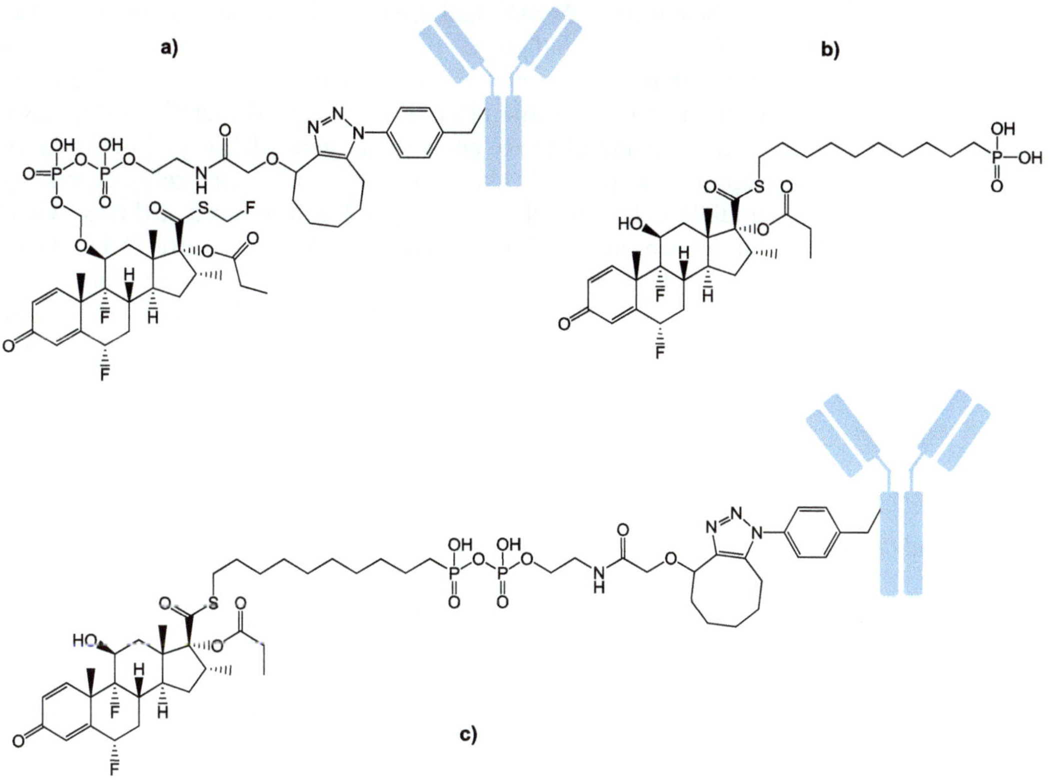

Fig. 4 (**a**) Anti-CD74 fluticasone propionate conjugate (**b**) Compound A (**c**) Anti-CD74-AXC496 conjugate

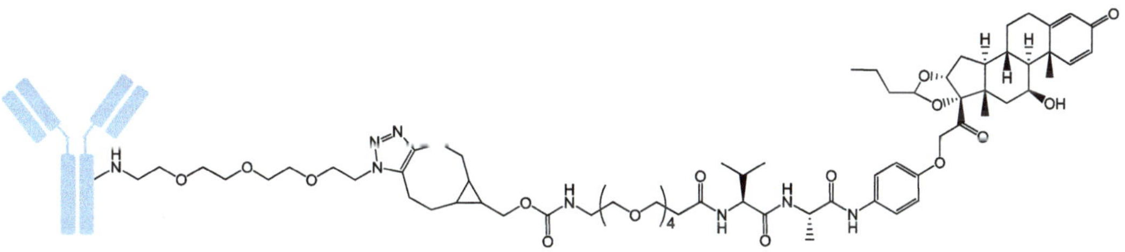

Fig. 5 Anti-PRLR glucocorticoid conjugate

2.1.6 Anti-TNFα Glucocorticoid Conjugate

Tumor Necrosis Factor alpha (TNFα) plays a central role in the pathophysiology of several human disorders [14, 15] and as such anti-TNFα agents (e.g., adalimumab, etanercept, infliximab) have clinically validated therapeutic utility in the treatment of autoimmune and inflammatory disorders such as rheumatoid arthritis, psoriasis, and inflammatory bowel disease [16]. Despite their success in the clinic, anti-TNFα biologics are still limited in the maximal efficacy they can achieve in patients [17] and a significant number of patients are refractory to anti-TNFα treatment necessitating the identification and development of more potent, broadly effective therapeutics.

Scientists at AbbVie had discovered that anti-TNFα mAbs, like adalimumab, could bind the transmembrane form of TNFα (tmTNFα) on activated immune cells, become internalized and traffic to the lysosome [18]. They reasoned that this mechanism could be manipulated to allow the targeted delivery of an immunosuppressive payload like glucocorticoids into cells expressing tmTNFα. Preclinical data in a collagen-induced arthritis (CIA) model demonstrated that just a single dose of an anti-TNFα glucocorticoid conjugate targeting mouse TNFα could completely inhibit disease for greater than 30 days [19, 20]. Additionally, the dose that generated maximal anti-inflammatory activity did not produce any unwanted GRM side effects. This most advanced antibody glucocorticoid conjugate to date has progressed into clinical trials for the treatment of autoimmune disease. (ClinicalTrials.gov Identifier: NCT03823391).

2.2 Payload Class: Antibiotic

2.2.1 Anti-*S. aureus* Antibiotic Conjugate

Scientists at Genentech have applied a novel application of ADC technology towards the treatment of infectious disease [21]. *Staphylococcus aureus* is a major bacterial pathogen whose emerging resistance to β-lactam antibiotics like methicillin has created a serious health crisis [22, 23]. Although phagocytic cells like neutrophils and macrophages can eliminate the majority of bacteria after infection, some pathogens survive within intracellular compartments where they remain resistant to conventional antibiotics and contribute to chronic or recurrent infections. An antibody antibiotic conjugate (AAC) designed to target the intracellular bacteria was identified by screening for anti-*S. aureus* antibodies from infected patients and mice. An antibody recognizing the bacterial cell wall glycopolymer β-O-linked *N*-acetylglucosamine wall-teichoic acid (β-GlcNAc WTA) was identified to have the highest specificity against the broadest spectrum of *S. aureus* strains. An analog of the bacterial RNA polymerase inhibitor rifampicin was designed to be proteolytically released within the phagolysosome and maintain potent bactericidal activity at lower pH (Fig. 6). The AAC has no direct anti-bacterial activity and requires the uptake of AAC-opsonized bacteria into host cells to release the antibiotic payload. Indeed, single-dose AAC treatment of MRSA-infected mice proved superior at eliminating bacteremia compared to twice daily vancomycin, and an AAC therapeutic (DSTA4637S) has now advanced into clinical trials (ClinicalTrials.gov Identifier NCT03162250). This novel approach to treat antibiotic-resistant infection may revive the effectiveness of other potent anti-bacterials that have limited utility as conventional drugs.

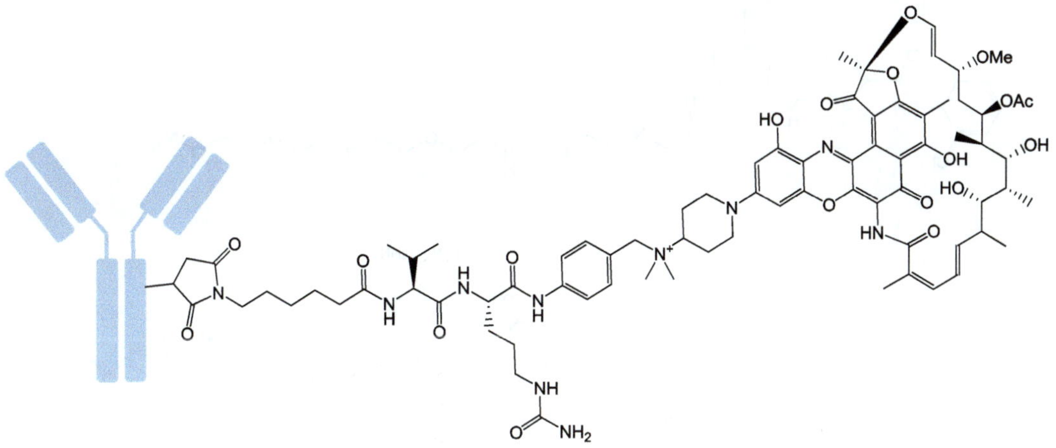

Fig. 6 Anti-*S. aureus* antibiotic conjugate

2.3 Payload Class: Kinase Inhibitor

2.3.1 Anti-CXCR4 Dasatinib Conjugate

Kinase inhibitors like dasatinib (Sprycel®; Bristol-Myers Squibb) are effective in the treatment of hematological disorders such as chronic myelogenous leukemia but their lack of selectivity against other kinase family members limits their therapeutic utility in other disease areas such as autoimmune diseases. These off-target activities lead to severe side effects including pulmonary hypertension, pleural effusions, and neutropenia [24]. In addition to its potent inhibition of Bcr-Abl, dasinitib also blocks Lck and Fyn, both important kinases in early T-cell Receptor (TCR) signaling during T cell activation [25, 26]. Researchers at the Scripps Research Institute and the California Institute for Biomedical Research (Calibr) explored the selective delivery of dasatinib directly to T lymphocytes via an ADC approach [27]. They identified the chemokine receptor CXCR4 as a highly expressed antigen on T cells with minimal to no expression on non-hematopoietic cells. Interestingly, the antibody scaffold used to target CXCR4 was generated by grafting a long bovine CDR3H loop containing a CXCR4 peptide antagonist onto CDR3H of trastuzumab [28] and internalization of this hybrid construct in human T cells was confirmed by confocal microscopy. Both cleavable and noncleavable dasatinib analog linkers were generated with payloads that retained Lck inhibitory activity similar to dasatinib. Two-step conjugation through primary amines on the anti-CXCR4 mAb afforded both ADCs with approximate DAR of three and low aggregation (Fig. 7a, b). Both ADCs demonstrated on-target delivery of their immunosuppressive dasatinib payloads to activated human T cells in vitro and effectively inhibited pro-inflammatory cytokine secretion. However, the lack of CXCR4 cross-reactivity limits evaluating the preclinical efficacy of these reagents in rodent models of T cell activation and inflammation.

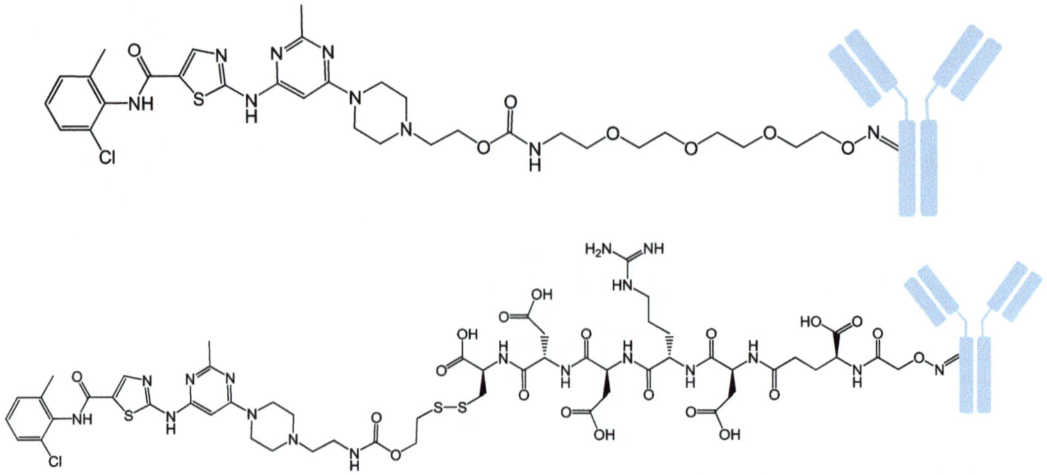

Fig. 7 (**a**) Noncleavable anti-CXCR4 dasatinib conjugate (**b**) Cleavable anti-CXCR4 dasatinib conjugate

2.4 Payload Class: Liver X Receptor (LXR) Agonist

2.4.1 Anti-CD11a LXR Agonist Conjugate

The Liver X receptor (LXR) family of nuclear receptors are important transcriptional regulators involved in lipid homeostasis and inflammation [29]. Indeed, efforts to exploit the therapeutic value of synthetic LXR agonists have been hampered due to unwanted on-target toxicities [30]. Therefore, an ADC strategy was evaluated to specifically target LXR agonist payload to pathogenic macrophages while sparing hepatocytes [31]. The leukocyte integrin CD11a was identified as a suitable target with a selective expression profile and an engineered anti-CD11a mAb was generated to allow for site-specific conjugation with an aminooxy-containing LXR agonist protease-sensitive linker (Fig. 8). The anti-CD11a LXR agonist conjugate demonstrated selective activation of LXR-dependent luciferase expression in a human monocytic cell line compared to a human hepatocyte cell line with same reporter system. As the authors expand on these initial, encouraging results through generation of a surrogate LXR agonist ADC that targets mouse CD11a, it will be interesting to see if ADC technology can spare the unwanted effects of LXR agonism in preclinical models of atherosclerosis and inflammation.

2.5 Payload Class: Phosphodiesterase 4 (PDE4) Inhibitor

2.5.1 Anti-CD11a PDE4 Inhibitor Conjugate

PDE4 is a key enzyme involved in the degradation of cyclic adenosine monophosphate (cAMP), an important second messenger of inflammatory signaling [32]. Inhibitors of PDE4 have progressed into the clinic to treat inflammatory disease [33] but dose-limiting toxicities have narrowed their therapeutic utility [34].

Expanding on their LXR agonist ADC work, scientists at Calibr identified an ADC-compatible analog of the potent PDE4 inhibitor GSK256066 to conjugate to their engineered anti-human CD11a mAb using the same site-specific conjugation chemistry as described previously [35] (Fig. 9a). The Fc region included

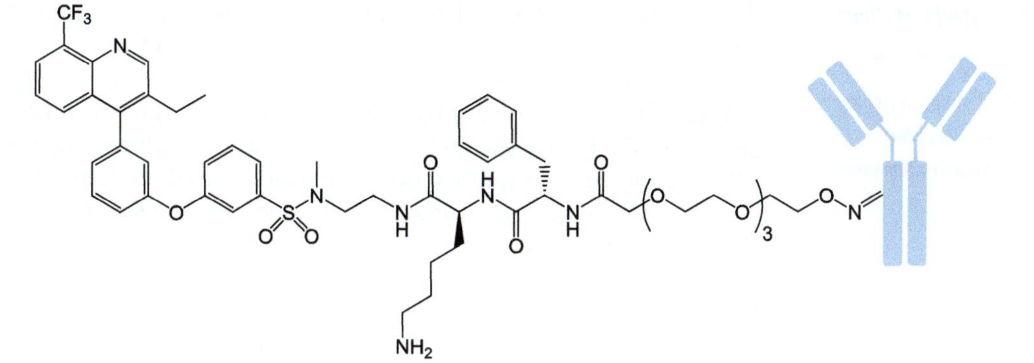

Fig. 8 Anti-CD11a LXR agonist conjugate

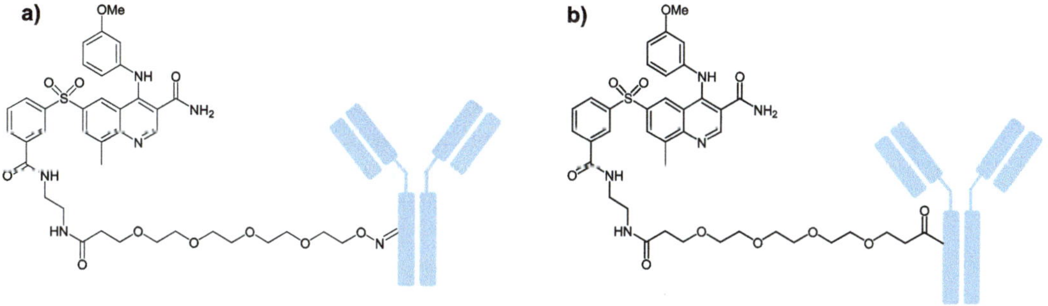

Fig. 9 (**a**) anti-human CD11a PDE4 inhibitor conjugate (**b**) anti-mouse CD11a PDE4 inhibitor conjugate

additional mutations to avoid Fcγ receptor uptake. An assessment of activity in LPS-stimulated PBMCs demonstrated potent inhibition of TNFα secretion with ADC treatment compared to unconjugated antibody. A surrogate ADC that binds mouse CD11a was also made using an NHS-ester analog of the PDE4 inhibitor to conjugate reactive amines on the antibody with an average DAR of three (Fig. 9b). Anti-inflammatory activity of this ADC was confirmed through attenuation of cytokine secretion from stimulated mouse peritoneal macrophages and its selectivity established through both competition with excess parental antibody and a lack of inhibitory activity on CD11a null cells. These in vitro ADC studies were translated into a mouse carrageenan air pouch model of inflammation where the anti-mCD11a PDE4 inhibitor conjugate had a modest but selective response in inhibiting pro-inflammatory cytokines within the air pouch exudate. As work in this area continues, it will be interesting to see the bioactivity of this tool reagent in chronic models of inflammation.

2.6 Payload Class: Bisphosphonate

2.6.1 Anti-Interleukin 6 (IL-6) Receptor Alendronate Conjugate

Tocilizumab (Actemra®; Roche) is an anti-IL-6 receptor antibody currently approved for the treatment of rheumatoid arthritis, an autoimmune disease involving severe inflammation with concomitant cartilage and bone destruction. Researchers sought to enhance the anti-inflammatory activity of tocilizumab through conjugation of alendronate, a bisphosphonate derivative used to treat bone disorders such as osteoporosis [36]. The mechanistic rationale was to capture the anti-inflammatory mechanism of IL-6 inhibition combined with the inhibitory activity of the bisphosphonate payload on activated macrophages within the inflamed joint. A disulfide-containing alendronate linker was conjugated selectively to the oxidized N-glycan on the constant region of tocilizumab which preserved anti-IL-6 receptor binding activity (Fig. 10). In a human macrophage viability assay, the anti-IL-6R alendronate conjugate demonstrated growth inhibitory activity compare to a nontargeted ADC control. Although an enhanced benefit was observed in a mouse model of arthritis both clinically and histologically with anti-IL-6R alendronate conjugate treatment compared to alendronate or parental mAb alone, the lack of a nontargeted alendronate conjugate control is this study does not exclude IL-6R-independent uptake mechanisms contributing to efficacy in this disease model.

2.7 Payload Class: Microtubule Inhibitor

2.7.1 Anti-CD30 Vedotin Conjugate (Adcetris)

Adcetris® (brentuximab vedotin) is an anti-CD30 conjugate carrying the anti-mitotic payload monomethyl auristatin (MMAE) (Fig. 11) and is approved for the treatment of relapsed Hodgkins lymphoma and systemic anaplastic large cell lymphoma [37]. As a member of the TNF receptor superfamily, CD30 is upregulated on activated B and T cells [38], Seattle Genetics has explored the therapeutic utility of Adcetris in the context of immune disease. A Phase I trial of brentuximab vedotin in patients with steroid refractory acute graft vs. host disease (GVHD) established tolerability and activity [39]; however, a Phase II study was withdrawn before enrollment (Clinicaltrials.gov Identifier NCT01616680). A phase II dose ranging study to evaluate brentuximab vedotin in adults with systemic lupus erythematosus (SLE) was also abandoned (Clinicaltrials.gov Identifier NCT02533570).

More recently, Phase II clinical trials have been initiated to study the efficacy of brentuximab vedotin in systemic sclerosis (Clinicaltrials.gov Identifiers NCT03198689 and NCT032222492), an autoimmune disease of the connective tissue. Considering the unmet medical need for patients with this disease, the potential for brentuximab vedotin to alleviate symptoms is highly anticipated.

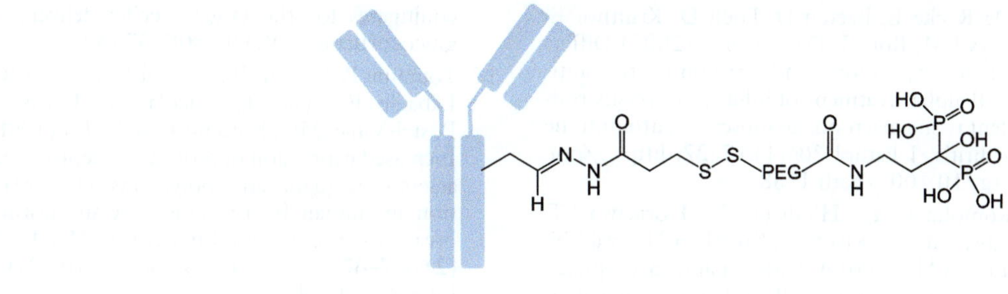

Fig. 10 Anti-interleukin 6 (IL-6) receptor alendronate conjugate

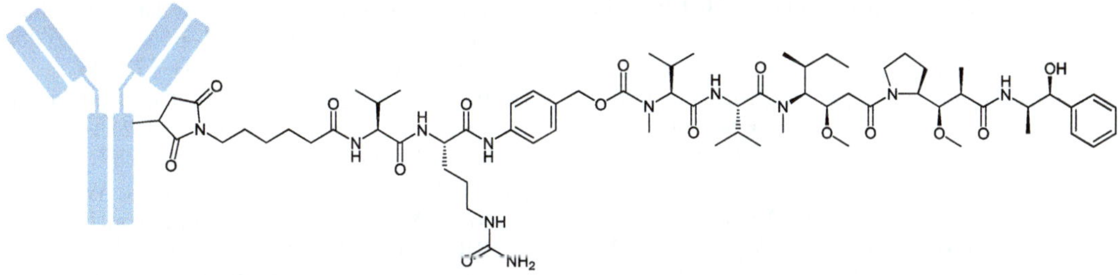

Fig. 11 Anti-CD30 MMAE conjugate (brentuximab vedotin; Adcetris®)

3 Concluding Remarks

Most of the ADCs described here are in the early stages of discovery and still exploring their potential to optimally modulate the activated phenotype of cells in disease. However, some ADCs have progressed into pivotal clinical trials that may prove whether this new therapeutic class can impact disease burden in patients outside of oncology indications. As we continue to build our ADC knowledge in both settings, there may also be opportunities for cross-over therapies. In conclusion, we are encouraged at the possibilities ADCs may hold for the treatment of a wide range of diseases and hope they will exhibit a significant advantage over conventional therapies.

References

1. Yu S, Lim A, Tremblay MS (2018) Next horizons: ADCs beyond oncology. In: Damelin M (ed) Innovations for next-generation antibody-drug conjugates. Springer International Publishing, Cham, pp 321–347. https://doi.org/10.1007/978-3-319-78154-9_14
2. Schacke H, Docke WD, Asadullah K (2002) Mechanisms involved in the side effects of glucocorticoids. Pharmacol Ther 96(1):23–43
3. Rosen J, Miner JN (2005) The search for safer glucocorticoid receptor ligands. Endocr Rev 26(3):452–464. https://doi.org/10.1210/er.2005-0002
4. Everts M, Kok RJ, Ásgeirsdóttir SA, Melgert BN, Moolenaar TJM, Koning GA, van Luyn MJA, Meijer DKF, Molema G (2002) Selective intracellular delivery of dexamethasone into activated endothelial cells using an E-Selectin-directed immunoconjugate. J Immunol 168 (2):883. https://doi.org/10.4049/jimmunol.168.2.883

5. De Rycke L, Baeten D, Foell D, Kruithof E, Veys EM, Roth J, De Keyser F (2005) Differential expression and response to anti-TNFalpha treatment of infiltrating versus resident tissue macrophage subsets in autoimmune arthritis. J Pathol 206(1):17–27. https://doi.org/10.1002/path.1758
6. Komohara Y, Hirahara J, Horikawa T, Kawamura K, Kiyota E, Sakashita N, Araki N, Takeya M (2006) AM-3K, an anti-macrophage antibody, recognizes CD163, a molecule associated with an anti-inflammatory macrophage phenotype. J Histochem Cytochem 54 (7):763–771. https://doi.org/10.1369/jhc.5A6871.2006
7. Li W, Xu LH, Yuan XM (2004) Macrophage hemoglobin scavenger receptor and ferritin accumulation in human atherosclerotic lesions. Ann N Y Acad Sci 1030:196–201. https://doi.org/10.1196/annals.1329.025
8. Graversen JH, Svendsen P, Dagnaes-Hansen F, Dal J, Anton G, Etzerodt A, Petersen MD, Christensen PA, Moller HJ, Moestrup SK (2012) Targeting the hemoglobin scavenger receptor CD163 in macrophages highly increases the anti-inflammatory potency of dexamethasone. Mol Ther 20(8):1550–1558. https://doi.org/10.1038/mt.2012.103
9. Tumey LN, Rago B, Han X (2015) In vivo biotransformations of antibody–drug conjugates. Bioanalysis 7(13):1649–1664. https://doi.org/10.4155/bio.15.84
10. Kern JC, Dooney D, Zhang R, Liang L, Brandish PE, Cheng M, Feng G, Beck A, Bresson D, Firdos J, Gately D, Knudsen N, Manibusan A, Sun Y, Garbaccio RM (2016) Novel phosphate modified cathepsin B linkers: improving aqueous solubility and enhancing payload scope of ADCs. Bioconjug Chem 27 (9):2081–2088. https://doi.org/10.1021/acs.bioconjchem.6b00337
11. Brandish PE, Palmieri A, Antonenko S, Beaumont M, Benso L, Cancilla M, Cheng M, Fayadat-Dilman L, Feng G, Figueroa I, Firdos J, Garbaccio R, Garvin-Queen L, Gately D, Geda P, Haines C, Hseih S, Hodges D, Kern J, Knudsen N, Kwasnjuk K, Liang L, Ma H, Manibusan A, Miller PL, Moy LY, Qu Y, Shah S, Shin JS, Stivers P, Sun Y, Tomazela D, Woo HC, Zaller D, Zhang S, Zhang Y, Zielstorff M (2018) Development of anti-CD74 antibody-drug conjugates to target glucocorticoids to immune cells. Bioconjug Chem 29 (7):2357–2369. https://doi.org/10.1021/acs.bioconjchem.8b00312
12. Han A, Olson W, Murphy AJ (2018) Preparation of novel steroids and their protein-conjugates for the target-specific delivery of glucocorticoids. WO2018089373A2
13. Touraine P, Martini JF, Zafrani B, Durand JC, Labaille F, Malet C, Nicolas A, Trivin C, Postel-Vinay MC, Kuttenn F, Kelly PA (1998) Increased expression of prolactin receptor gene assessed by quantitative polymerase chain reaction in human breast tumors versus normal breast tissues. J Clin Endocrinol Metab 83 (2):667–674. https://doi.org/10.1210/jcem.83.2.4564
14. Aggarwal BB, Gupta SC, Kim JH (2012) Historical perspectives on tumor necrosis factor and its superfamily: 25 years later, a golden journey. Blood 119(3):651–665. https://doi.org/10.1182/blood-2011-04-325225
15. Bradley JR (2008) TNF-mediated inflammatory disease. J Pathol 214(2):149–160. https://doi.org/10.1002/path.2287
16. Lin J, Ziring D, Desai S, Kim S, Wong M, Korin Y, Braun J, Reed E, Gjertson D, Singh RR (2008) TNFalpha blockade in human diseases: an overview of efficacy and safety. Clin Immunol 126(1):13–30. https://doi.org/10.1016/j.clim.2007.08.012
17. Breedveld FC, Weisman MH, Kavanaugh AF, Cohen SB, Pavelka K, van Vollenhoven R, Sharp J, Perez JL, Spencer-Green GT (2006) The PREMIER study: a multicenter, randomized, double-blind clinical trial of combination therapy with adalimumab plus methotrexate versus methotrexate alone or adalimumab alone in patients with early, aggressive rheumatoid arthritis who had not had previous methotrexate treatment. Arthritis Rheum 54(1):26–37. https://doi.org/10.1002/art.21519
18. Deora A, Hegde S, Lee J, Choi CH, Chang Q, Lee C, Eaton L, Tang H, Wang D, Lee D, Michalak M, Tomlinson M, Tao Q, Gaur N, Harvey B, McLoughlin S, Labkovsky B, Ghayur T (2017) Transmembrane TNF-dependent uptake of anti-TNF antibodies. MAbs 9(4):680–695. https://doi.org/10.1080/19420862.2017.1304869
19. Waegell W BS, Mathieu S, Phillips L, Goess C, Hobson A, McPherson M, Stoffel R (2018) Development of a novel therapeutic antibody drug conjugate for the treatment of autoimmune disease. In: The resolution of inflammation in health and disease, Dublin, Ireland, Mar 24–28
20. McPherson MJ, Hobson AD, Hayes ME, Marvin CC, Schmidt D, Waegell W, Goess C, Oh JZ, Hernandez A, Jr., Randolph JT (2017) Preparation of glucocorticoid receptor agonist and immunoconjugates thereof. WO2017210471A1

21. Lehar SM, Pillow T, Xu M, Staben L, Kajihara KK, Vandlen R, DePalatis L, Raab H, Hazenbos WL, Morisaki JH, Kim J, Park S, Darwish M, Lee BC, Hernandez H, Loyet KM, Lupardus P, Fong R, Yan D, Chalouni C, Luis E, Khalfin Y, Plise E, Cheong J, Lyssikatos JP, Strandh M, Koefoed K, Andersen PS, Flygare JA, Wah Tan M, Brown EJ, Mariathasan S (2015) Novel antibody-antibiotic conjugate eliminates intracellular S. aureus. Nature 527 (7578):323–328. https://doi.org/10.1038/nature16057
22. Boucher HW, Talbot GH, Bradley JS, Edwards JE, Gilbert D, Rice LB, Scheld M, Spellberg B, Bartlett J (2009) Bad bugs, no drugs: no ESKAPE! An update from the Infectious Diseases Society of America. Clin Infect Dis 48 (1):1–12. https://doi.org/10.1086/595011
23. Nannini E, Murray BE, Arias CA (2010) Resistance or decreased susceptibility to glycopeptides, daptomycin, and linezolid in methicillin-resistant Staphylococcus aureus. Curr Opin Pharmacol 10(5):516–521. https://doi.org/10.1016/j.coph.2010.06.006
24. Caldemeyer L, Dugan M, Edwards J, Akard L (2016) Long-term side effects of tyrosine kinase inhibitors in chronic myeloid Leukemia. Curr Hematol Malig Rep 11(2):71–79. https://doi.org/10.1007/s11899-016-0309-2
25. Blake S, Hughes TP, Mayrhofer G, Lyons AB (2008) The Src/ABL kinase inhibitor dasatinib (BMS-354825) inhibits function of normal human T-lymphocytes in vitro. Clin Immunol 127(3):330–339. https://doi.org/10.1016/j.clim.2008.02.006
26. Schade AE, Schieven GL, Townsend R, Jankowska AM, Susulic V, Zhang R, Szpurka H, Maciejewski JP (2008) Dasatinib, a small-molecule protein tyrosine kinase inhibitor, inhibits T-cell activation and proliferation. Blood 111(3):1366–1377. https://doi.org/10.1182/blood-2007-04-084814
27. Wang RE, Liu T, Wang Y, Cao Y, Du J, Luo X, Deshmukh V, Kim CH, Lawson BR, Tremblay MS, Young TS, Kazane SA, Wang F, Schultz PG (2015) An immunosuppressive antibody-drug conjugate. J Am Chem Soc 137 (9):3229–3232. https://doi.org/10.1021/jacs.5b00620
28. Liu T, Liu Y, Wang Y, Hull M, Schultz PG, Wang F (2014) Rational design of CXCR4 specific antibodies with elongated CDRs. J Am Chem Soc 136(30):10557–10560. https://doi.org/10.1021/ja5042447
29. Joseph SB, Castrillo A, Laffitte BA, Mangelsdorf DJ, Tontonoz P (2003) Reciprocal regulation of inflammation and lipid metabolism by liver X receptors. Nat Med 9 (2):213–219. https://doi.org/10.1038/nm820
30. Kirchgessner TG, Sleph P, Ostrowski J, Lupisella J, Ryan CS, Liu X, Fernando G, Grimm D, Shipkova P, Zhang R, Garcia R, Zhu J, He A, Malone H, Martin R, Behnia K, Wang Z, Barrett YC, Garmise RJ, Yuan L, Zhang J, Gandhi MD, Wastall P, Li T, Du S, Salvador L, Mohan R, Cantor GH, Kick E, Lee J, Frost RJ (2016) Beneficial and adverse effects of an LXR agonist on human lipid and lipoprotein metabolism and circulating neutrophils. Cell Metab 24(2):223–233. https://doi.org/10.1016/j.cmet.2016.07.016
31. Lim RK, Yu S, Cheng B, Li S, Kim NJ, Cao Y, Chi V, Kim JY, Chatterjee AK, Schultz PG, Tremblay MS, Kazane SA (2015) Targeted delivery of LXR agonist using a site-specific antibody-drug conjugate. Bioconjug Chem 26(11):2216–2222. https://doi.org/10.1021/acs.bioconjchem.5b00203
32. Yan K, Gao L-N, Cui Y-L, Zhang Y, Zhou X (2016) The cyclic AMP signaling pathway: exploring targets for successful drug discovery (review). Mol Med Rep 13(5):3715–3723. https://doi.org/10.3892/mmr.2016.5005
33. Jin SL, Ding SL, Lin SC (2012) Phosphodiesterase 4 and its inhibitors in inflammatory diseases. Chang Gung Med J 35(3):197–210
34. Spina D (2008) PDE4 inhibitors: current status. Br J Pharmacol 155(3):308–315. https://doi.org/10.1038/bjp.2008.307
35. Yu S, Pearson AD, Lim RK, Rodgers DT, Li S, Parker HB, Weglarz M, Hampton EN, Bollong MJ, Shen J, Zambaldo C, Wang D, Woods AK, Wright TM, Schultz PG, Kazane SA, Young TS, Tremblay MS (2016) Targeted delivery of an anti-inflammatory PDE4 inhibitor to immune cells via an antibody-drug conjugate. Mol Ther 24(12):2078–2089. https://doi.org/10.1038/mt.2016.175
36. Lee H, Bhang SH, Lee JH, Kim H, Hahn SK (2017) Tocilizumab-alendronate conjugate for treatment of rheumatoid arthritis. Bioconjug Chem 28(4):1084–1092. https://doi.org/10.1021/acs.bioconjchem.7b00008
37. Senter PD, Sievers EL (2012) The discovery and development of brentuximab vedotin for use in relapsed Hodgkin lymphoma and systemic anaplastic large cell lymphoma. Nat Biotechnol 30(7):631–637. https://doi.org/10.1038/nbt.2289
38. Granados S, Hwang ST (2004) Roles for CD30 in the biology and treatment of CD30 lymphoproliferative diseases. J Invest Dermatol

122(6):1345–1347. https://doi.org/10.1111/j.0022-202X.2004.22616.x
39. Chen YB, Perales MA, Li S, Kempner M, Reynolds C, Brown J, Efebera YA, Devine SM, El-Jawahri A, McAfee SL, Spitzer TR, Soiffer RJ, Ritz J, Cutler C (2017) Phase 1 multicenter trial of brentuximab vedotin for steroid-refractory acute graft-versus-host disease. Blood 129(24):3256–3261. https://doi.org/10.1182/blood-2017-03-772210

Chapter 3

Conjugations to Endogenous Cysteine Residues

Durgesh V. Nadkarni

Abstract

Interchain disulfide bonds of antibodies can be reduced by agents such as TCEP or DTT to form reactive cysteine residues. These endogenous cysteines are used for conjugation to biologically active drugs either directly or via linkers to prepare antibody drug conjugates (ADCs). The anti-notch 3 ADC described here is being evaluated in the early clinical development program as a potential treatment for a variety of cancers. The ADC is composed of an IgG1 mAb that is conjugated by endogenous cysteines to a cytotoxic microtubulin inhibitor via a maleimide-containing linker. The endogenous cysteine residues are produced by partial reduction of the mAb with TCEP reducing agent. The conjugation results in the formation of a mixture of 2, 4, 6, and 8 loaded ADC species. In addition to the desired product, several product-related impurities such as aggregates are generated during the conjugation reaction. The product- and process-related impurities are separated from the monomeric ADC by column chromatography and ultrafiltration-diafiltration techniques. The temperature of TCEP reduction step has an impact on the level of aggregates produced in the reaction. The temperature also impacts the isomeric composition of the 4 loaded ADC species.

Key words Notch 3 ADC, Conjugation, TCEP, Payload, Aggregates, Auristatin

1 Introduction

Several methods exist for the covalent conjugation of small molecule drugs to monoclonal antibodies. The most common methods employ conjugation of the drug via a linker to either lysines or endogenous cysteine residues on the mAb [1]. Several newer techniques utilize site-specific conjugation of the drug to engineered functional groups on the antibodies [2]. Direct conjugation of the linker-drug (payload) to reactive lysine residues on the surface of the IgGs leads to the formation of heterogeneous mixture of numerous ADC species in stochastic distribution. The resulting conjugate contains the linker-drug that is covalently attached to the mAb by a stable amide bond linkage. The average drug loading on the ADC is controlled by the stoichiometric ratio of the drug/mAb. Each ADC species may have different physical and pharmacokinetic properties. This method is employed for the production

L. Nathan Tumey (ed.), *Antibody-Drug Conjugates: Methods and Protocols*, Methods in Molecular Biology, vol. 2078, https://doi.org/10.1007/978-1-4939-9929-3_3, © Springer Science+Business Media, LLC, part of Springer Nature 2020

of clinically approved ADCs such as Besponsa® and Mylotarg® [3]. A variation of this approach was used for the preparation of Kadcyla® where in the first step the linker is conjugated to surface lysines on the mAb followed by coupling of the drug to the linker conjugated to mAb [4].

In another conjugation approach, the interchain disulfide bonds of IgGs are first reduced in a controlled manner by reducing agents such as Tris(2-carboxyethyl)phosphine (TCEP) or Dithiothreitol (DTT) to form endogenous cysteine residues. The linker-drug containing a reactive functional group such as maleimide, halo acetamide or other functional group is then conjugated to the interchain cysteine residues. This technique also results in the generation of a heterogeneous mixture of ADC species with variable drug loadings, typically exhibiting a drug-to-antibody ratio (DAR) of 0–8. The average drug loading on the ADC is controlled by the ratio of the reducing agent to mAb during the disulfide reduction step and the stoichiometric ratio of the drug to antibody. In contrast to lysine conjugations, in conventional cysteine conjugation, drug is conjugated to the mAb either in the hinge region of the mAb between two heavy chains or between the light and the heavy chains. In this chapter we describe the detailed methodology employed for the conventional cysteine conjugation used for the large-scale preparation of an anti-Notch 3 targeted ADC. This conjugation approach was also used for the preparation of ADC Adcetris® by Seattle Genetics [5].

More recently several conjugation techniques have been developed that employ site-specific conjugation of drug-likers to specific residues (native or engineered amino acids, unnatural amino acids, and glycans) on the mAb. The ADCs prepared by site-specific conjugation techniques yield more homogeneous conjugates. The conjugations can be carried out with more control to produce the desired ADC species as the major product with specific drug loading (DAR). The site of conjugation is known to impact stability, pharmacokinetics (PK), and overall efficacy of ADCs. The specific sites on the mAb are selected for conjugation based on initial screening of several ADC species for these quality attributes [6]. The conjugation methods used for site-specific conjugations are described in several other chapters in this volume.

The structure of the anti-notch 3 ADC is shown in Fig. 1 below. The ADC is composed of an IgG1 monoclonal antibody that is conjugated via interchain cysteines, produced after partial reduction of interchain disulfides, to an auristatin-containing linker-payload PF-06424469 [7]. The conjugation to the auristatin linker-payload results in the formation of cysteine conjugated species from DAR 0–8 as shown in Fig. 1. During early preclinical investigations of the PK, safety, and efficacy the ADC mixture with an average DAR of ~4 exhibited optimum performance [8].

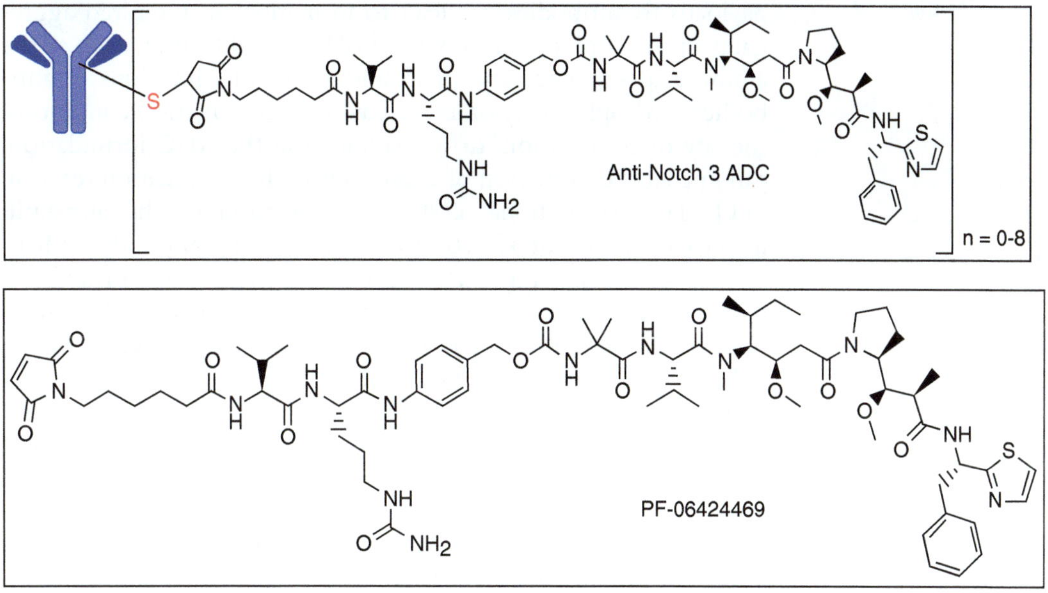

Fig. 1 Chemical structures of anti-notch 3 ADC and the linker-payload PF-06424469

In the first step the interchain disulfides of the anti-notch 3 mAb are reduced by an aqueous solution of TCEP (2.2–2.5 equivalent) at 37 °C. This is followed by addition of the solution of linker-payload (PF-06424469) to the reaction mixture. The linker-payload is added in sufficient stoichiometric excess to the mAb in order to conjugate the interchain cysteines produced in the TCEP reduction step. If the payload is not soluble in buffer solutions then it is typically dissolved in an organic solvent such as DMSO or *N*,*N*-dimethylacetamide. For the method described herein we used DMSO to dissolve PF-06424469 prior to its addition to the conjugation mixture. At the end of conjugation, the reaction mixture contains the desired ADC species as well as the product- and process-related impurities. The crude ADC mixture is generally purified by using either column chromatography or ultrafiltration-diafiltration (UF-DF) or combination of the two techniques [9]. During the initial discovery stage there may be a need for preparation of small quantities of several ADC molecules with different mAbs and linker-payload combination for screening studies. During these studies it is convenient to purify the crude ADC mixtures by size exclusion chromatography (SEC), and if needed followed by UF-DF or dialysis. For clinical and manufacturing scale preparation of many conjugates, purification of the crude reaction mixture by UF-DF is often sufficient to remove process-related impurities [5]. Crude ADC mixtures are purified by column chromatography when certain impurities such as aggregates or other product- and process-related impurities cannot be removed by UF-DF alone. The conjugation of linker-payloads to antibodies can lead to formation of undesired aggregates in the conjugation mixture [10]. Several factors, such as the amino acid sequence and posttranslational modifications of antibodies, hydrophobicity of linker-payloads, conjugation conditions, the site of conjugation, drug loading, and the ADC formulation, can impact the formation of aggregates in the conjugation reaction [11]. The conventional cysteine conjugation of the auristatin linker-payload PF-06424469 to an anti-notch 3 antibody leads to formation of some aggregates (4–6%). Aggregates are formed primarily after conjugation of the partially reduced mAb to the linker-payload PF-06424469. The temperature of the reduction of the mAb by TCEP impacts the level of aggregate formation after conjugation with PF-06424469. Under standard reduction-conjugation protocol, the mAb is treated with the reducing agent at 37 °C. Following the reduction, the mixture is cooled to 25 °C and then treated with the linker-payload. Lowering the temperature of the TCEP reduction step to 0–5 °C followed by conjugation to PF-06424469 at 25 °C leads to formation of the ADC with lower level of aggregates (~1–2%) [9].

Conjugation of linker-payload to endogenous cysteines of the mAb by the procedure described here leads to the formation of a mixture of regioisomers of 2, 4, and 6 loaded conjugated species. The temperature of the TCEP reduction step was found to impact the relative composition of the regioisomers of the 4 loaded species. The ADC material prepared by the process where the mAb is partially reduced by TCEP at 37 °C followed by conjugation to PF-06424469 at 25 °C leads to formation 4 loaded species containing a mixture of the regioisomers as shown in Fig. 2. The isomer with more hinge conjugated species is the major component of the mixture of 4 loaded species. In contrast, when the ADC is prepared by the procedure where the temperature of the TCEP reduction step is 0–5 °C, a change in the composition of the regioisomers of 4 loaded species is observed. In this case the isomer with conjugation between light and heavy chains is obtained as the major component of the 4 loaded species. The other regioisomers are formed at trace levels [9].

The crude conjugation reaction mixture contains other process-related impurities; excess quenching agent, linker-payload-related species, buffer salts, and other agents used in the formulation of the mAb such as EDTA and sucrose. The monomeric Notch 3 ADC material is separated from impurities by purification of ADC mixture on a ceramic hydroxyapatite resin column [12]. All product- and process-related impurities can be separated from the desired monomeric ADC during this purification process [13]. After purification, the selected fractions are pooled and further purified by UF-DF to concentrate the ADC solution to the desired concentration and replace the buffer of the pooled fractions with the final formulation buffer.

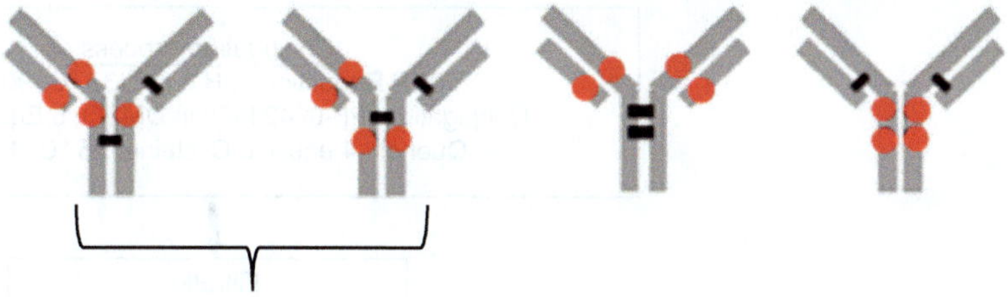

Temperature of TCEP reduction step				
	37 °C	trace	minor	major
	0-5 °C	trace	major	minor

Fig. 2 Regioisomers of 4 loaded species

The overall conjugation and purification process is shown below in Fig. 3.

2 Materials

2.1 Raw Materials

1. Dimethyl sulfoxide (DMSO).
2. Water for injection (WFI).
3. Solution of 10 N sodium hydroxide.
4. Tris(2-carboxyethyl)phosphine hydrochloride TCEP HCl (0.5 M solution, Sigma Aldrich).
5. Sucrose (Low Endotoxin).
6. L-Histidine.
7. L-Histidine monohydrochloride monohydrate.
8. Polysorbate-80.
9. Disodium EDTA dihydrate.
10. 20 mM sodium phosphate buffer (pH 7.2), 400 mM sodium chloride.
11. Mobile phase A: Ammonium sulfate (1.5 M) solution, 50 mM potassium phosphate dibasic, pH 7 and mobile phase B: 10% isopropanol, 50 mM potassium phosphate dibasic, pH 7.

2.2 Starting Materials

1. PF-06424469 Linker-Payload (*see* **Note 1**).
2. Anti-notch 3 IgG1 monoclonal antibody stock solution (*see* **Note 2**).

2.3 Critical Equipment

1. 4 L Glass reactor with an impeller.
2. 2 L Glass reactor with an impeller.
3. Circulating bath.
4. pH meter.
5. Temperature probe (thermocouple).

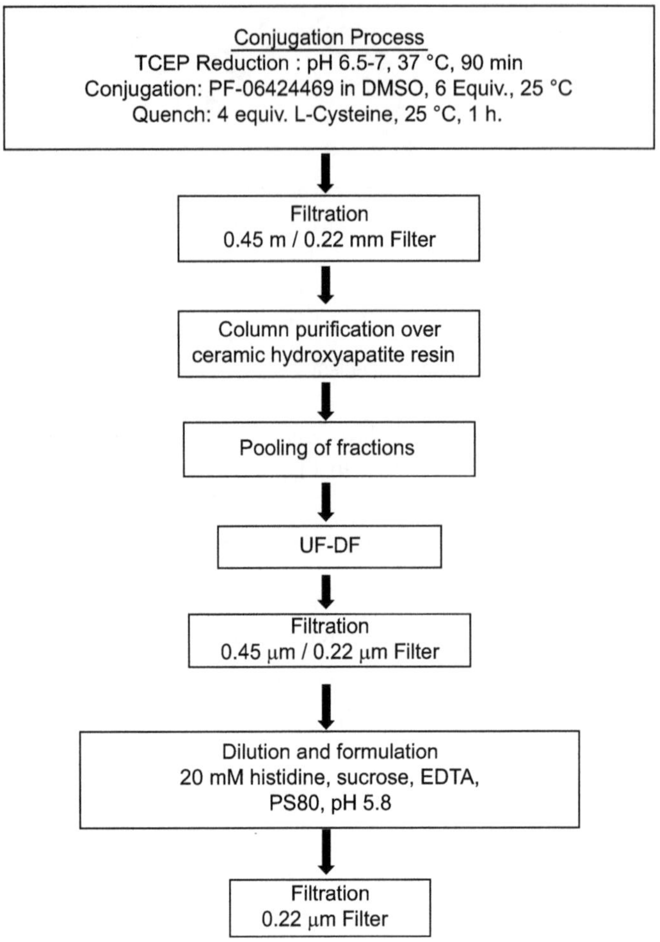

Fig. 3 Overall process for the preparation of Notch 3 ADC

6. UF/DF system.
7. Weighing balance.
8. Glove box balance for weighing PF-06424469 (*see* **Note 3**).
9. Axichrom™ 70/300 purification column (GE Lifesciences).
10. YMC-Pack Diol-200 (300 × 8 mm ID).
11. Thermo Propac HIC10 column (4.6 mm × 10 cm, 5 μm).

2.4 Consumable Items

1. Tubing (Masterflex® Platinum cured silicon tubing (50 A), L/S® 24).
2. Tubing (Masterflex® Platinum cured silicon tubing (50 A), L/S® 35).
3. Peristaltic pump.
4. PETG bottles.
5. Glass bottles used for buffers.

6. Sterile Biotainer bottles.
7. CryoTube vials.
8. Serological pipettes (50 mL, 20 mL, 10 mL).
9. Pellicon 3 UF/DF Ultracel Membrane (30 kD MWCO) (0.11 cm^2) (Millipore).
10. Sartobran 300 sterile filter (0.45 + 0.22 μm) (Sartorius).
11. Sartobran 150 sterile filter (0.45 + 0.22 μm) (Sartorius).

3 Methods

3.1 Conjugation of Anti-notch 3 mAb to PF-06424469 Linker-Payload

1. A solution of an anti-notch 3 antibody (1 equivalent) is placed in a jacketed reactor equipped with either a magnetic stir bar or an overhead agitator. The pH of the solution of anti-Notch 3 antibody is adjusted to 6.5–7 (*see* **Note 4**). The solution of the antibody is warmed to 37 °C. An aqueous solution of TCEP hydrochloride (2.2 equiv.) is added to the antibody solution (*see* **Note 5**). The resulting solution is stirred for 90 min at 37 °C (*see* **Note 6**).
2. The solution is then cooled to 25 °C. The solution of PF-06424469 (6 equivalent) in DMSO (7.7 mg/mL) is added slowly to the antibody solution over 10–15 min (7.7 mg/mL) (*see* **Note 7**). The reaction mixture is stirred for 1 h. The mixture is quenched by addition of L-cysteine (4 equivalents) (*see* **Note 8**) and stirred for 30 min at 25 °C. The reaction mixture is filtered through 0.2 μm filter. The resulting unpurified product consists of an ADC with an average DAR of ~4 as evaluated by hydrophobic interaction chromatography (HIC) and aggregate level of ~ 5% (by size exclusion chromatography).

3.2 Purification of the Reaction Mixture

1. The ADC mixture is purified by column chromatography over ceramic hydroxyapatite resin (type 1, 40 μm), column volume = 7.5 mL (*see* **Note 9**).
2. The following purification parameters are used for separation of aggregates from the monomer species, Mobile phase A: 5 mM sodium phosphate, pH 7; Mobile phase B: 200 mM sodium phosphate, pH 7; buffer gradient = 10–70% mobile phase B over 20 column volumes, protein loading on the column = 15 mg/mL, flow rate = 1 mL/min, column bed height = 22 cm.
3. The first fraction is collected from the beginning of the main peak through to the next 6.9 column volume followed by fraction every 1/3 column volume for the next three fractions. The fractions are analyzed by in-process UV assay for values of

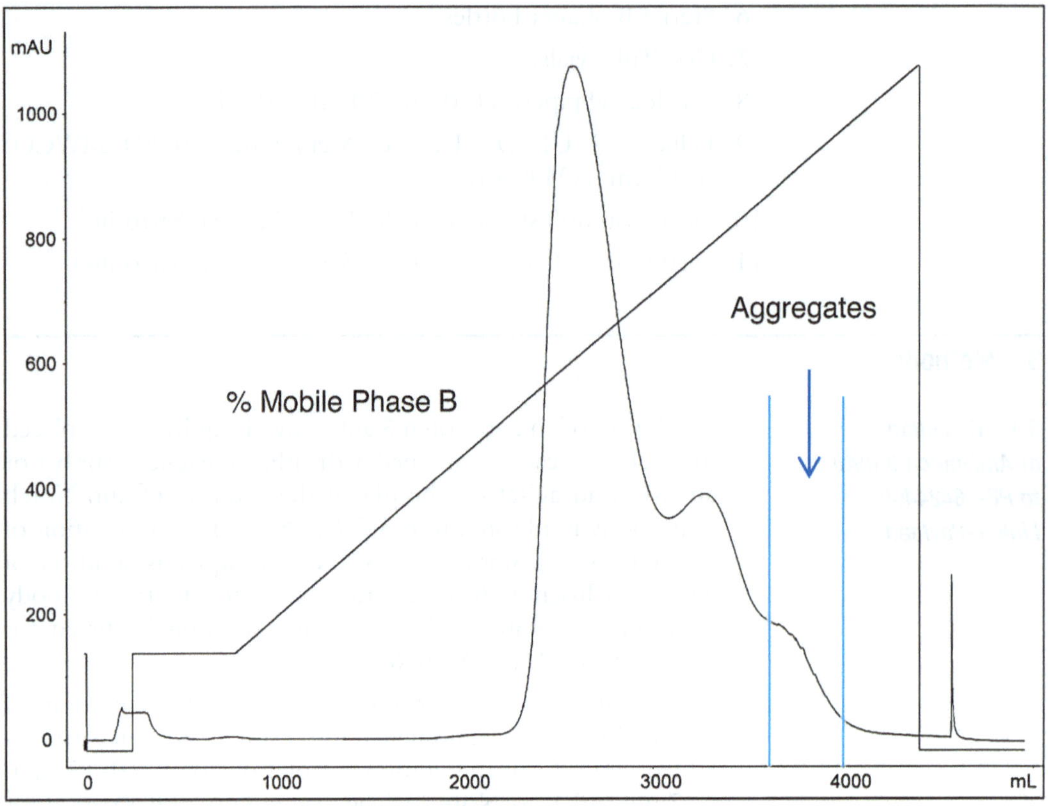

Fig. 4 Purification profile of Notch 3 ADC on the hydroxyapatite resin column with phosphate buffer as an eluent (UV detection at 280 nm)

the DAR and by SEC analytical method for aggregates. Most of the monomer elutes in fraction 1 of the collected set of fractions affording ADC product in 85–88% yield (based on the protein yield). The aggregates are in the last peak as shown in the chromatogram (*see* Fig. 4). The isolated ADC material has the average DAR of 3.6 (HIC assay) and aggregate content of ~1% (SEC assay).

3.3 Concentration

1. The ADC material obtained after column chromatography is further purified and buffer exchanged by ultrafiltration/diafiltration process (UF-DF) using Ultracel membrane cartridges (30 kD) and 20 mM histidine buffer as diafiltration buffer (pH 5.8). The retentate solution is collected and filtered through 0.2 μm filter.

3.4 ADC Formulation and Storage

1. The purified ADC material is formulated using standard formulation excipients such as sucrose, EDTA, and PS 80. The formulated ADC solution is stored frozen for long-term storage.

3.5 Determination of Average Drug Loading and Drug Distribution of the ADC

1. An analytical HIC method is used to determine the drug loading and the drug load distribution of the ADC as follows. The reference material (25 μL) and test samples are diluted to 2 mg/mL with diluent (half strength of the mobile phase A) and injected onto a Thermo Propac HIC10 column (4.6 mm × 10 cm, 5 μm).
2. The mobile phase A is 1.5 M ammonium sulfate, 50 mM potassium phosphate dibasic, pH 7 and mobile phase B is 10% isopropanol, 50 mM potassium phosphate dibasic, pH 7.
3. The samples are eluted with the flow rate of 0.8 mL/min and at the column temperature of 30 °C. Species of different DAR are separated using a salt gradient and detected by UV absorbance at 280 nm. The average DAR and distribution profile are determined by peak area percentage of each species (Fig. 5).

3.6 Determination of Aggregate Content by Analytical SEC

1. The SEC method is used to determine product purity and aggregate content. The test samples are diluted with the mobile phase (20 mM sodium phosphate, 400 mM sodium chloride, pH 7.2) at the concentration of 2 mg/mL and injected onto the YMC-Pack Diol-200 (300 × 8 mm ID) column at 0.75 mL/min for 20 min. The aggregate and monomer species in the crude ADC preparation are reported as the percent of the total area for all protein-related peaks (Fig. 6).

3.7 Determination of Average Drug Loading (DAR) by Reduced Reverse Phase HPLC

1. The sample is denatured in 4 M guanidine-HCl, 50 mM Tris, pH 7.8 and of 20 mM DTT at 37 °C for about 30 min. The reduced samples (10 μL) are separated and monitored at 214 nm by using an Agilent HPLC with a Agilent Zorbax 300SB-CN column (150 × 4.6 mm, 3.5 μm) at the column temperature of 75 °C. The samples are eluted using the mobile phase A (0.1% TFA in water) and mobile phase B (80% acetonitrile, 20% isopropanol and 0.1% TFA) with the flow rate of 0.75 mL/min (Fig. 7).

4 Notes

1. The linker-payload PF-06424469 is prepared by procedures listed in reference 7.
2. The anti-notch 3 antibody is prepared using mammalian cell lines by standard recombinant monoclonal antibody preparation and purification techniques.
3. The linker-payload PF-06424469 is extremely toxic. Use of glove box or other engineering controls is recommended during weighing operation of the powder. Precaution should be taken to wear appropriate PPE during all operations.

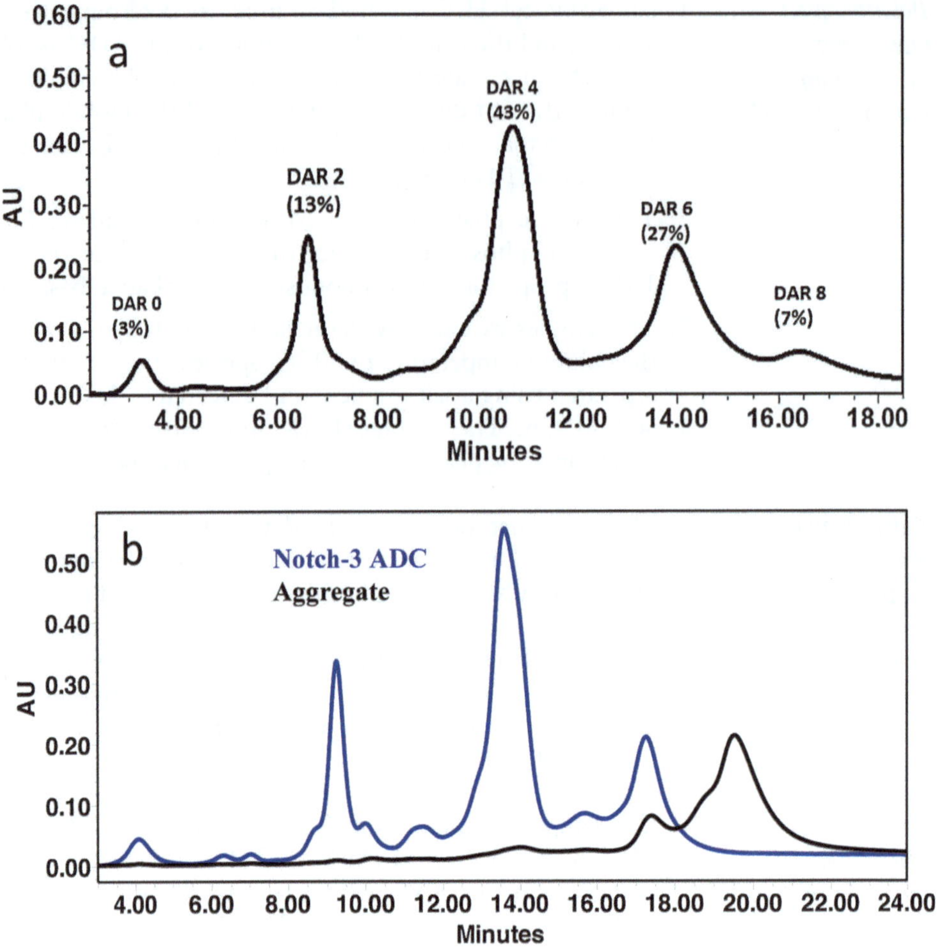

Fig. 5 Analytical HIC chromatograms of Notch 3 ADC (**a**) before purification and (**b**) after purification by column chromatography (blue) and isolated aggregates (black)

4. The anti-notch 3 antibody is formulated in 20 mM histidine buffer, pH 5–6. The pH of the antibody solution is adjusted with 200 mM histidine buffer solution, pH 7.8. The final concentration of histidine in the reaction mixture is 100 mM.

5. During TCEP addition, the rate of agitation should be controlled to obtain homogeneous solution of the antibody. The stoichiometric ratio of TCEP to mAb is critical for the formation of the conjugate with the desired DAR value. Before performing scale up of this conjugation, the correct charge of the TCEP should be determined by performing small-scale titration experiments with the TCEP and mAb samples. The thiol content of the mAb formed after the reduction can be evaluated using Ellman's reagent (bis-dithionitrobenzoic acid, DTNB). Alternatively, the reduced mAb samples can be conjugated to excess linker-payload. The DAR of the reaction

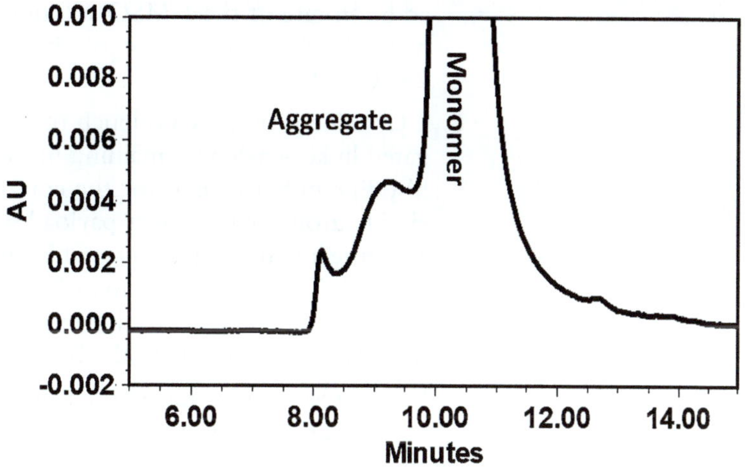

Fig. 6 SEC chromatograph of unpurified Notch 3 ADC

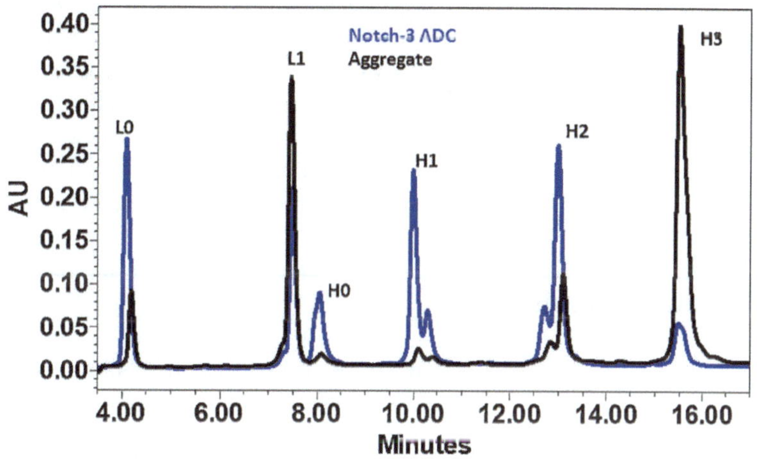

Fig. 7 Analytical RP-HPLC chromatogram of Notch 3 ADC purified by column chromatography. *L* light chain, *H* heavy chain. L0, L1, H0, H1, H2, and H3 represent the number of drug-related species conjugated to the light or the heavy chain

mixture sample after conjugation is determined by using either analytical HIC or reduced reverse phase HPLC assay.

6. It is a good practice to perform reduction and conjugation reactions under an inert atmosphere (either nitrogen or argon). However, we have not observed any significant difference in DAR values or other quality attributes of conjugates when the reduction-conjugation steps were performed in the presence of air.

7. Final concentration of DMSO in the reaction mixture is 11.3% (v/v). The addition of DMSO to the solution of antibody in histidine buffer solution is moderately exothermic. The

addition rate of the DMSO solution is controlled in order to maintain the temperature of the reaction mixture between 23 °C and 27 °C.

8. L-Cysteine is used as a quench reagent to react with unconjugated linker-payload remaining in the reaction mixture. When histidine buffer is used for the conjugation reaction, the maleimide group of the linker-payload slowly reacts with histidine resulting in the formation of histidine adduct of the linker-payload. The rate of reaction of cysteines on the mAb or as a quench reagent with the linker-payload is significantly faster than with the histidine in the buffer at pH 6–7.
9. Several resins and elution buffers were screened for purification of this ADC. Best results were obtained with ceramic hydroxyapatite resin with the sodium phosphate gradient reported in this procedure. For the Notch 3 ADC described here we were unable to purify the ADC only with ultrafiltration-diafiltration step. Purification by column chromatography successfully separated aggregates, residual-free drug (eluted in flow through), and solvent DMSO (eluted in flow through). For many other ADC preparations, where the formation of product-related impurities such as aggregates is minimal, purification by UF-DF alone is usually sufficient to separate ADC species from small molecule process-related impurities.

Acknowledgement

The author thanks Qingping Jiang, He Meng, Jeffry Borgmeyer, Nataliya Bazhina, and Olga Friese for their contributions during the development of this work. The author also thanks Leo Letendre, Heyi Li, Bo Arve, and Aparna Deora for their support and encouragement.

References

1. Mallory RG, Mine C, Longyu L, Jiaming Z, Barbara O, Thayumanavan S (2015) Field guide to challenges and opportunities in antibody-drug conjugates for chemists. Bioconjug Chem 26(11):2198–2215
2. Zhou Q (2017) Site-specific antibody conjugation for ADC and beyond. Biomedicine 5:64
3. Hamann PR (2011) In: Barrish JC, Carter PH, Cheng PTW, Zahler R (eds) Accounts in drug discovery: case studies in medicinal chemistry. The genesis of the antibody conjugate gemtuzumab ozogamicin (Mylotarg®) for acute myeloid leukemia. Chapter 5: 103–119
4. Chen Y, Kim MT, Zheng L, Deperalta G, Jacobson F (2016) Structural characterization of cross-linked species in Trastuzumab Emtansine (Kadcyla). Bioconjug Chem 27:2037–2047
5. Lyon RP, Meyer DL, Setter JR, Senter PD (2012) Conjugation of anticancer drugs through endogenous monoclonal antibody cysteine residues. Methods Enzymol 502:123–138
6. Behrens CR, Liu B (2014) Methods for site-specific drug conjugation to antibodies. MAbs 6(1):46–53

7. Geles KG, Gao Y, Sapra P, Tchitstiakova LG, Zhou SB (2014) Anti-notch 3 antibodies and antibody drug conjugates. Pfizer Inc., New York, NY. Patent 0127211A1
8. Hamblett KJ, Senter PD, Chace DF, Sun MMC, Lenox J, Cerveny CG, Kissler KM, Bernhardt SX, Kopcha AK, Zabinski RF, Meyer DL, Francisco JA (2004) Effects of drug loading on the antitumor activity of a monoclonal antibody drug conjugate. Clin Cancer Res 10:7063–7070
9. Nadkarni DV, Jiang Q, Friese O, Bazhina N, Meng H, Guo J, Kutlik R, Borgmeyer J (2018) Process development and structural characterization of an anti-notch 3 antibody–drug conjugate. Org Process Res Dev 22:286–295
10. Hollander I, Kunz A, Hamann PR (2008) Selection of reaction additives used in the preparation of monomeric antibody–Calicheamicin conjugates. Bioconjug Chem 19:358–361
11. Li W, Prabakaran P, Chen W, Zhu Z, Feng Y, Dimitrov DS (2016) Antibody aggregation: insights from sequence and structure. Antibodies 5:19–23
12. Gagnon P, Beam K (2009) Antibody aggregate removal by hydroxyapatite chromatography. Curr Pharm Biotechnol 10:440–446
13. Nadkarni DV, Borgmeyer J, Meng H, Jiang Q (2017) Purification of antibody drug conjugates using a sodium phosphate gradient. Pfizer Inc., New York, NY. Patent WO 2017/109619 Al

Chapter 4

Site-Specific Conjugation to Cys-Engineered THIOMAB™ Antibodies

Pragya Adhikari, Neelie Zacharias, Rachana Ohri, and Jack Sadowsky

Abstract

Antibodies bearing engineered cysteine residues (termed THIOMAB™ antibodies) enable the site-selective attachment of a drug, label or other payload for specific delivery to certain tissues (e.g., tumors). This Chapter describes detailed methods we have developed and optimized for the conjugation, purification and analysis of THIOMAB™ antibody drug conjugates (TDCs).

Key words Maleimide, Disulfide, ADC, Engineered cysteine, THIOMAB, Site-specific conjugation

1 Introduction

Of the various methods available to chemically attach small molecule payloads or imaging probes to antibodies, site-specific conjugation methods have clear advantages in that they generate more homogeneous products and may result in improved therapeutic or diagnostic outcomes (e.g., improved safety and enhanced image contrast, respectively) [1, 2]. Most site-specific conjugation strategies require recombinant incorporation into the antibody of one or more amino acid residues or peptide segments that can be reacted selectively versus endogenous residues with an appropriately functionalized small molecule via either a chemical or enzymatic process. Arguably, the simplest and most well-validated such approach to date involves recombinant mutation of one or more amino acids to an engineered cysteine, a residue which has been known for at least 70 years to be chemoselectively reactive toward certain electrophilic functionalities (e.g., maleimides and haloacetamides) [3]. Genentech was the first to report the successful deployment of an engineered Cys approach to generate homogeneous antibody–drug conjugates (ADCs), highlighting improvements in pharmacokinetics and safety concomitant with site-specific conjugation [2, 4]. Since those initial reports, much has been learned

L. Nathan Tumey (ed.), *Antibody-Drug Conjugates: Methods and Protocols*, Methods in Molecular Biology, vol. 2078,
https://doi.org/10.1007/978-1-4939-9929-3_4,

regarding optimal sites at which to place the engineered Cys residue to achieve optimal stability both of the direct connection to the antibody as well as the more distal payload in biological milieu [5, 6]. A previous report in this journal presented basic methods for conjugation, purification, and analysis of THIOMAB™ antibody–drug conjugates [7]. In this chapter, we describe further details, additional methods, tips, and tricks developed over the years since that initial report, aiming to give the reader a more comprehensive understanding of the processes involved in THIOMAB™ antibody conjugate preparation for in vitro and in vivo studies.

2 Materials

2.1 THIOMAB™ Antibody Deblocking

1. *THIOMAB™ antibody*: Expressed and purified from an appropriate host cell line, as described previously [7].
2. *1 M Tris pH 8.0 stock solution*: Dissolve 88.8 g of TRIS HCL and 53.0 g of TRIS base in 1 L of sterile water. Bring the pH to 8.0 with 37% hydrochloric acid. Filter the buffer. This solution can be stored at room temperature for at least 6 months.
3. *1 M Tris, pH 7.5 stock solution*: Dissolve 134.5 g of TRIS HCL and 18.0 g of TRIS Base in 1 L of sterile water. Bring the pH to 7.5 with 37% hydrochloric acid. Filter the buffer. This solution can be stored at room temperature for at least 6 months.
4. *100 mM DTT stock solution*: Dissolve 154.2 mg of dithiothreitol (DTT) in 10 mL of sterile water. This solution can be stored as aliquots at −20 °C. Once the aliquot is thawed it should be used within approximately 30 min.
5. *0.2 M EDTA, pH 8.0 stock solution*: Dissolve 56.52 g of EDTA (tetrasodium tetrahydrate salt) in 1 L of sterile water. Bring the pH to 8.0 with 50% NaOH. Filter the buffer. This solution can be stored at room temperature for at least 6 months.
6. *50 mM Tris, pH 7.5*: Dilute 50 mL of 1 M Tris, pH 7.5 (from above) in 950 mL of sterile water. Filter the buffer. This solution can be stored at room temperature for at least 6 months.
7. *200 mM Succinate, pH 5.0 stock solution*: Dissolve 23.32 g of succinic acid in 1 L of sterile water. Bring the pH to 5.0 with 50% NaOH. Filter the buffer. This solution can be stored at room temperature for at least 6 months.
8. *5 M NaCl*: Dissolve 292.2 g of NaCl in 1 L of sterile water. Filter the buffer. This solution can be stored at room temperature for at least 6 months.
9. *Loading Buffer (20 mM succinate, pH 5.0)*: Dilute 10 mL of 200 mM succinate, pH 5.0 stock solution (above) in 990 mL of

sterile water. Filter the buffer. This solution can be stored at room temperature for at least 6 months.

10. *Elution Buffer (50 mM Tris pH 7.5, 150 mM NaCl)*: Dilute 50 mL of 1 M Tris, pH 7.5 stock solution (above) and 30 mL of 5 M NaCl (above) in 920 mL of sterile water. Filter the buffer. This solution can be stored at room temperature for at least 6 months.
11. *10% acetic acid*: Dilute 1 mL of glacial acetic acid in 9 mL of sterile water in a glass vial. Filter the buffer. This solution can be stored at room temperature for at least 6 months.
12. *100 mM DHAA*: Dissolve 174.11 mg of dehydroascorbic acid (DHAA) in 10 mL of *N,N'*-dimethylacetamide (DMA). Heating at 37 °C or sonication speeds dissolution. DHAA is sensitive to light; solutions should be kept covered in foil and used fresh.
13. SP-HP cation exchange column (GE healthcare).
14. Akta or other FPLC purification system.

2.2 Conjugation to THIOMAB™ Antibody Cysteines

1. Deblocked THIOMAB™ antibody (in 20 mM succinate, pH 5.0, 2 mM EDTA).
2. Linker-payload (10 mM stock in *N,N'*-dimethylformamide, DMF, or other suitable cosolvent).
3. DMF (or other suitable cosolvent).
4. 1 M Tris, pH 7.5 buffer.
5. 1 M Tris, pH 8.0 buffer.
6. Polypropylene tubes (e.g., 1.5-mL snap-cap, 15-mL conical or 50-mL conical).

2.3 Conjugate Purification (See Note 1)

1. Desalting (spin column method):
   (a) Zeba™ Spin Desalting Columns, 7 K MWCO, 5 mL (Thermo Scientific, Prod #: 89892).
   (b) 15 mL or 50 mL tubes (Fisher Scientific).
   (c) Bench top centrifuge.
   (d) 0.5 N Sodium Hydroxide (NaOH): 50 mL 10 N NaOH in 950 mL Milli-Q ultrapure water. Filter through 0.2 μm filter.
2. Cation exchange (FPLC method).
   (a) AKTA purification system (GE).
   (b) SPHP column: HiLoad 26/10 SP Sephorose High Performance (GE Healthcare, Prod #: 17-1138-01).

(c) Buffer A (10 mM succinate, pH 5): 50 mL 200 mM succinate, pH 5 in 950 mL Milli-Q ultrapure water. Filter through 0.2 μm filter.

(d) Buffer B (10 mM succinate, 300 mM NaCl, pH 5): 50 mL 200 mM succinate, pH 5, 60 mL 5 M NaCl in 890 mL Milli-Q ultrapure water. Filter through 0.2 μm filter.

(e) 500 mL bottle to collect flow-through.

(f) 2 mL 96-well plates for fraction collection.

3. Dialysis

(a) Slide-A-Lyzer Gamma Irradiated Dialysis Cassette Extra-Strength, 10,000 MWCO, 3–12 mL capacity (Thermo Scientific, Prod #: 66453).

(b) Beaker (autoclaved).

(c) Syringe and needle.

(d) Foam floater.

(e) Magnetic stir plate.

(f) Cold room or deli case.

(g) Formulation buffer (20 mM histidine-acetate, 240 mM sucrose, pH 5.5): 3.1 g histidine, 1.03 mL glacial acetic acid, 82.1 g sucrose NF grade, adjust pH to 5.5, make up volume to 1 L using Milli-Q ultrapure water. Filter through 0.2 μm filter.

4. Removal of free linker-payload (charcoal method).

(a) Dextran-coated activated charcoal (Sigma-Aldrich, Prod #: C6241).

(b) 0.2 μm spin filter: Spin-X Centrifuge Tube Filter, 0.22 μm cellulose acetate (Costar, Prod #: 8160). For larger volumes: Ultrafree-CL GV 0.22 μm sterile filters (Merck Millipore, Prod #: UFC40GV0S).

(c) Bench top centrifuge.

(d) Formulation buffer (20 mM histidine-acetate, 240 mM sucrose, pH 5.5): 3.1 g histidine, 1.03 mL glacial acetic acid, 82.1 g sucrose NF grade, adjust pH to 5.5, make up volume to 1 L using Milli-Q ultrapure water. Filter through 0.2 μm filter.

(e) Rotator.

5. Cation exchange (spin column method):

(a) S maxi columns: Pierce® Strong Cation Exchange Spin Columns, Maxi (Thermo Scientific, Prod #: 90009).

(b) 50 mL tubes (Fisher Scientific)

(c) Bench top centrifuge.

(d) Wash buffer (20 mM Histidine-Acetate, pH 5.5): 3.1 g histidine, 1.03 mL glacial acetic acid, adjust pH to 5.5, make up volume to 1 L using Milli-Q ultrapure water. Filter through 0.2 μm filter.

(e) Elution buffer (20 mM Histidine-Acetate, 300 mM NaCl, pH 5.5): 3.1 g histidine, 1.03 mL glacial acetic acid, 60 mL 5 M NaCl, adjust pH to 5.5, make up volume to 1 L using Milli-Q ultrapure water. Filter through 0.2 μm filter.

6. Size-exclusion chromatography (FPLC method).

(a) AKTA purification system (GE).

(b) S200 column: HiPrep 16/60 Sephacryl S-200 HR (maximum 5 mL sample volume) (GE Healthcare, Prod #: 17116601) or a HiPrep 26/60 Sephacryl S-200 HR (maximum 13 mL sample volume) (GE Healthcare, Prod #: 17119501).

(c) Luer-lok Syringe: Disposable Syringes with Luer-Lok Tips, sterile, 5 mL (BD, Prod #: 309646).

(d) Buffer (20 mM Histidine-Acetate, 300 mM NaCl, pH 5.5): 3.1 g histidine, 1.03 mL glacial acetic acid, 60 mL 5 M NaCl, adjust pH to 5.5, make up volume to 1 L using Milli-Q ultrapure water. Filter through 0.2 μm filter.

(e) 2 mL 96-well plates and lids for fraction collection: 96-well deep well plates (VWR, Prod #: 10755-250) and 96-well sterile sealing cap, square well (Labnet, Prod #: P9639).

7. Endotoxin removal (Triton precipitation method).

(a) Ice bucket.

(b) Ice.

(c) 10% Triton X-114: Triton® X-114, 10% aqueous solution, proteomic grade, 10 mL, sterile (GBiosciences, Prod #: DG009).

(d) Incubator.

(e) Bench top, fixed angle centrifuge.

(f) 0.2 μm spin filter.

2.4 Conjugate Analysis

1. Agilent 1260 series LCMS (or other LCMS system).
2. PLRP-S column (Agilent product # PL1912-1802, 1000 angstroms, 8 μm, 50 × 2.1 mm) (*see* **Note 2**).
3. Buffer A: Milli-Q Ultrapure Water with 0.05% LCMS-grade TFA (Sigma-Aldrich product # 302031-10 × 1 mL).
4. Buffer B: Chromasolv-grade Acetonitrile (Sigma-Aldrich product # 34967-1L) with 0.05% LCMS-grade TFA.

5. Deglycosylation: PNGase F (New England Biolabs product # P0710S).
6. LysC digestion: Lysyl endopeptidase (Wako product # 129-02541). Make 1 mg/mL stock solution in water, which may be stored as aliquots at −78 °C.
7. IdeS digestion: IdeS "Fabricator" enzyme (Genovis product # A0-FR1-050).
8. DTT reduction: DTT (Sigma-Aldrich product #D9779-10 g). Make 1 M solution in water, which may be stored as aliquots at − 20 °C.
9. LCMS vials with plastic low-volume inserts (Agilent product # 5182-0715).
10. (For SEC measurements) Agilent 1260 Infinity HPLC.
11. SEC buffer: 0.2 M potassium phosphate pH 6.2 with 0.25 mM potassium chloride and 15% IPA is used as mobile phase.
12. *SEC column*: TSKgel G3000SWXL (Tosoh product # 808541).
13. Conjugate concentration determination.

    BCA:

    (a) Microplate Reader capable of reading at 562 nm.
    (b) BCA kit (Thermo Scientific product #23225).
    (c) 96-well clear plate, flat bottom, 400 μL well (sterile) (Nunc product #156545
    (d) Appropriate antibody standard at known concentration.

    Ides:

    (a) Agilent 1200 series HPLC.
    (b) Buffers: Same as LCMS buffers.
14. Endotoxin measurement.
    (a) Endosafe LAL reader (Charles River).
    (b) LAL cartilages (Charles River product # PTS20F).

3 Methods

THIOMAB™ antibodies were prepared by expression in Chinese hamster ovary (CHO) cells followed by purification via standard techniques, which are not described below, but are described in the literature [7]. The incorporated cysteines in THIOMAB™ antibody preparations are initially present as mixed disulfides with cysteine or glutathione and are thus not initially reactive toward thiol-reactive payloads. The procedures described below therefore begin with the processing ("deblocking") required to make the free thiol of the incorporated Cys fully available for conjugation (Fig. 1).

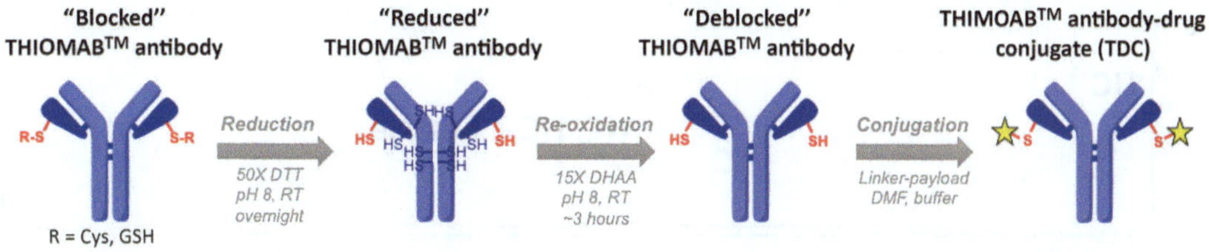

Fig. 1 Scheme for "deblocking" a THIOMAB™ antibody to enable subsequent conjugation to a thiol-reactive linker-drug moiety

3.1 Deblocking

1. Determine the concentration of the THIOMAB™ antibody (e.g., using absorbance at 280 nm or a BCA assay).
2. Dilute the antibody to <10 mg/mL using 50 mM Tris pH 7.5 and adjust pH to ~7.5 by adding 1 M Tris, pH 8.0 to a final Tris concentration of 100 mM.
3. Add 0.2 M EDTA, pH 8.0 solution to a final EDTA concentration of 2 mM.
4. Add 100 mM DTT to a final concentration at least 100 times that of the antibody.
5. Allow antibody to react with DTT at room temperature overnight to ensure complete reduction of interchain disulfides and removal of glutathione/cysteine adducts, the latter of which appear by mass spectrometry as additions of 121 Da (cysteine) or 304 Da (glutathione) to the mass of the chain into which the engineered Cys has been incorporated (Fig. 2) (*see* **Note 3**).
6. Dilute the reduced THIOMAB™ antibody solution at least fivefold with Loading Buffer (20 mM succinate pH 5), ensuring final salt concentration is less than 15 mM and final pH is approximately 5.0. Add 10% acetic acid to the mixture to adjust pH, if necessary.
7. Load the THIOMAB™ antibody onto a pre-equilibrated SP-HP cation exchange column using an FPLC instrument.
8. Wash the column with 5–10 column volumes of Loading Buffer to remove excess DTT.
9. Elute the bound antibody with Elution Buffer (50 mM Tris pH 7.5, 150 mM NaCl), monitoring UV signal at 280 nm.
10. Measure the pH of the eluted THIOMAB™ antibody solution, adjusting to 7.5 with 1 M Tris, pH 8.0 if necessary.
11. Using the 100 mM DHAA stock solution, add 15 equivalents of DHAA to the antibody solution to initiate reoxidation of the interchain Cys disulfides.
12. Monitor reoxidation of the antibody by DHAA by LCMS. A convenient way to do this is to track the disappearance of free light chain, which can often be chromatographically separated

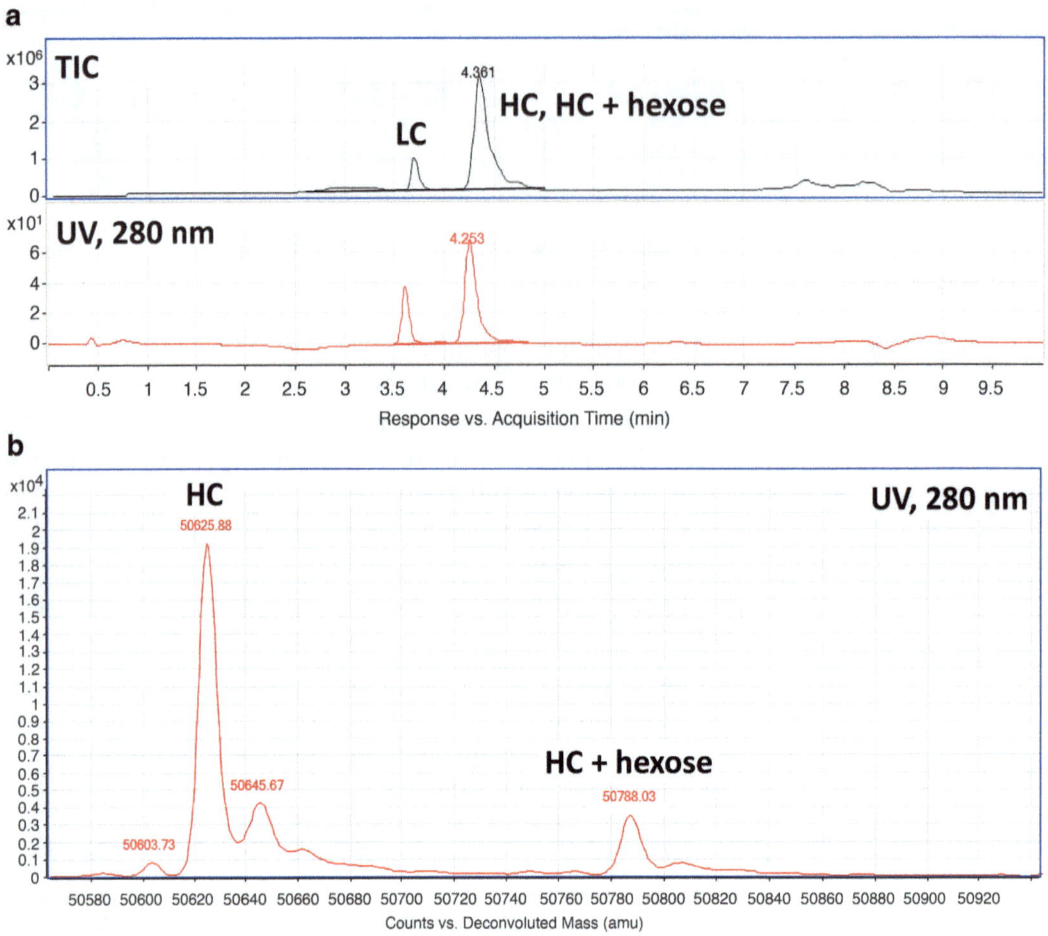

Fig. 2 (**a**) Reverse-phase LCMS total ion chromatogram (TIC) and UV spectra at 280 nm of a reduced THIOMAB™ antibody which shows separation of HC (late-eluting peak) and LC (early-eluting peak). (**b**) Deconvoluted spectra of the HC peak shows no presence of HC + cysteine (+121 Da) or HC + glutathione (+304 Da), indicating that purification and reoxidation can proceed

from intact antibody on LCMS (Fig. 3). We consider reoxidation "complete" when the area of the UV peak (at 280 nm) corresponding to the free light chain is <3% that of the intact antibody peak. Add additional DHAA if reoxidation is incomplete after 3 h and follow the reaction closely thereafter (*see* **Note 4**).

13. Dilute the reoxidized THIOMAB™ antibody solution at least fivefold with Loading Buffer, ensuring salt concentration is less than 15 mM and pH is approximately 5.0. Add 10% acetic acid to adjust pH if necessary.
14. Load diluted antibody onto a pre-equilibrated SP-HP cation exchange column using an FPLC instrument.

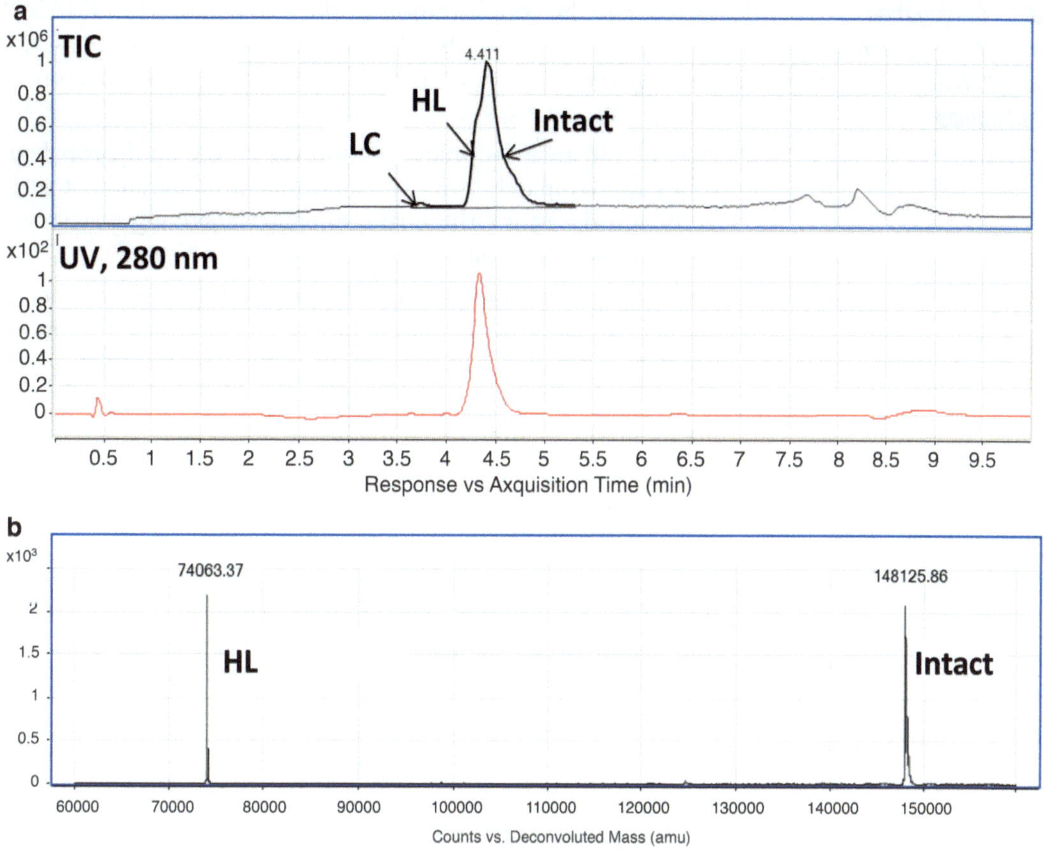

Fig. 3 (**a**) Reverse-phase LCMS TIC and UV (at 280 nm) spectra of the reoxidized antibody shows that the light-chain (LC) peak area is <3% that of the intact antibody peak. An additional shoulder corresponding to a heavy chain-light chain (HL) "half-antibody" in which the hinge disulfides on the heavy chain are intramolecularly crosslinked may also be present. (**b**) Deconvoluted mass spectrum showing the HL and intact antibody peaks. The HL species ionizes more efficiently than the intact antibody; when measured by independent means, the HL species is generally <5% of the reoxidized antibody preparation

15. Wash the column with 5–10 column volumes of Loading Buffer to remove DHAA.
16. Elute the bound antibody with a gradient of 30–100% Elution Buffer in Loading Buffer over 15 column volumes. Monitor protein elution by UV at 280 nm.
17. Pool fractions corresponding to intact, reoxidized, and monomeric (by SEC) THIOMAB™ antibody and concentrate if desired.
18. The THIOMAB™ antibody may be used immediately for conjugation reactions or, for future use, may be dialyzed in 20 mM succinate, pH 5.0, 150 mM NaCl, 2 mM EDTA, sterile-filtered, aliquoted, and stored at −80°C for at least 2 years prior to performing conjugation reactions.

3.2 Conjugation of Linker-Payloads to THIOMAB™ Antibodies

1. Determine the concentration of the deblocked THIOMAB™ antibody (e.g., using absorbance at 280 nm or a BCA assay). Subsequent calculations assume an antibody concentration of 10 mg/mL (~68 μM).
2. Pipette into an appropriate reaction vessel (e.g., polypropylene tube) approximately twice the amount, in milligrams, of antibody you desire for the final conjugate, assuming (conservatively) a 50% yield following purification (*see* **Note 5**).
3. For conjugation of maleimides to the THIOMAB™ antibody, add 75 μL of 1 M Tris, pH 7.5 to a final concentration of 75 mM Tris. For conjugation of activated disulfides (e.g., nitro-pyridyldisulfide), add 75 μL of 1 M Tris, pH 8.5 to a final concentration of 75 mM Tris (*see* **Note 6**).
4. Prepare an intermediate dilution of the linker-payload in DMF to 670 μM or 10 times the final concentration of the antibody (*see* **Notes** 7 and **8**).
5. Add 0.1 mL of the intermediate dilution of maleimide compound to the antibody/Tris mixture, ensuring complete mixing by pipetting up and down and ensuring no unmixed antibody or linker-payload solution remains on the sides of the tube or tube cap. Do not vortex (*see* **Note 9**).
6. Generally, the reaction may be allowed to sit at room temperature, ideally in the dark, and can be monitored (ideally, by LCMS) to ensure completion before purification (*see* **Note 10**).
7. When complete, the reaction may be diluted in a buffer suitable for the subsequent purification method desired (e.g., with >5× volume of 20 mM histidine acetate, pH 5.5 for loading onto a cation exchange column). Alternatively, the reaction may be loaded directly onto an appropriate column without dilution (e.g., gel filtration column connected to an Akta purification system).

3.3 Conjugate Purification by Disposable Gel Filtration Columns (See Note 11)

1. Snap off bottom seal of Zeba desalting column, unscrew cap slightly so loose but not falling off and put column in falcon tube.
2. Centrifuge at 1000 × *g* for 2 min.
3. Discard flow-through and add 0.5 N NaOH to resin to sanitize column and fill to top. Let sit for 30 min.
4. Centrifuge at 1000 × *g* for 2 min.
5. Discard flow-through and add desired formulation buffer to the resin (filled to top), screwing cap on loosely.
6. Centrifuge at 1000 × *g* for 2 min.

7. Repeat **steps 5** and **6** until flow-through is pH of buffer. Verify appropriate pH in flow-through using pH strips.
8. Add 500–2000 μL of sample to resin (depending on Zeba column size) and place column in a new, pre-weighed falcon tube.
9. Centrifuge at 1000 × *g* for 2 min to elute conjugate.

3.4 Conjugate Purification by Disposable Cation Exchange Columns (See Note 12)

1. Add 20 mM histidine-acetate pH 5.5 buffer to the column vessel, fill to top.
2. Centrifuge at 500 × *g* for 3 min.
3. Discard flow-through.
4. Repeat **steps 1** to **3** once (for a total of two washes).
5. Add <2 mL of conjugate solution to the top of the cation exchange column and fill the column vessel with 20 mM histidine-acetate pH 5.5 buffer up to the top (for a >fivefold dilution). This will result in a diluted conjugate with pH 5.5 and sufficiently low salt concentration (<20 mM) to enable efficient binding of the conjugate to the cation exchange resin.
6. Centrifuge at 500 × *g* for 3 min.
7. Collect sample loading flow-through just in case sample does not bind. Save and set aside until desired conjugate is isolated after the procedure.
8. Repeat **steps 5** to 7 until all of sample is loaded on column.
9. Add 20 mM histidine-acetate pH 5.5 buffer to column, fill to top.
10. Centrifuge at 500 × *g* for 3 min.
11. Discard flow-through.
12. Repeat **steps 9** to **11** twice for a total of three washes (*see* **Note 13**).
13. Add 5 mL 20 mM histidine-acetate, pH 5.5, 300 mM NaCl and place column vessel into new, pre-weighed 50 mL falcon tube.
14. Centrifuge at 500 × *g* for 3 min.
15. A second elution step with higher salt concentration can be done, but collect the eluate in a new tube since this second elution will likely contain more aggregate.

3.5 Conjugate Purification by Cation Exchange Using FPLC System (See Note 14)

1. Dilute conjugate sample by tenfold using buffer A (10 mM succinate pH 5) and check the pH. Adjust pH with 10% acetic acid if necessary to achieve pH 5.
2. Load sample onto SPHP column (GE Healthcare) using a sample line connected to sample pump (instead of using a syringe and sample loop).

3. Collect load flow-through in case sample loading was inefficient. Discard at the end of this procedure if successful in isolating the desired conjugate.
4. Wash column with 5–10 column volumes of buffer A.
5. Elute with a gradient 30–100% of buffer B (10 mM succinate, pH 5, 300 mM NaCl).
6. Collect 1.5–2 mL fractions in 96-well plates throughout method. Pool and concentrate fractions (e.g., using Amicon spin-tubes with a 10,000 MW cutoff) as appropriate.

3.6 Conjugate Purification by Size-Exclusion Chromatography Using FPLC System (See Note 15)

1. Sanitize the AKTA system without the column attached with 0.5 N NaOH by flushing all buffer lines, ports, column lines, sample line or loop, and outlet lines with NaOH and letting the solution sit for 30 min.
2. Flush whole system and lines with water then buffer that will be used on size-exclusion column (e.g., 20 mM histidine-acetate, pH 5.5).
3. Attach and sanitize column by loading the maximum sample volume of 0.5 N NaOH to column followed by 1 column volume of water then 1.25 column volume of buffer (make sure pH and conductivity at the end point corresponds to expected buffer pH and conductivity).
4. Load sample using sample loop on injection valve. Draw up sample using needle and luer-loc syringe. Remove needle and knockout all air bubbles. Screw syringe into syringe port on AKTA injection valve and inject sample into sample loop.
5. Run 5 times the sample loop volume of buffer through loop when loading sample onto column to completely flush out sample loop.
6. Change injection valve to "manual load" and start fraction collection.
7. Flow at least 1.25 CV of buffer over column before initiating another injection.

3.7 Conjugate Purification and Reformulation by Dialysis (See Note 16)

1. Add desired formulation buffer to a large beaker. A 200-fold dilution for the buffer volume is recommended (For example: A 3 mL sample would require at least 600 mL of buffer. Therefore, the dialysis would be carried out in 1 L of buffer in a 1 L beaker).
2. Hydrate the membrane by putting the cassette in buffer for 2 min.
3. Draw up sample in syringe with a needle, knockout and remove all bubbles in syringe.

4. Push needle through membrane in one of the four ports (do not use/puncture a port more than once).
5. Add sample from syringe into cassette slowly to prevent bubbles from forming inside cassette. Angle cassette diagonally so that sample is dripping into pool forming inside cassette.
6. When all of the sample is inside the cassette, draw up all the remaining air inside the cassette (without taking out needle form port).
7. Draw air until there is only a small air bubble left.
8. Add a foam floater to the top of cassette and put in beaker already filled with desired formulation buffer. Cover the beaker with aluminum foil.
9. Put covered dialysis beaker in deli case refrigerator or cold room for refrigerated dialysis. If faster dialysis is desired then dialyze at room temperature.
10. After dialyzing for a minimum of 2 h, the buffer can be changed out for another round of dialysis so as to reach a minimum of 40,000-fold dilution by dialysis.
11. Dialysis may go on overnight or over the weekend (refrigeration is recommended for these long dialysis times).

3.8 Conjugate Purification Using Activated Charcoal (See Note 17)

1. Weigh out 100 mg of activated charcoal.
2. Add charcoal and sterile water to 0.2 μm spin filter.
3. Centrifuge until all the water has flowed through.
4. Repeat **steps 2** and **3** twice for a total of three rinses.
5. Resuspend the charcoal in 1000 μL of formulation buffer by pipetting up and down.
6. Add 1/10 (by volume) of charcoal slurry to conjugate (e.g., Add 30 μL of slurry to 300 μL of conjugate).
7. Incubate with gentle agitation or rotation at room temperature for 30 min or longer.
8. Add charcoal conjugate solution to a rinsed 0.2 μm spin filter.
9. Centrifuge.
10. Flow-through contains the purified conjugate.
11. Process can be repeated again with remaining, unused charcoal slurry or fresh slurry to remove more free linker-payload.

3.9 Precipitation and Removal of Endotoxin (See Note 18)

1. Chill conjugate on ice or an hour (unless sample is already cold due to storage in fridge overnight).
2. Add 10% Triton X114 (stored in fridge) to a final concentration of 0.1–0.5% to sample (e.g., If 0.1% Triton X114 is desired in sample, add 5.1 μL of 10% Triton X114 to 0.5 mL of sample).

3. Mix well by pipetting up and down.
4. Incubate mixture on ice for 1 h minimum.
5. Incubate at 37 °C for 15 min (bring sample up to room temperature).
6. Centrifuge at 20800 × *g* at 30 °C for 5 min.
7. Draw the supernatant carefully into new tube. Pellet is easily disturbed and looks like an oil drop. Best to leave some supernatant behind to avoid having triton in sample.
8. Filter drawn supernatant through 0.2 μm filter.

3.10 Conjugate LCMS (DAR) Analysis (See Note 19)

1. Deglycosylation (removal of Fc glycans on N297; Fig. 4a): Dilute 5 μL of THIOMAB™ antibody conjugate into 30 μL PBS and add 1 μL PNGase F (5000 U/mL). Incubate the sample mixture at 37 °C overnight. This method is generally useful when minimal chemical perturbation of the antibody conjugate is desired prior to analysis.
2. Reduction (cleavage of interchain disulfides to give separated heavy and light chains; Fig. 4b, **Note 20**): Mix solution containing 20 μg of conjugate with 1 M Tris, pH 8.0 to give a final Tris concentration of 100 mM. Add 100 mM DTT to a final concentration of 10 mM. React at 37 °C for at least 15 min.
3. LysC partial digestion (proteolytic cleavage after Lys-225, giving separated Fab and Fc domains; Fig. 4c, **Note 21**): Mix

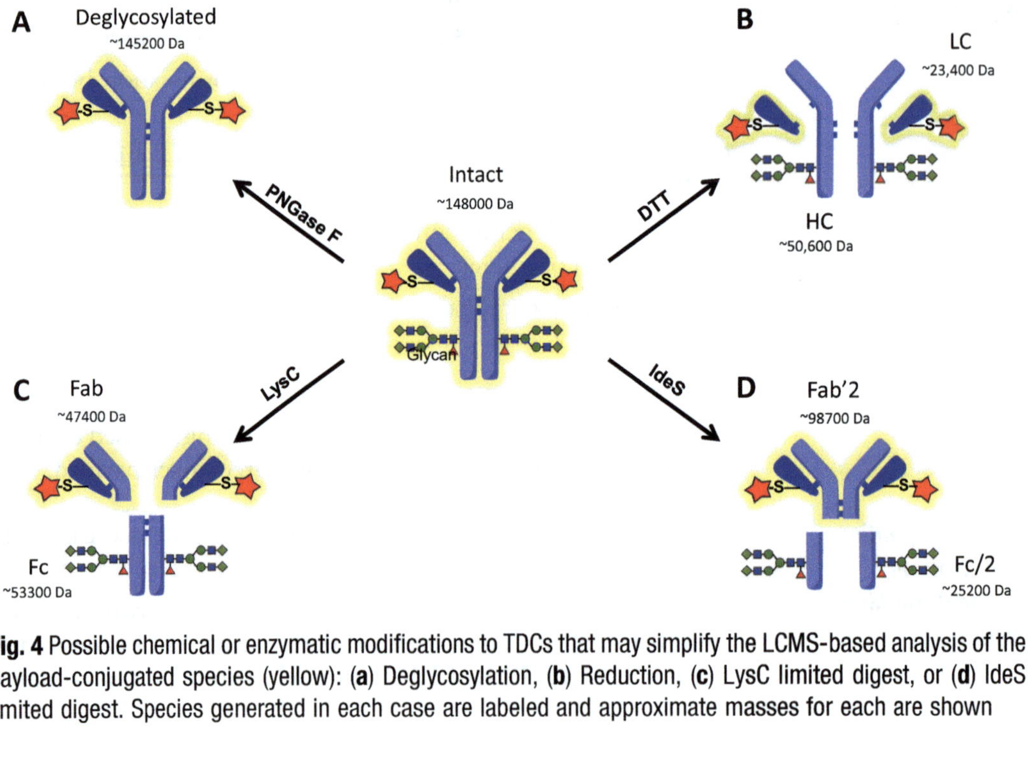

Fig. 4 Possible chemical or enzymatic modifications to TDCs that may simplify the LCMS-based analysis of the payload-conjugated species (yellow): (**a**) Deglycosylation, (**b**) Reduction, (**c**) LysC limited digest, or (**d**) IdeS limited digest. Species generated in each case are labeled and approximate masses for each are shown

solution containing 20 μg of antibody conjugate with 1 M Tris, pH 8.0 to give a final Tris concentration of 100 mM. Add 0.5 μL of 0.5 mg/mL lysyl endopeptidase (Wako, Product #129-02541). Incubate at 37 °C for no more than 15 min since prolonged incubation will result in nonspecific degradation of the conjugate.

4. IdeS partial digestion (proteolytic cleavage after Gly-239, giving separated Fab'2 and Fc/2 domains; Fig. 4d, **Note 22**): Dilute 10 μL of the conjugate (from 1 to 10 mg/mL) in 39 μL of PBS and add 1 μL of 30 units/μL IdeS enzyme (Fabricator, Genovis). Incubate at least 1 h (longer incubation times are acceptable as no over-digestion by IdeS occurs).

3.11 Conjugate SEC Analysis (Aggregation State)

1. THIOMAB™ antibody drug conjugates may aggregate due to the hydrophobic properties of the linker-payload. Analysis of aggregation state can be performed by injection of a small amount of conjugate (e.g., 1–20 μg) onto an appropriate analytical size-exclusion chromatography (SEC) column (*see* **Note 23**).

3.12 Free Linker-Payload Analysis (in Purified Conjugates)

1. To ensure no remaining linker-payload is present in purified conjugates, we perform LCMS analysis of the conjugate, monitoring presence of the free linker-payload (or known byproducts thereof) by extracted ion. A standard curve with the unconjugated linker-payload in conjugate formulation buffer enables quantitation in conjugate samples.

3.13 Conjugate Concentration Determination

1. BCA assay: Follow the manufacturer's instructions to perform a BCA assay using an antibody (ideally, the antibody from which the conjugate was made) as a standard at a known concentration (e.g., determined by UV) to determine the concentration of the conjugate (*see* **Note 24**).
2. IdeS method: For IgG1-based conjugates, digestion with IdeS using the method described above produces cleanly two identical Fc/2 fragments and one Fab'2 fragment. If the linker payload was conjugated to a THIOMAB™ site in the Fab region, the peak area of the Fc/2 fragment, as eluted on an HPLC column, can be compared to that of an antibody with known concentration to determine the concentration of the conjugate (*see* **Note 25**).

3.14 Endotoxin Measurement

1. For in vivo studies, it is important to ensure endotoxin levels in the final, purified conjugate are low. We use equipment from Charles River that employ the limulus amoebocyte lysate (LAL) assay for highly sensitive detection of endotoxin in conjugate samples. Use manufacturer's instructions to determine levels of endotoxin in conjugate samples, paying

particular attention to the requirement that introduced samples be of sufficiently high pH and omit bubbles to ensure consistent and accurate endotoxin readings.

4 Notes

1. All buffers should be sterile-filtered and reagents should be analytical grade to avoid introduction of endotoxin or other impurities into the final conjugate.
2. For analysis of antibodies and fragments thereof, heating the column to 80 °C is necessary to obtain acceptable elution from the PLRP-S column.
3. It is critical that glutathione and cysteine adducts are completely removed as their presence will negatively impact subsequent conjugation reactions.
4. Allowing reoxidation to go too long can cause covalent cross-linking of THIOMAB™ antibody species, which manifests as high-order aggregates that must be removed in the final preparation and thus reduces overall intact antibody yield. The methods described here for the reoxidation step should be considered guidelines; careful optimization of DHAA equivalents added, reagent concentrations, reaction time, temperature, and other reaction parameters is required to maximize yield of desired reoxidized intact antibody.
5. Appropriate reaction vessels include any polypropylene tube, vial, or bottle with a volume capacity at least 110% that of the volume of antibody added in this step. For a 10 mg-scale reaction, for example, pipette 1 mL of the 10 mg/mL antibody stock into a 1.5-mL Eppendorf tube.
6. For reaction of linker-payloads with other thiol-reactive handles, buffer added for pH adjustment may need optimization. We have found, for example, that exchange of the THIOMAB™ antibody into an inorganic buffer (e.g., 50 mM borate, pH 8.0, 2 mM EDTA) is an attractive starting point when considering conjugation of non-maleimide/non-disulfide linker-payloads. Since maleimide reactions are reasonably efficient at pH 5 (the pH of the deblocked THIOMAB™ antibody storage buffer), it is not absolutely necessary to adjust the pH of the antibody stock solution prior to addition of a maleimide-bearing payload. However, we have found that addition of 1 M Tris, pH 7.5 to the antibody to a final concentration of ~10–100 mM Tris (pH ~7.5) accelerates reaction with maleimides and does not generally result in over-modification of the antibody. Conjugation of activated disulfides is not efficient below pH 8.0.

7. Other suitable cosolvents include water, *N*,*N*-dimethylacetamide (DMA), propylene glycol (PG) and dimethylsulfoxide (DMSO). Higher or lower stock concentrations, depending on compound solubility, are also acceptable if desired.
8. The optimal concentration of the intermediate dilution and therefore the number of equivalents of linker-payload added to the antibody in this step can be determined from a small-scale pilot reaction (e.g., with 0.1 mg antibody), conducted with various linker-payload-to-antibody ratios. For especially hydrophobic compounds, dilution of the stock material in more DMF or in propylene glycol to give final reaction solutions that contain a lower concentration of linker-payload and/or up to 20% DMF (v/v) or 50% propylene glycol (v/v) is often possible without affecting aggregation state of the antibody.
9. Solution temperature may increase somewhat following addition of linker-payload due to heat of dilution of DMF or other organic cosolvent in the aqueous antibody solution.
10. Alternatively, the reaction temperature can be 37 °C to accelerate the reaction rate and enhance linker-payload solubility, albeit with a possible negative consequence on antibody aggregation state.
11. This method is useful for quick purification of conjugate reactions or for final formulation of conjugates that have undergone other purification steps. Purification of crude conjugation reactions by this method does not always remove free linker-payload completely; the user is therefore advised to test for the presence of free linker-payload, especially in conjugates that have undergone only this purification step (*see* Subheading 3.12).
12. This method is effective for quick purification of conjugates from free linker-payload and does not result in extensive dilution of the sample provided that the original sample volume is equal to or greater than the dilution volume. However, formulation in a buffer of choice may be desired post-elution. The column described has, conservatively, a binding capacity of 40 mg for THIOMAB™ antibody drug conjugates in our experience.
13. If there is concern that the conjugate will be contaminated with unacceptable levels of endotoxin, the resin-bound conjugate may be washed with Triton solution and then by 20 mM histidine-acetate, pH 5.5 prior to elution in the next step.
14. This method is useful for removing both free linker-payload and aggregated conjugate, the former of which generally elutes earlier and the latter of which elutes later than the desired monomeric conjugate. Dilution of the conjugate across several

fractions in a buffer that is a mixture of buffer A and B is expected, which may necessitate concentration and reformulation in a buffer of choice.

15. This method is useful for removal of free linker-payload and other small molecule impurities as well as aggregated conjugate. Eluted conjugate is generally diluted in the running buffer, which may necessitate concentration and exchange into a formulation buffer of choice prior to biological testing.
16. This method is useful for exchange of conjugates into a formulation buffer suitable for subsequent biological or other testing and removal of small molecule impurities (e.g., free linker-payload). Some concentration of the conjugate in the dialysis membrane occurs.
17. This method is useful for removal of especially hydrophobic or otherwise difficult-to-remove linker-payloads or other impurities from purified conjugate samples. The method is less effective in conjugate reactions with 10% or above of organic solvent (e.g., DMF).
18. This method is useful for removal of endotoxin if present in the purified conjugate. We have found that this method is effective for this purpose, but even if performed carefully, results in significant reductions of final conjugate yield (especially at small scales) and introduction of a detectable (by MS) level of Triton detergent.
19. To determine the drug-to-antibody ratio (DAR) and identify and quantify undesired byproducts or impurities, conjugates in crude or purified form should be analyzed by LCMS. Because of the large size of intact antibodies (~148,000 Da) and their often heterogeneous glycosylation pattern, we have found that analysis of antibody fragments (e.g., reduced or partially digested by one of various proteases) is often preferred for atomic level characterization of THIOMAB™ antibody conjugates. We describe briefly below methods for analytical-scale generation of THIOMAB™ antibody fragments that we have found most useful.
20. This method is generally useful for maleimide-linked THIOMAB™ antibody conjugates, but is not advised for disulfide-linked conjugates or for conjugates involving payloads that are sensitive to DTT.
21. This method is generally useful when the engineered Cys residue is present in the Fab region. The LysC method is not advised when the linker-payload bears a lysine residue (e.g., Phe-Lys-PAB) as the enzyme is specific for cleavage after lysine.
22. This method is useful when the engineered THIOMAB™ antibody cysteine is in the Fc domain since the Fc/2 fragments

generated are small in size (~25 kDa), bearing only the glycans. Since IdeS is a cysteine protease, this method is not generally effective when performed on crude THIOMAB™ antibody reaction mixtures containing excess (Cys-reactive) linker-payload.

23. We have found that the Shodex KW802.5 or TSKgelG3000SWXL column with a running buffer of 0.2 M potassium phosphate, pH 6.2, 0.25 mM potassium chloride and 15% isopropanol is an effective way to monitor conjugate aggregation of both crude and purified conjugates.
24. We have found this method to be highly robust and accurate for most conjugate samples, with the exception of those bearing a payload that absorbs near 562 nm, the wavelength used for BCA assays.
25. We have found this method to be highly effective, even for conjugates that bear payloads with strong UV absorbance.

Acknowledgements

We acknowledge Martine Darwish, Breanna Vollmar, and Richard Vandlen for helpful comments.

References

1. Agarwal P, Bertozzi CR (2015) Site-specific antibody-drug conjugates: the nexus of bioorthogonal chemistry, protein engineering, and drug development. Bioconjug Chem 26 (2):176–192. https://doi.org/10.1021/bc5004982
2. Junutula JR, Raab H, Clark S, Bhakta S, Leipold DD, Weir S, Chen Y, Simpson M, Tsai SP, Dennis MS et al (2008) Site-specific conjugation of a cytotoxic drug to an antibody improves the therapeutic index. Nat Biotechnol 26(8):925–932. https://doi.org/10.1038/nbt.1480
3. Gunnoo SB, Madder A (2016) Chemical protein modification through cysteine. Chembiochem 17(7):529–553. https://doi.org/10.1002/cbic.201500667
4. Shen B-Q, Xu K, Liu L, Raab H, Bhakta S, Kenrick M, Parsons-Reponte KL, Tien J, Yu SF, Mai E et al (2012) Conjugation site modulates the in vivo stability and therapeutic activity of antibody-drug conjugates. Nat Biotechnol 30 (2):184–189. https://doi.org/10.1038/nbt.2108
5. Ohri R, Bhakta S, Fourie-O'Donohue A, Dela Cruz-Chuh J, Tsai SP, Cook R, Wei B, Ng C, Wong AW, Bos AB et al (2018) High-throughput cysteine scanning to identify stable antibody conjugation sites for maleimide- and disulfide-based linkers. Bioconjug Chem 29 (2):473–485. https://doi.org/10.1021/acs.bioconjchem.7b00791
6. Su D, Kozak KR, Sadowsky J, Yu SF, Fourie-O'Donohue A, Nelson C, Vandlen R, Ohri R, Liu L, Ng C et al (2018) Modulating antibody--drug conjugate payload metabolism by conjugation site and linker modification. Bioconjug Chem 29(4):1155–1167. https://doi.org/10.1021/acs.bioconjchem.7b00785
7. Bhakta S, Raab H, Junutula JR (2013) Engineering THIOMABs for site-specific conjugation of Thiol-reactive linkers. Humana Press, Totowa, NJ, pp 189–203. https://doi.org/10.1007/978-1-62703-541-5_11

Chapter 5

Transglutaminase-Mediated Conjugations

Yasuaki Anami and Kyoji Tsuchikama

Abstract

Microbial transglutaminase (MTGase) catalyzes site-specific transpeptidation between a primary amine within linkers and the side chain of glutamine 295 within deglycosylated chimeric, humanized, and human IgG1s, affording homogeneous antibody–drug conjugates (ADCs). This method can be empowered by mutation of asparagine 297, insertion of a glutamine-containing peptide tag, and the use of branched linkers. Such modifications facilitate the conjugation process and provide flexibility in adjusting the conjugation site and drug-to-antibody ratio (DAR). Here, we present a protocol optimized in our group for MTGase-mediated linker incorporation and subsequent click chemistry-based payload installation. Both small linear linkers and bulky branched linkers can be incorporated into the Fc moiety within various antibodies, affording homogeneous ADCs with defined DARs. Thanks to the high homogeneity, ADCs constructed using this method can be analyzed using a single-quadrupole electrospray ionization (ESI) mass spectrometer, which many laboratories own for regular analysis of small molecules and peptides. The approach presented here allows for facile and cost-effective production of various homogeneous ADCs and other antibody conjugates for research and clinical purposes.

Key words Antibodies, Antibody–drug conjugates, Cancer, Chemotherapy, Conjugation, Homogeneous, Linker, Payload, Site-specific, Transglutaminase

1 Introduction

Linker conjugation chemistry is a critical component for successfully constructing antibody–drug conjugates (ADCs) [1–4]. ADC linkers are introduced onto monoclonal antibodies (mAbs) through a covalent bond using a variety of chemical or enzymatic reactions. As exemplified by the FDA-approved Adcetris® and Kadcyla® [5, 6], amide coupling with lysine residues and maleimide alkylation with reduced cysteine residues are most commonly used for linker installation [3, 7, 8]. While technically simple, these conjugation reactions occur on multiple lysine or cysteine residues in a nonspecific manner, resulting in heterogeneous mixtures of ADCs that differ in drug-to-antibody ratios (DARs) and linker installation sites.

L. Nathan Tumey (ed.), *Antibody-Drug Conjugates: Methods and Protocols*, Methods in Molecular Biology, vol. 2078, https://doi.org/10.1007/978-1-4939-9929-3_5,

ADC heterogeneity often leads to reduced therapeutic efficacy, accelerated clearance, and narrow therapeutic window [9–11]. Using these stochastic reactions also creates a challenge for minimizing lot-to-lot variation in production, which is required for clinical applications and commercialization. To solve the issues associated with ADC heterogeneity, many types of site-specific conjugation methods have been developed. One such method is incorporation of additional cysteine residues (THIOMAB technology) [10, 12] or azide-containing amino acids [13–15] into mAbs by genetic engineering. Cysteine rebridging using dibromo- or dithiophenolmaleimide (next-generation maleimide) is another method for site-specific conjugation [16–20]. In addition, (chemo)enzymatic linker conjugation is a powerful approach to producing homogeneous ADCs with defined DARs and conjugation sites. A variety of enzymes are used for this purpose, including sortase [21, 22], formylglycine-generating enzyme (SMARTag technology) [23, 24], β-1,4-galactosyltransferase [25], endoglycosidase (GlycoConnect technology) [26], and phosphopantetheinyl transferase [27].

Microbial transglutaminase (MTGase) catalyzes transpeptidation between an exogenous primary amine and the side chain of glutamine 295 (Q295) within deglycosylated chimeric, humanized, and human IgG1s, enabling site-specific conjugation of two linker units per mAb [28, 29] (Fig. 1a). This method provides a number of advantages in ADC construction as follows: (1) Linker and payload are installed onto the Fc moiety, minimizing the risk of impairment in binding affinity or specificity by the added components. (2) Only removal of *N*-glycan chains from a mAb using peptide-*N*-glycosidase F (PNGase F) is required prior to mAb–linker conjugation. Therefore, native antibodies can be used without genetic engineering. (3) Recombinant engineering can empower MTGase-mediated transpeptidation in various ways. For example, mutation of asparagine 297 to alanine, serine, or glutamine (N297A, N297S, or N297Q) allows omission of the deglycosylation step [30, 31] (Fig. 1b). In particular, N297Q mutation provides additional sites for linker conjugation, allowing for the installation of four linker units per mAb [28, 32, 33]. Incorporation of a LLQG peptide tag (Q-tag) also allows for payload installation at desired sites other than Q295 (Fig. 1c) [34]. (4) MTGase is commercially available not only as a research-grade pure enzyme but also as a food processing agent known as Activa TI® (a mixture of MTGase and maltodextrin). The use of Activa TI® can significantly reduce the production costs because of its affordability (100–150 US dollars/kg as of February 2019).

In this chapter, we describe a protocol optimized in our laboratory for MTGase-mediated linker incorporation and subsequent click chemistry-based payload installation. Dennler and coworkers have described a similar protocol in detail [35]. However, only the

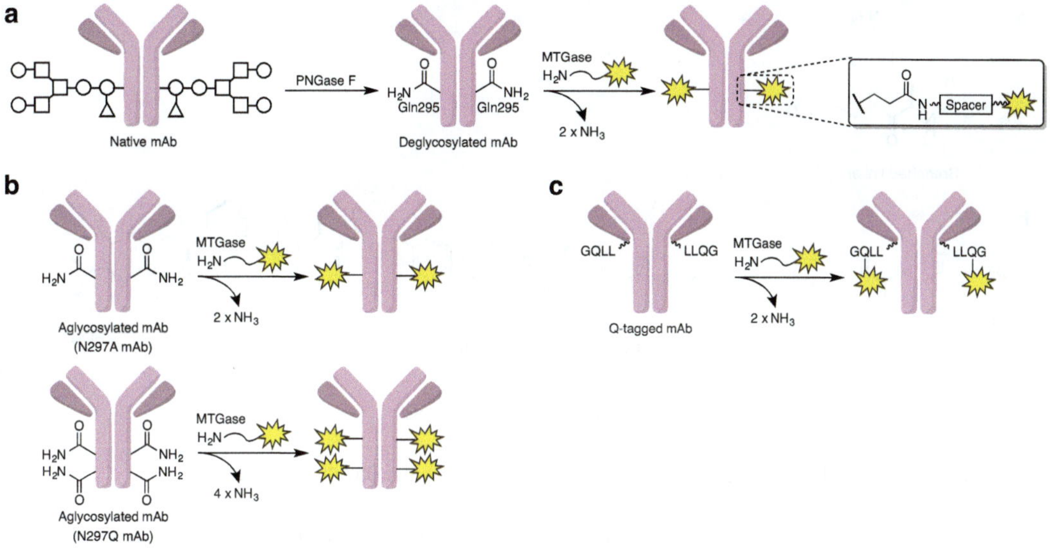

Fig. 1 Antibody–drug conjugation through microbial transglutaminase (MTGase)-mediated transpeptidation. Conjugation of linkers to a native mAb after deglycosylation by PNGase F (**a**), an aglycosylated mAb with a mutation at N297 (**b**) and a Q-tagged mAb (**c**)

use of small linear linkers was demonstrated and incorporation of bulky linker units can be difficult using this method [35–37]. We have shown that under optimal conditions MTGase-mediated transpeptidation enables quantitative installation of both linear linkers and branched linkers [30, 38]. The use of branched linkers affords homogeneous ADCs with higher DARs [30].

2 Materials

2.1 Deglycosylation

1. Human or humanized IgG1 (2 mg/mL in PBS) (*see* **Notes 1** and **2**).
2. PNGase F (500 units/μL, New England Biolabs).
3. Molecular weight cut-off filter: Amicon® Ultra-4 Centrifugal Filter Units (50 kDa MWCO).

2.2 MTGase-Mediated Antibody–Linker Conjugation

1. Deglycosylated humanized or human IgG1 (5–15 mg/mL in PBS) stored at 4 °C. Alternatively, humanized or human IgG1 with a N297A, N297S, or N297Q mutation.
2. MTGase: 40% (w/v) Activa TI® in PBS (Ajinomoto, available from Modernist Pantry) or recombinant MTGase in PBS (Zedira, reconstituted at 250 units/mL). These solutions should be stored at −20 °C until use (*see* **Note 3**).
3. Branched linker containing reaction handles for click reaction: L-lysine capped with two azide groups (Fig. 2a), dissolved in

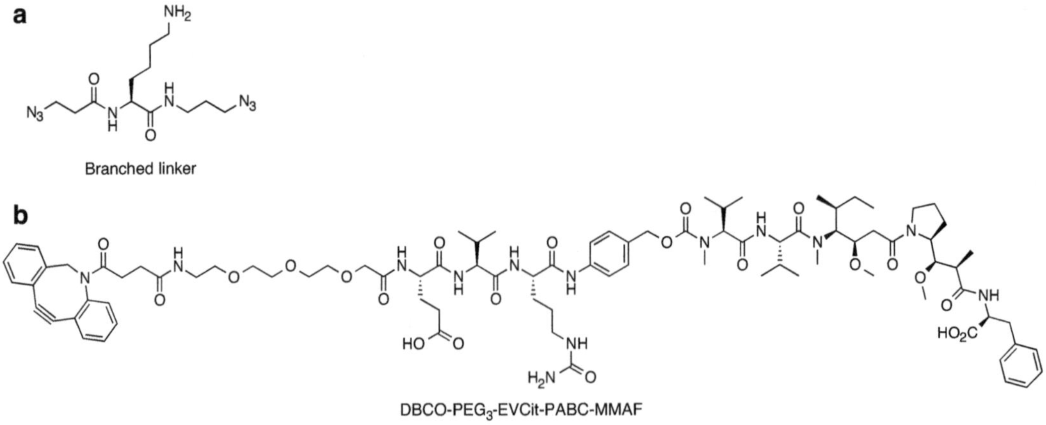

Fig. 2 Chemical structures of representative branched linker (**a**) and payload modules (**b**)

Milli-Q water at 100 mM (*see* **Note 4**). Alternatively, linear linkers such as 11-azido-3,6,9-trioxaundecan-1-amine.

4. Centrifugal filter: Corning™ Costar™ Spin-X™ Centrifuge Tube Filters (0.22 μm).
5. Column for size-exclusion chromatography (SEC): Superdex 200 increase 10/300 GL (GE Healthcare).
6. Eluent for SEC purification: PBS.

2.3 Payload Installation

1. Payload module containing a reaction handle for click reaction such as DBCO-spacer-MMAF (4 mM in DMSO, spacer: PEG_3-glutamic acid-valine-citrulline-*p*-aminobenzyloxycarbonyl) [38] (Fig. 2b) (*see* **Notes 5** and **6**). This solution should be stored at −20 °C or −80 °C until use.
2. Column for SEC: Superdex 200 increase 10/300 GL (GE Healthcare).
3. Eluent for SEC purification: PBS.

2.4 LC/MS Analysis

1. Reducing agent: 100 mM dithiothreitol (DTT) in water.
2. LC-MS system: Agilent 1100 HPLC connected to an Agilent 1946D single quadrupole electrospray ionization (ESI) mass spectrometer (*see* **Note 7**). Fragmentor voltage: 350 V (for intact analysis) or 200 V (for heavy and light chain analysis). Capillary voltage: 5500 V. Drying gas temperature: 350 °C. Drying gas flow: 13 L/min. Nebulizer pressure: 60 psig. Step size: 0.05. Mass scan range: 1400–3000 *m*/*z* (for intact analysis) or 900–2500 *m*/*z* (for heavy and light chain analysis).
3. Reverse-phase HPLC column: MabPac RP column 3 × 50 mm, 4 μm (Thermo Scientific). Column temperature: 80 °C.

4. Eluent for intact analysis: mobile phase A = water (0.1% formic acid); mobile phase B = acetonitrile (0.1% formic acid); gradient over 6.8 min from A:B = 75:25 to 1:99; flow rate = 0.4 mL/min.
5. Eluent for heavy and light chain analysis: mobile phase A = water (0.1% formic acid); mobile phase B = acetonitrile (0.1% formic acid); gradient over 10.25 min from A:B = 80:20 to 1:99; flow rate = 0.4 mL/min.
6. Analysis software: Agilent ChemStation and MassHunter with Bioconfirm Software, and ESIprot [39] (optional, available from http://www.lababi.bioprocess.org/index.php/lababi-software/84-esiprot).

2.5 Hydrophobic Interaction Chromatography (HIC) Analysis

1. Agilent 1100 HPLC system.
2. HIC column: MAbPac HIC-Butyl column 4.6 × 100 mm, 5 μm (Thermo Scientific).
3. Column temperature: room temperature.
4. Eluent: mobile phase A = 50 mM sodium phosphate containing ammonium sulfate (1.5 M) and 5% isopropanol (pH 7.4); mobile phase B = 50 mM sodium phosphate containing 20% isopropanol (pH 7.4); gradient over 30 min from A:B = 99:1 to 1:99; flow rate = 0.5 mL/min.

3 Method

3.1 Deglycosylation

1. If mAb is frozen, thaw quickly in a water bath at 37 °C and keep the solution on ice.
2. Adjust the mAb concentration to 2 mg/mL with PBS.
3. Add 2 μL of PNGase F (500 units/μL) to a solution of mAb in PBS (2 mg/mL, 1 mL) (*see* **Note 8**).
4. Incubate the mixture at 37 °C overnight (16–20 h).
5. To monitor the reaction, dilute 5 μL of the reaction mixture with 5 μL PBS. For intact analysis, do not add DTT. For heavy and light chain analysis, add 1 μL of 100 mM DTT and incubate at room temperature for 5–20 min to completely reduce interchain disulfide bonds. Finally, inject 10 μL of the diluted sample into LC/MS (*see* **Note 9**). Analysis conditions are described in Subheading 2.4. Process the raw data using Agilent ChemStation and MassHunter software. Generate and analyze deconvoluted mass spectra using Agilent Bioconfirm Software. Alternatively, use ESIprot software [39] for manual deconvolution. We routinely use this software for quick data evaluation.

6. Remove the PNGase F by centrifugal filtration. Load the reaction mixture onto a molecular weight cut-off filter (50 kDa) and centrifuge at 4000 × *g* for 20 min at 4 °C. Wash the sample three times or more with PBS (*see* **Note 10**).

3.2 MTGase-Mediated Antibody–Linker Conjugation

1. Concentrate the deglycosylated or mutated mAb by centrifugal filtration using a molecular weight cut-off filter (50 kDa) to approximately 10 mg/mL (*see* **Note 11**).
2. Mix the deglycosylated or mutated mAb (final concentration, >5 mg/mL), branched linker (40 equivalent per reaction site), and Activa TI® (final concentration, 8% (w/v)) or recombinant MTGase (6.7 units per 1 mg of mAb). Incubate the mixture at room temperature overnight without shaking or inversion (*see* **Note 12**). If MTGase precipitates during conjugation, remove the viscous sediment by filtration using a centrifuge tube filter (15,000 × *g* at 4 °C, for 30 min or longer until supernatant is completely collected).
3. Monitor the reaction by LC/MS as described in Subheading 3.1, **step 5** (Figs. 3a, b and 4a, b).
4. Purify the linker conjugate by SEC purification (eluent: PBS, flow rate = 0.6 mL/min). Purity of the product should be >95%. Concentrate the mAb–linker conjugate using a molecular weight cut-off filter (50 kDa) to 4 mg/mL or higher. The solution can be stored at 4 °C until use (*see* **Note 13**).

3.3 Strain-Promoted Azide–Alkyne Cycloaddition for Payload Installation

1. Mix DBCO–spacer–MMAF (4 mM stock solution in DMSO, 1.5 equivalent per azide group) with the mAb–linker conjugate in PBS (final concentration: 4 mg/mL, DMSO level is 10% or lower).
2. Incubate the mixture at room temperature for 1 h.
3. Monitor the reaction by LC/MS as described in Subheading 3.1, **step 5** (Figs. 3c, d and 4c) (*see* **Note 14**). If the reaction is not completed, add the payload module (1.5 equivalent per azide group, keep DMSO concentration under 10%) and incubate the reaction mixture at room temperature for additional 1 h.
4. Purify the sample by SEC (flow rate = 0.6 mL/min) to afford an ADC (Fig. 3e). Purity of the product should be >95%. Concentrate the ADC using a molecular weight cut-off filter (50 kDa) to 1 mg/mL or higher. The solution can be stored at 4 °C until use.
5. Analyze the purified ADC by LC/MS as described in Subheading 3.1, **step 5**. Determine the average DAR value based on UV peak areas. HIC analysis is an alternative method to determine the ADC hydrophobicity and average DAR (analysis conditions are described in Subheading 2.5).

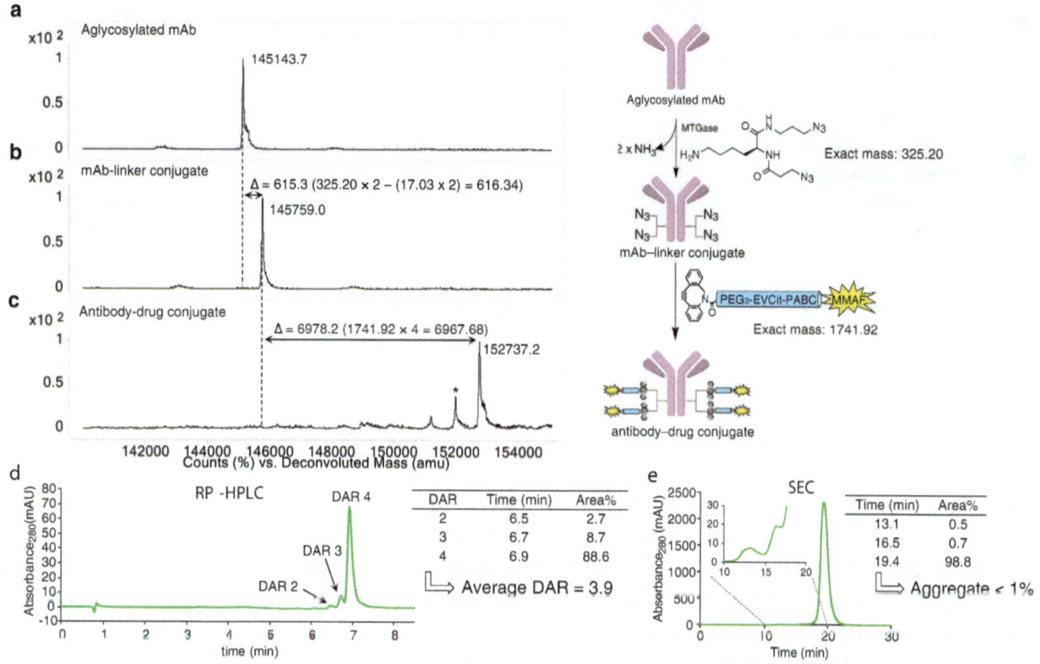

Fig. 3 Construction and characterization of an ADC. Deconvoluted ESI-mass spectra of aglycosylated N297A mAb (**a**), antibody-branched linker conjugate (**b**), and ADC (**c**). (**b**) The mass difference between aglycosylated mAb and mAb-linker conjugate is 615.3 Da, which corresponds to two branched linker units (exact mass: 325.20 Da, $2 \times 325.20 = 650.40$ Da) along with the loss of two ammonia molecules ($2 \times 17.03 = 34.06$ Da). (**c**) The mass difference between mAb–linker conjugate and ADC is 6978.2 Da, which corresponds to four payload modules (exact mass: 1741.92 Da, $4 \times 1741.92 = 6967.68$ Da). Asterisk (∗) indicates a fragment ion detected in ESI-MS analysis. (**d**) The reverse-phase HPLC trace (UV: 280 nm) of an ADC. The average DAR was determined to be 3.9 based on the peak areas of each DAR species. (**e**) The SEC trace (UV: 280 nm) of the same ADC

4 Notes

1. Although human IgG1s are used in this protocol, other subclasses and mAbs derived from non-human host animals may also be used in MTGase-mediated linker conjugation.
2. Depending on the amino acid sequence of the variable region or host species used for mAb production, glutamine residues other than Q295 may be reactive in MTGase-mediated conjugation. Indeed, we have observed that a rat IgG2a accepts linker units not only at conserved Q295 [40] but also at another unidentified glutamine based on the protocol described here, affording a conjugate with a DAR of 4. Therefore, it is strongly recommended to verify whether this method is applicable for a mAb of interest by performing a small-scale

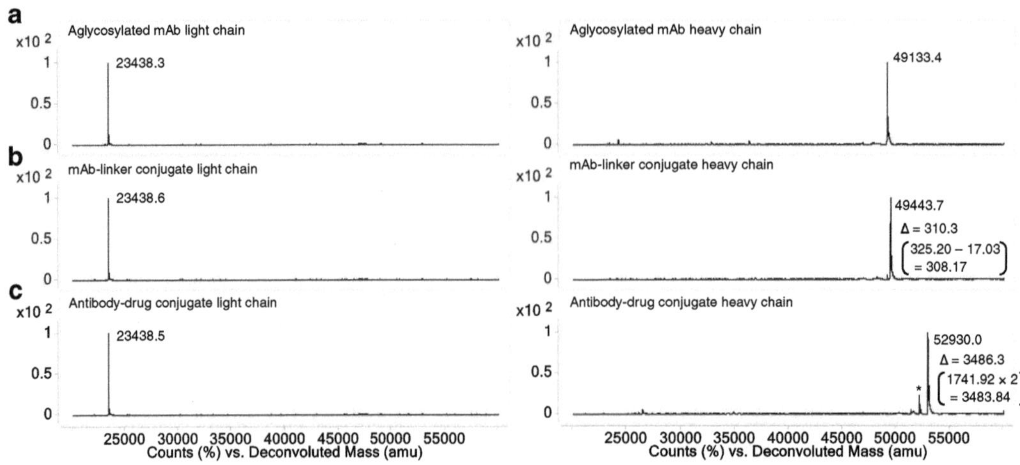

Fig. 4 Deconvoluted ESI-mass spectra of light and heavy chain of aglycosylated N297A mAb (**a**), mAb–-branched linker conjugate (**b**), and ADC (**c**). (**b**) The mass difference between heavy chains of aglycosylated mAb and mAb-linker conjugate is 310.3 Da, which corresponds to a branched linker (exact mass: 325.20 Da) along with the loss of an ammonia molecule (17.03 Da). (**c**) The mass difference between heavy chains of mAb-linker conjugate and ADC is 3486.3 Da, which corresponds to two payload modules (exact mass: 1741.92 Da, $2 \times 1741.92 = 3483.84$ Da). Asterisk (∗) indicates a fragment ion detected in ESI-MS analysis

test conjugation and following validation for DAR, homogeneity, binding affinity, and specificity.

3. Sonication is necessary to completely dissolve Activa TI® in PBS. Once a stock solution is aliquoted and frozen for storage, avoid repeated freeze–thaw cycles.
4. Water is most recommended for preparing a linker solution. DMSO can also be used as long as the final DMSO concentration is limited to less than 10%. To this end, dissolve a linker in DMSO at a high concentration (>1 M). We have confirmed that 10% DMSO neither impairs MTGase's activity nor denatures IgG1s during conjugation.
5. As proposed by Schibli and coworkers [29], we usually employ a two-step conjugation that relies on MTGase-mediated linker incorporation and following click coupling for installing payload molecules. As previously reported [34], payload molecules can be directly installed onto mAbs by MTGase conjugation. However, as described in Subheading 3.2, a large number of linkers (40–200 equivalent per reaction site) are generally required to achieve quantitative conjugation at Q295 (and Q297 if incorporated by mutation). Most ADC payload molecules are expensive and thus direct installation using MTGase can be not cost-effective in large-scale production.
6. We routinely use 4 mM payload stock solutions. However, they may be further concentrated if necessary.

7. Thanks to the site-specificity of the MTGase-mediated conjugation and high homogeneity of the products, a single-quadrupole LCMS system can provide sensitivity and resolution high enough to characterize the conjugates generated by this protocol. Note that about half of the mass peaks are outside the scan range and not detectable in the case of whole IgG and ADC analysis. However, peak deconvolution can be performed only with the peaks detected.
8. We found that the ratio of mAb/PNGase F (2 mg:1000 units) is optimal for this reaction. The concentrations of mAb and PNGase F may be increased as long as this ratio is unchanged.
9. If the deglycosylation is not completed, add additional PNGase F (2 μL) and incubate the reaction mixture at 37 °C until maximum conversion is achieved. Based on our experience, additional incubation for 16–20 h is sufficient to complete deglycosylation of most mAbs with low reactivity.
10. Centrifugation conditions may need to be modified for each sample depending on the antibody concentration and the volume loaded onto a filter. Purification by SEC is another option at this step.
11. A high mAb concentration is a key to achieve quantitative mAb–branched linker conjugation. Therefore, adjust the mAb concentration to 5–20 mg/mL. We routinely prepare mAb solutions approximately at 10 mg/mL.
12. Though the method described here is optimized for connecting the bulky branched linkers developed by our group [30, 38] as well as simple linear linkers, the linker structure can impact the conjugation efficiency. Therefore, conjugation conditions may need to be optimized to achieve complete conversion in each case. Parameters that should be optimized include the MTGase concentration, pH, temperature, and incubation time.
13. Complete removal of MTGase using a SEC or protein A column is strongly recommended at this step. We have experienced incomplete removal of MTGase (38 kDa) using molecular weight cut-off filters (50 and 100 kDa), leading to linker deconjugation by residual MTGase during storage.
14. The enzymatically cleavable spacer valine–citrulline–*p*-aminobenzyloxycarbonyl can undergo fragmentation in ESI-MS analysis as shown in Fig. 3c. This issue may be circumvented by fine-tuning ESI parameters, in particular the fragmentor voltage. The use of DBCO-payload modules without this spacer (noncleavable variant) is an alternative approach to verifying the conjugation efficiency.

Acknowledgements

The authors would like to thank Dr. Aiko Yamaguchi for her constructive input and Dr. Georgina T. Salazar for editing the manuscript.

References

1. McCombs JR, Owen SC (2015) Antibody drug conjugates: design and selection of linker, payload and conjugation chemistry. AAPS J 17:339–351. https://doi.org/10.1208/s12248-014-9710-8
2. Dennler P, Fischer E, Schibli R (2015) Antibody conjugates: from heterogeneous populations to defined reagents. Antibodies 4:197–224. https://doi.org/10.3390/antib4030197
3. Tsuchikama K, An Z (2018) Antibody-drug conjugates: recent advances in conjugation and linker chemistries. Protein Cell 9:33–46. https://doi.org/10.1007/s13238-016-0323-0
4. Dan N, Setua S, Kashyap VK et al (2018) Antibody-drug conjugates for cancer therapy: chemistry to clinical implications. Pharmaceuticals (Basel) 11:32. https://doi.org/10.3390/ph11020032
5. Lewis Phillips GD, Li G, Dugger DL et al (2008) Targeting HER2-positive breast cancer with trastuzumab-DM1, an antibody-cytotoxic drug conjugate. Cancer Res 68:9280–9290. https://doi.org/10.1158/0008-5472.CAN-08-1776
6. Katz J, Janik JE, Younes A (2011) Brentuximab vedotin (SGN-35). Clin Cancer Res 17:6428–6436. https://doi.org/10.1158/1078-0432.CCR-11-0488
7. Agarwal P, Bertozzi CR (2015) Site-specific antibody-drug conjugates: the nexus of bioorthogonal chemistry, protein engineering, and drug development. Bioconjug Chem 26:176–192. https://doi.org/10.1021/bc5004982
8. Chudasama V, Maruani A, Caddick S (2016) Recent advances in the construction of antibody-drug conjugates. Nat Chem 8:114–119. https://doi.org/10.1038/nchem.2415
9. Hamblett KJ, Senter PD, Chace DF et al (2004) Effects of drug loading on the antitumor activity of a monoclonal antibody drug conjugate. Clin Cancer Res 10:7063–7070. https://doi.org/10.1158/1078-0432.CCR-04-0789
10. Junutula JR, Raab H, Clark S et al (2008) Site-specific conjugation of a cytotoxic drug to an antibody improves the therapeutic index. Nat Biotechnol 26:925–932. https://doi.org/10.1038/nbt.1480
11. van Berkel SS, van Delft FL (2018) Enzymatic strategies for (near) clinical development of antibody-drug conjugates. Drug Discov Today Technol 30:3–10. https://doi.org/10.1016/j.ddtec.2018.09.005
12. Shen B-Q, Xu K, Liu L et al (2012) Conjugation site modulates the in vivo stability and therapeutic activity of antibody-drug conjugates. Nat Biotechnol 30:184–189. https://doi.org/10.1038/nbt.2108
13. Axup JY, Bajjuri KM, Ritland M et al (2012) Synthesis of site-specific antibody-drug conjugates using unnatural amino acids. Proc Natl Acad Sci U S A 109:16101–16106. https://doi.org/10.1073/pnas.1211023109
14. Zimmerman ES, Heibeck TH, Gill A et al (2014) Production of site-specific antibody-drug conjugates using optimized non-natural amino acids in a cell-free expression system. Bioconjug Chem 25:351–361. https://doi.org/10.1021/bc400490z
15. VanBrunt MP, Shanebeck K, Caldwell Z et al (2015) Genetically encoded azide containing amino acid in mammalian cells enables site-specific antibody-drug conjugates using click cycloaddition chemistry. Bioconjug Chem 26:2249–2260. https://doi.org/10.1021/acs.bioconjchem.5b00359
16. Bryden F, Maruani A, Savoie H et al (2014) Regioselective and stoichiometrically controlled conjugation of photodynamic sensitizers to a HER2 targeting antibody fragment. Bioconjug Chem 25:611–617. https://doi.org/10.1021/bc5000324
17. Schumacher FF, Nunes JPM, Maruani A et al (2014) Next generation maleimides enable the controlled assembly of antibody-drug conjugates via native disulfide bond bridging. Org Biomol Chem 12:7261–7269. https://doi.org/10.1039/c4ob01550a
18. Behrens CR, Ha EH, Chinn LL et al (2015) Antibody-drug conjugates (ADCs) derived from interchain cysteine cross-linking

demonstrate improved homogeneity and other pharmacological properties over conventional heterogeneous ADCs. Mol Pharm 12:3986–3998. https://doi.org/10.1021/acs.molpharmaceut.5b00432

19. Maruani A, Smith MEB, Miranda E et al (2015) A plug-and-play approach to antibody-based therapeutics via a chemoselective dual click strategy. Nat Commun 6:6645. https://doi.org/10.1038/ncomms7645
20. Forte N, Chudasama V, Baker JR (2018) Homogeneous antibody-drug conjugates via site-selective disulfide bridging. Drug Discov Today Technol 30:11–20. https://doi.org/10.1016/j.ddtec.2018.09.004
21. Popp MW-L, Antos JM, Ploegh HL (2009) Site-specific protein labeling via sortase-mediated transpeptidation. Curr Protoc Protein Sci 56:15.3.1–15.3.9. https://doi.org/10.1002/0471140864.ps1503s56
22. Beerli RR, Hell T, Merkel AS, Grawunder U (2015) Sortase enzyme-mediated generation of site-specifically conjugated antibody drug conjugates with high in vitro and in vivo potency. PLoS One 10:e0131177. https://doi.org/10.1371/journal.pone.0131177
23. Rabuka D, Rush JS, deHart GW et al (2012) Site-specific chemical protein conjugation using genetically encoded aldehyde tags. Nat Protoc 7:1052–1067. https://doi.org/10.1038/nprot.2012.045
24. Drake PM, Albers AE, Baker J et al (2014) Aldehyde tag coupled with HIPS chemistry enables the production of ADCs conjugated site-specifically to different antibody regions with distinct in vivo efficacy and PK outcomes. Bioconjug Chem 25:1331–1341. https://doi.org/10.1021/bc500189z
25. Zhou Q, Stefano JE, Manning C et al (2014) Site-specific antibody-drug conjugation through glycoengineering. Bioconjug Chem 25:510–520. https://doi.org/10.1021/bc400505q
26. van Geel R, Wijdeven MA, Heesbeen R et al (2015) Chemoenzymatic conjugation of toxic payloads to the globally conserved N-glycan of native mAbs provides homogeneous and highly efficacious antibody-drug conjugates. Bioconjug Chem 26:2233–2242. https://doi.org/10.1021/acs.bioconjchem.5b00224
27. Grünewald J, Klock HE, Cellitti SE et al (2015) Efficient preparation of site-specific antibody–drug conjugates using phosphopantetheinyl transferases. Bioconjug Chem 26:2554–2562. https://doi.org/10.1021/acs.bioconjchem.5b00558
28. Jeger S, Zimmermann K, Blanc A et al (2010) Site-specific and stoichiometric modification of antibodies by bacterial transglutaminase. Angew Chem Int Ed 49:9995–9997. https://doi.org/10.1002/anie.201004243
29. Dennler P, Chiotellis A, Fischer E et al (2014) Transglutaminase-based chemo-enzymatic conjugation approach yields homogeneous antibody-drug conjugates. Bioconjug Chem 25:569–578. https://doi.org/10.1021/bc400574z
30. Anami Y, Xiong W, Gui X et al (2017) Enzymatic conjugation using branched linkers for constructing homogeneous antibody-drug conjugates with high potency. Org Biomol Chem 15:5635–5642. https://doi.org/10.1039/c7ob01027c
31. Spycher PR, Amann CA, Wehrmüller JE et al (2017) Dual, site-specific modification of antibodies by using solid-phase immobilized microbial transglutaminase. Chembiochem 18:1923–1927. https://doi.org/10.1002/cbic.201700188
32. Lhospice F, Brégeon D, Belmant C et al (2015) Site-specific conjugation of monomethyl Auristatin E to Anti-CD30 Antibodies Improves Their Pharmacokinetics and Therapeutic Index in Rodent Models. Mol Pharm 12:1863–1871. https://doi.org/10.1021/mp500666j
33. DeVay RM, Delaria K, Zhu G et al (2017) Improved Lysosomal Trafficking Can Modulate the Potency of Antibody Drug Conjugates. Bioconjug Chem 28:1102–1114. https://doi.org/10.1021/acs.bioconjchem.7b00013
34. Strop P, Liu S-H, Dorywalska M et al (2013) Location matters: site of conjugation modulates stability and pharmacokinetics of antibody drug conjugates. Chem Biol 20:161–167. https://doi.org/10.1016/j.chembiol.2013.01.010
35. Dennler P, Schibli R, Fischer E (2013) Enzymatic Antibody Modification by Bacterial Transglutaminase. In: Ducry L (ed) Antibody-Drug Conjugates. Humana Press, Totowa, NJ, pp 205–215
36. Gundersen MT, Keillor JW, Pelletier JN (2013) Microbial transglutaminase displays broad acyl-acceptor substrate specificity. Appl Microbiol Biotechnol 98:219–230. https://doi.org/10.1007/s00253-013-4886-x
37. Dennler P, Bailey LK, Spycher PR et al (2015) Microbial transglutaminase and c-myc-tag: a strong couple for the functionalization of antibody-like protein scaffolds from discovery platforms. Chembiochem 16:861–867. https://doi.org/10.1002/cbic.201500009

38. Anami Y, Yamazaki CM, Xiong W et al (2018) Glutamic acid-valine-citrulline linkers ensure stability and efficacy of antibody-drug conjugates in mice. Nat Commun 9:2512. https://doi.org/10.1038/s41467-018-04982-3
39. Winkler R (2010) ESIprot: a universal tool for charge state determination and molecular weight calculation of proteins from electrospray ionization mass spectrometry data. Rapid Commun Mass Spectrom 24:285–294. https://doi.org/10.1002/rcm.4384
40. Miyakawa S, Nomura Y, Sakamoto T et al (2008) Structural and molecular basis for hyperspecificity of RNA aptamer to human immunoglobulin G. RNA 14:1154–1163. https://doi.org/10.1261/rna.1005808

Chapter 6

Click Chemistry Conjugations

Tak Ian Chio and Susan L. Bane

Abstract

Click chemistry has found wide application in bioconjugation, enabling control over the site of modification in biomolecules. Demonstrations of this chemistry to construct chemically defined antibody–drug conjugates (ADCs) have increased in recent years, following studies that support benefits of homogeneity and site-specificity of drug placement on the antibody. In this chapter, a brief history of early applications of this chemistry in ADCs is presented. Examples of click chemistries that are utilized for ADC synthesis, including those currently undergoing clinical investigations, are enumerated. Protocols for two common conjugation methods based on carbonyl-aminooxy coupling and strain-promoted azide–alkyne cycloaddition are described.

Key words Click chemistry, Site-specific, Antibody–drug conjugates (ADCs), Aldehyde, Oxime, Strain-promoted azide–alkyne cycloaddition (SPAAC), Bioconjugation

1 Introduction

The bioconjugation strategy to connect a drug molecule to an antibody continues to be an active area of research in the field of antibody–drug conjugates (ADCs) [1]. Among the four ADCs currently approved by the U.S. Food and Drug Administration (FDA), all of them (Mylotarg, Adcetris, Kadcyla, and Besponsa) are made using stochastic conjugation chemistries that target native lysine or cysteine residues of the antibody. Consequently, these ADCs have heterogeneous drug-to-antibody ratios (DARs) and conjugation sites. For instance, Mylotarg (gemtuzumab ozogamicin), the first FDA-approved ADC, is composed of a mixture of antibodies with a range of DARs, of which ~50% remains unconjugated and can compete with the active ADC for target cell uptake [2]. In addition, the ADCs with variable DARs can possess differential pharmacological properties. Indeed, corroborative studies over the past decade have reached a consensus that the DAR and the site of drug conjugation can have an impact on the pharmacokinetics and the therapeutic index of ADCs [3–5]. Therefore,

L. Nathan Tumey (ed.), *Antibody-Drug Conjugates: Methods and Protocols*, Methods in Molecular Biology, vol. 2078, https://doi.org/10.1007/978-1-4939-9929-3_6, © Springer Science+Business Media, LLC, part of Springer Nature 2020

methods and conjugation chemistries that enable the synthesis of homogeneous, site-specific ADCs are desired.

One seminal method for creating site-specific ADCs is the THIOMABs technology from Genentech [3]. In this approach, the antibody is engineered with cysteine residues at particular sites, to which cysteine-reactive (often maleimide-functionalized) drug-linkers will solely attach if the interchain disulfides are left unreduced. A revolving concern regarding this approach is the stability of the conjugation, namely that the thiosuccinimidyl linkage formed from the reaction of cysteine with maleimide is reversible and can thus undergo premature cleavage upon exchange with circulating thiols in vivo. Continued research for stability improvement notwithstanding [4, 6–8], interests in other conjugation chemistries forge another front working in parallel toward chemically defined and stable ADCs.

Concurrent development in bioorthogonal chemistries has provided a number of chemical strategies for ADC applications [9]. Often referred interchangeably to as click chemistries, these reactions involve the selective coupling of two unnatural functionalities that are orthogonal, or inert, to other biological functional groups. The product of these reactions should be stable in the biological milieu. The preconditions to be classified as bioorthogonal thus coincide with the attributes that are presently in demand for bioconjugation in ADC production.

While extended exploration of click chemistries for site-specific antibody–drug conjugation is relatively recent, examples of utility of such chemistry can be found even in early-generation ADCs, including Mylotarg [10]. Mylotarg contains a hydrazone bond, formed via one of the earliest bioorthogonal reactions—condensation of a carbonyl (aldehyde/ketone) with an α-effect amine. In this case, the carbonyl is an aromatic ketone installed in a lysine-targeted linker to the antibody and the α-effect amine is a hydrazide derivatized on the calicheamicin payload. It should be noted that the conjugation to the antibody still stems from the lysine-reactive component of the linker, hence the aforementioned heterogeneity of this ADC. The purpose of the hydrazone, which is acid-labile, is to render the ADC susceptible to drug cleavage upon cellular internationalization to the acidic lysosomal compartment. The same pH-sensitive linker is also present in the recently approved ADC, Besponsa (inotuzumab ozogamicin). Outside of serving as a cleavable linker, hydrazone ligation has also been applied for direct conjugation to antibodies that include predecessors of Mylotarg [10–12]. However, the conjugates lacked homogeneity, as the number of aldehydes introduced to the antibody through oxidation of the attached glycan was heterogeneous. Although site-specific ADCs using hydrazone ligation has subsequently been demonstrated [13], the hydrazone linkage has generally been deemed not sufficiently stable to avoid off-target cleavage under physiological conditions [14].

Application of carbonyl-based chemistry with α-effect amine continues as the field shifts toward site-specific conjugation. Alkoxyamine is a common choice for the α-effect nucleophile. The condensation product, an oxime, is hydrolytically more stable than a hydrazone [15]. Some site-specific ADCs generated via oxime ligation are currently undergoing clinical development (e.g. ARX788 from Ambrx) [16] or preclinical assessment (e.g. LCB14-0110 from LegoChem Biosciences) [17].

Variations of the carbonyl-based chemistry have also been developed to improve from deficiencies of oxime ligation. Oxime formation suffers from slow kinetics and necessitates acidic condition as well as high concentration of reactants (or large excess of one) to reach appreciable conversion [18, 19]. Hydrazino *iso*-Pictet-Spengler (HIPS) ligation, which pairs an aldehyde with an alkylhydrazine-functionalized indole, has been shown to perform optimally at near-neutral pH (pH 6) [20]. The product contains a newly formed C–C bond and is reportedly more stable than the corresponding oxime. Utility of this chemistry for site-specific ADCs has been demonstrated [21] and one (Trph-222 from Triphase—licensed from Catalent) has recently entered clinical trials [22].

In addition to HIPS, other aldehyde-based chemistries have also been reported for ADC synthesis. In a direct comparison of the rate of antibody–drug conjugation, the trapped-Knoevenagel ligation has a reported rate of 0.4 M^{-1} s^{-1} at pH 7, compared to 0.03 M^{-1} s^{-1} at pH 4.6 for oxime ligation [23]. Despite the improvement, the rate is still considered relatively slow. A substantially faster aldehyde-based reaction, with rate constants in the order of 10^3 M^{-1} s^{-1} at neutral pH, involves an aromatic aldehyde with a boronic acid at the *ortho* position [24–27]. We have demonstrated that coupling this moiety with an α-amino-hydrazide as the nucleophile produces a unique zwitterionic boron–nitrogen heterocycle, a 2,3,1-benzodiazaborine (DAB) derivative, that is stable across a wide range of pH [28]. We have recently applied this chemistry to generate site-specific antibody conjugates [29]. Although the work presented thus far has used fluorophore payloads as proof-of-principle, the conjugate's stability in human serum and its preservation of antibody function show promise for the utility of this developing chemistry for efficient ADC production.

Aside from carbonyl condensation chemistries, another class of click chemistry that is widely employed in the development of site-specific ADCs is the azide–alkyne cycloaddition (AAC) reaction. Two major types that have been widely used for bioconjugation are the copper-catalyzed AAC (CuAAC) and the strain-promoted AAC (SPAAC). The former involves the coupling of an azide with a linear alkyne and the latter with a cyclooctyne. As the names suggest, CuAAC is catalyzed by copper while SPAAC relies on the ring strain on the cyclooctyne for its reactivity. Both reactions produce a

1,4-substituted triazole, though only the CuAAC product is regiospecific [30]. Site-specific ADCs conjugated via CuAAC and SPAAC have both been demonstrated [31–37] and some of them are currently under clinical evaluation (e.g. STRO-001 from Sutro Biopharma [38] and ADCT-601 from ADC Therapeutics [39]). For CuAAC, oxidation of certain amino acids on the antibody by copper has been observed and is a factor to consider, as oxidized proteins may cause an immunogenic response [34].

Application of the inverse-electron-demand Diels Alder (IEDDA) reactions to construct site-specific ADCs has also been demonstrated. The IEDDA reactions involve the ligation of a strained alkene with a tetrazine and constitute some of the fastest bioorthogonal reactions to date [40]. In particular, in a recent study, an antibody equipped with a cyclopropene was site-specifically conjugated to a tetrazine-functionalized payload [41]. The conjugation was reportedly faster than most of the conjugations that made use of other bioorthogonal handles.

Table 1 illustrates the various click chemistries that have been applied for the generation of homogeneous, site-specific ADCs. At present, two of the most common click chemistries reported for antibody–drug conjugation are the oxime and the SPAAC ligations. Therefore, this chapter will focus on the specific methodology for these two chemistries, even as others may assume a broader role in the future.

To implement these chemistries for ADC assembly, the bioorthogonal reactive groups need to be introduced to the antibody and the payload. In general, for oxime and SPAAC ligations, the carbonyl or the azide, respectively, is installed on the antibody while the aminooxy or the cyclooctyne is placed on the drug-linker. Tables 2 and 3 list select methods that have been developed to enable site-specific incorporation of the carbonyl/azide handle onto the antibody. A collection of previously synthesized drug-linkers that carry the complementary reactive group is also included. Readers are encouraged to refer to the cited references for detailed instructions on the derivatization process prior to conjugation. The method section will concentrate on the procedure to perform the conjugation using oxime and SPAAC chemistries.

2 Materials

2.1 General

1. Dimethyl sulfoxide (DMSO)/dimethylformamide (DMF)/dimethylacetamide (DMA).
2. Desalting column.
3. 30 or 50 kDa MWCO ultracentrifugal filter.
4. 0.2 μm syringe filter.

Table 1
Click chemistries for site-specific antibody–drug conjugation

Click chemistry	Reaction scheme	Ref. (Year)
Oxime	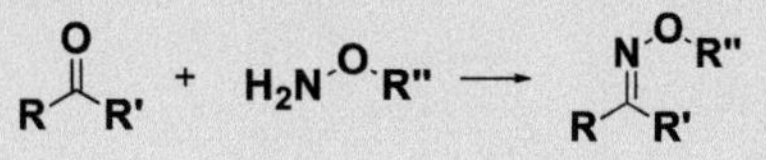	[42] (2012) [43–45] (2014) [46, 47] (2015)
Hydrazino-*iso*-Pictet-Spengler (HIPS)	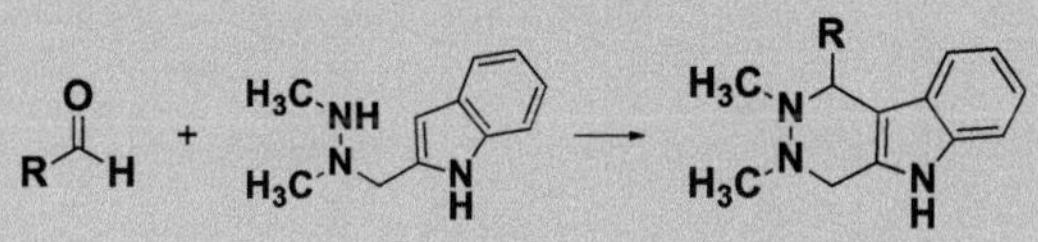	[21] (2014)
Trapped-Knoevenagel	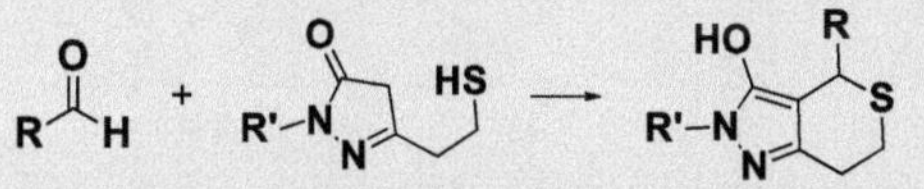	[23] (2015)
Tandem Knoevenagel condensation-Michael addition	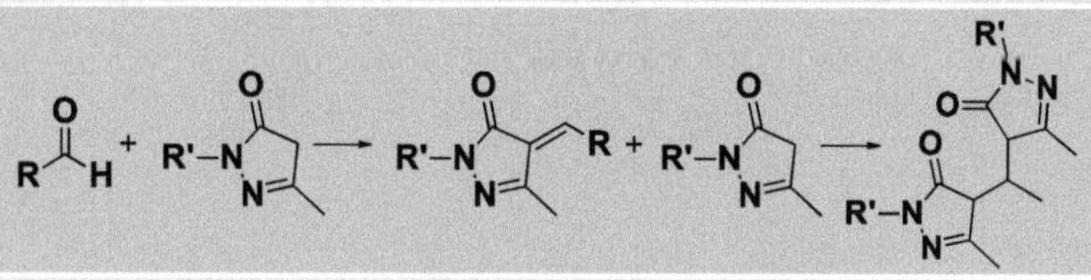	[48] (2016)
Copper-catalyzed azide–alkyne cycloaddition (CuAAC)	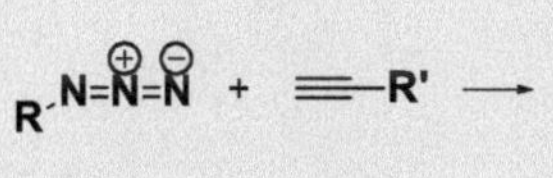	[34] (2015) [37] (2016)
Strain-promoted azide–alkyne cycloaddition (SPAAC)	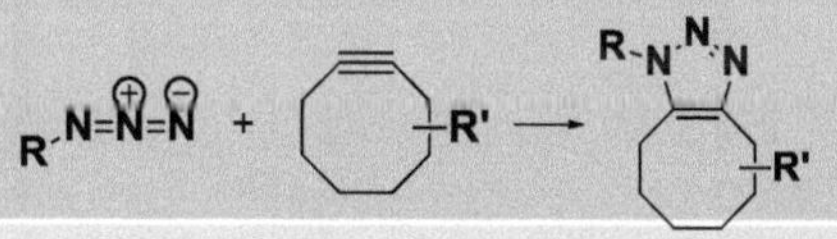	[31–33] (2014) [34, 35] (2015) [49] (2017)
Inverse-electron-demand Diels Alder cycloaddition (IEDDA)	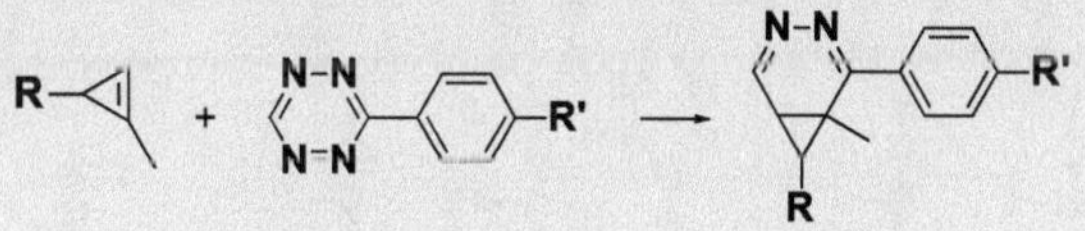	[40] (2018)
Diazaborine (DAB)	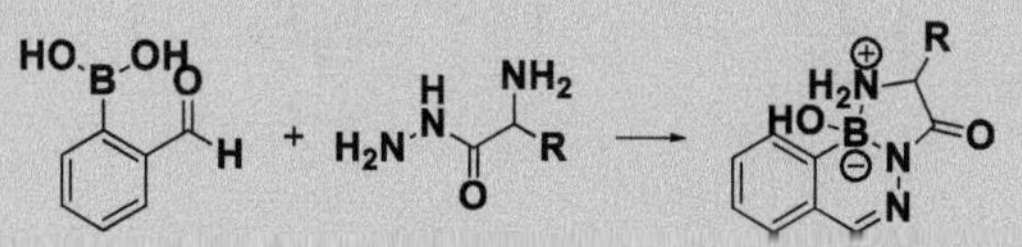	[29] (2019)

Table 2
Methods for site-specific incorporation of a carbonyl handle onto an antibody

Approach	Scheme[a]	Click chemistry	Drug-linker[b]	Reported DAR (Expected DAR)	Ref.
Glycan remodeling	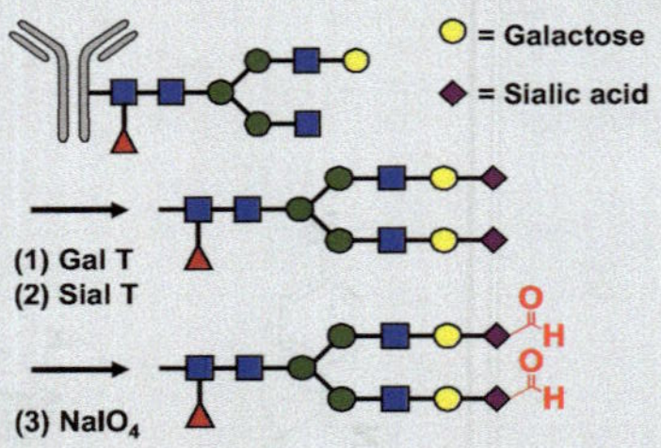	Oxime	Aminooxy-MMAE Aminooxy-Dol10	1.3–1.9 (4)	[44]
Glycan remodeling	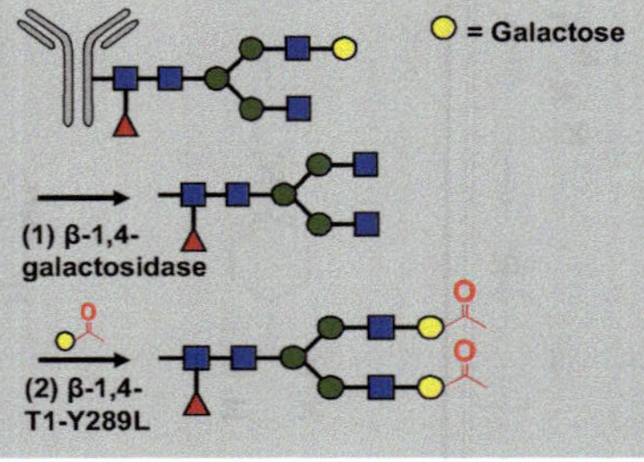	Oxime	Aminooxy-AF	4 (4)	[45]
Unnatural amino acid (UAA) mutagenesis	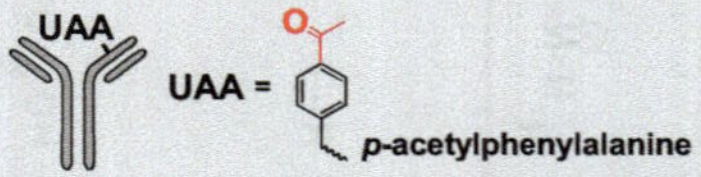	Oxime	Aminooxy-AF Aminooxy-MMAD	>1.9 (2)	[42] [43]
N-terminal serine engineering	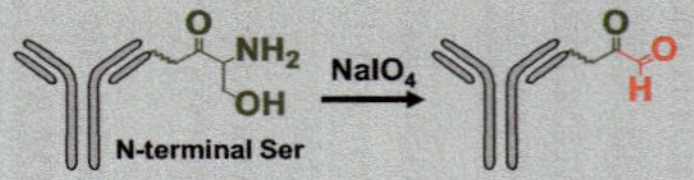	Oxime	Aminooxy-MMAE	1.9 (2)	[46]

Enzymatic modification of a peptide tag	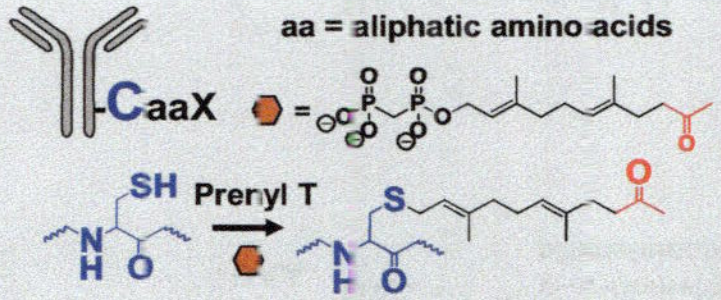	Oxime	Aminooxy-MMAF	2 (2)[c]	[47, 50]
Enzymatic modification of a peptide tag	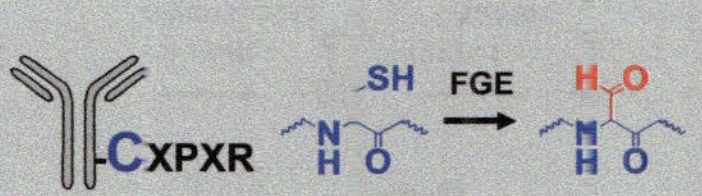	HIPS Knoevenagel	HIPS-maytansine thioPz-maytansine Pz-maytansine	1.5 – >1.8 (2) 2 (2)[c] 4 (4)[c]	[21] [23] [48]
Enzymatic modification of a peptide tag	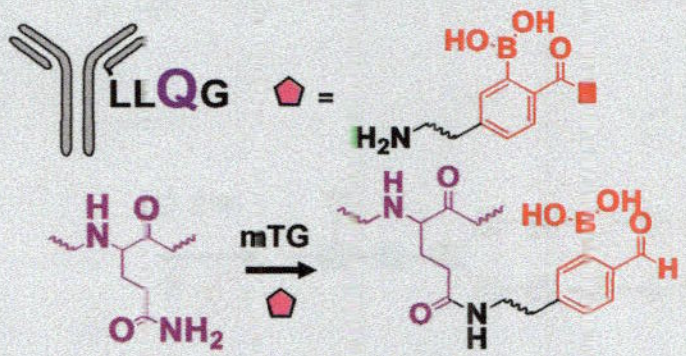	DAB	N/A	1.6 – >1.9 (2)	[29]

[a]Gal T: β-1,4-galactosyltransferase, Sial T: α-2,6-sialyltransferase, $NaIO_4$: sodium periodate, β-1,4-T1-Y289L: Y289 mutant of β-1,4-galactosyltransferase, Prenyl T: prenyl transferase, FGE: formylglycine-generating enzyme, mTG: microbial transglutaminase
[b]MMAD/MMAE/MMAF: monomethyl auristatin D/E/F, Dol 10: dolastatin 10, AF: auristatin F, thioPz: thiopyrazolone, Pz: pyrazolone. Regarding the drug-linkers listed, only the functional group and the drug are specified. The linker connecting these two moieties may vary.
[c]DAR not explicitly stated

Table 3
Methods for site-specific incorporation of an azide handle onto an antibody

Approach	Scheme[a]	Click chemistry	Drug-linker[b]	Reported DAR (Expected DAR)	Ref.
Glycan remodeling	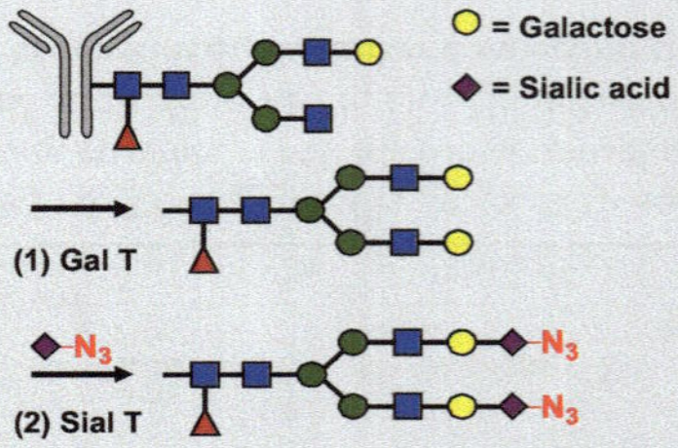	SPAAC	DIBO-Dox	4.5 (4)	[31]
Glycan remodeling	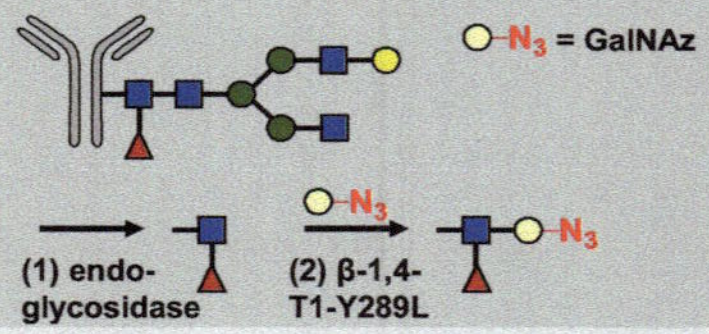	SPAAC CuAAC	BCN-Dox BCN-MMAE BCN-MMAF BCN-maytansine BCN DUMSA Alkyne-PBD	>1.9 (2) >1.9 (2) 3.8 (4)	[34] [37]
Unnatural amino acid (UAA) mutagenesis	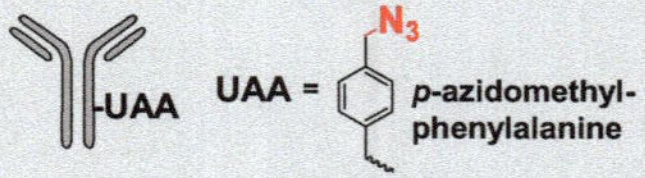	SPAAC	DBCO-MMAF	1.2–1.9 (2)	[32]
UAA mutagenesis	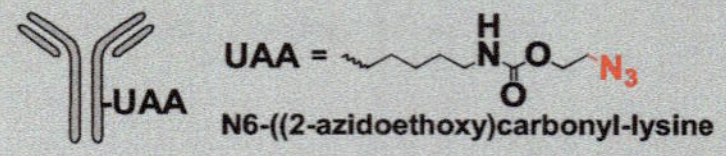	CuAAC SPAAC	Alkyne-PBD Alkyne-AF BCN-AF	1.8 – >1.9 (2)	[35]

Enzymatic modification of a peptide tag	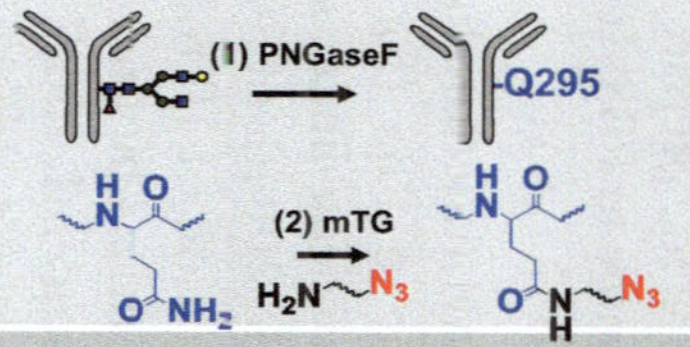	SPAAC	DBCO-MMAE	>1.9 (2)	[33]
Enzymatic modification of a peptide tag	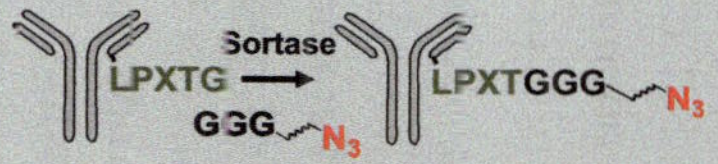	SPAAC	DBCO-MMAE	3.3 (4)	[49]

[a]GalNAz: azido-modified *N*-acetyl-D-galactosamine, PNGase F: *N*-glycosidase F

[b]DIBO: dibenzocyclooctyne, BCN: bicyclo[6.1.0]nonyne, DUMSA: duocarmycin SA, PBD: pyrrolobenzodiazepine dimer, DBCO: aza-dibenzocyclooctyne. Regarding the drug-linkers listed, only the functional group and the drug are specified. The linker connecting these two moieties may vary.

2.2 Oxime Ligation

1. Acetate buffer, pH 4.5: 0.1 M sodium acetate, pH 4.5.
2. PBS: 10 mM sodium phosphate, 150 mM NaCl, pH 7.4.
3. Aldehyde/ketone-functionalized antibody.
4. Aminooxy-functionalized drug-linker.
5. 4-amino-DL-phenylalanine.
6. 37 °C incubator/water bath.

2.3 SPAAC Ligation

1. PBS: 10 mM sodium phosphate, 150 mM NaCl, pH 7.4.
2. Azide-functionalized antibody.
3. Aza-dibenzocyclooctyne (DBCO)-functionalized drug-linker.

3 Method

3.1 Oxime Ligation

1. The conjugation reaction can be performed either at acidic pH (method A) or in the presence of a catalyst at neutral pH (method B). Depending on the method selected, buffer exchange the purified carbonyl-functionalized antibody into a buffer of appropriate pH using a desalting column (e.g. PD-10 column containing Sephadex G-25 resin, GE Healthcare). For method A, 0.1 M acetate buffer, pH 4.5 can be used. For method B, PBS can be used (*see* **Note 1**).
2. Prepare a 26.7 mM stock solution of an aminooxy-functionalized drug-linker in DMSO (*see* **Note 2**).
3. If method B is applied, prepare a 50 mM stock solution of 4-amino-phenylalanine in PBS. If method A is applied, skip this step and proceed to the next.
4. To 10 mg of carbonyl-functionalized antibody in acetate buffer (for method A) or in PBS (for method B), add 50 μL of 26.7 mM aminooxy drug-linker stock (*see* **Note 3**). If method B is applied, also add 200 μL of 50 mM 4-amino-phenylalanine for a final concentration of 10 mM. Make up the final volume of the sample to 1 mL. The final composition of the sample is the following: 10 mg/mL (66.7 μM) antibody and 1.33 mM aminooxy-functionalized drug-linker in the buffer of choice containing 5% DMSO (and 10 mM 4-amino-phenylalanine if method B is used) (*see* **Notes 4–7**).
5. For method A, allow the sample to incubate at 37 °C for 1–4 days. For method B, allow the sample to incubate at 4 °C overnight (*see* **Note 8**).
6. Remove excess drug-linkers by subjecting the sample to a desalting column equilibrated with PBS (*see* **Note 9**).
7. The resultant ADC sample may be concentrated using a 30 or 50 kDa MWCO protein concentrator (e.g. Amicon Ultra centrifugal filter).

8. Filter the purified ADC with a 0.2 μm syringe filter.
9. The ADC sample can be stored at −20 °C to −80 °C until use.

3.2 SPAAC Ligation

1. Take the purified antibody functionalized with azide, buffer exchange using a desalting column equilibrated with PBS (*see* **Note 10**).
2. Prepare a 26.7 mM stock solution of a DBCO-functionalized drug-linker in DMSO (*see* **Notes 2** and **11**).
3. To 10 mg of azide-functionalized antibody in PBS, add 50 μL of 26.7 mM DBCO drug-linker stock (*see* **Note 3**). Make up the final volume of the sample to 1 mL. The final composition of the sample is the following: 10 mg/mL (66.7 μM) antibody and 1.33 mM DBCO-functionalized drug-linker in PBS containing 5% DMSO (*see* **Notes 4–6**).
4. Allow the sample to incubate at room temperature for 2 h (*see* **Note 8**).
5. Remove excess drug-linkers by subjecting the sample to a desalting column equilibrated with PBS (*see* **Note 9**).
6. The resultant ADC sample may be concentrated using a 30 or 50 kDa MWCO protein concentrator (e.g. Amicon Ultra centrifugal filter).
7. Filter the purified ADC with a 0.2 μm syringe filter.
8. The ADC sample can be stored at −20 °C to −80 °C until use.

4 Notes

1. Avoid amine-containing buffers, such as Tris or glycine.
2. Drug-linker may be dissolved in organic solvents other than DMSO, typically DMF or DMA.
3. The protocol here is for a scale of 10 mg antibody.
4. Here the antibody is assumed to have one reactive group on each light or heavy chain for a total of two reactive groups per antibody. The concentration of the drug-linker selected here (1.33 mM) corresponds to ten equivalents relative to the number of reactive group on the antibody.
5. The conjugation is reported to be more efficient with higher reactant concentrations [18, 51].
6. The percentage of organic cosolvent is dependent on the solubility of the drug-linker. A less-soluble drug-linker would require a higher percentage of organic cosolvent.
7. Aniline or other aniline derivatives may be used as alternative catalysts, which are commonly used at 10 mM to 100 mM range [19, 46, 52–54]. We use 4-amino-phenylalanine for

catalysis, which is more biocompatible than aniline and accelerates the conjugation reaction rate at low temperature and neutral pH [55].

8. Analysis by LC-MS or hydrophobic interaction chromatography (HIC) is recommended to ensure that the conjugation is complete within the suggested time frame.
9. ADC can be further purified using HIC if the conjugation does not reach 100%.
10. Avoid azide (such as sodium azide)-containing buffers. Buffers other than PBS with a buffer range near neutral pH may be used [56].
11. Other cyclooctyne-functionalized drug-linkers may be considered. Reported examples include dibenzocyclooctyne derivatives, such as DIBO, [31] and bicyclo[6.1.0]nonyne (BCN) [34, 35]. BCN is reportedly able to conjugate with an azide-functionalized antibody more efficiently and is considered a less-hydrophobic alternative to DBCO [34].

References

1. Beck A, Goetsch L, Dumontet C, Corvaia N (2017) Strategies and challenges for the next generation of antibody-drug conjugates. Nat Rev Drug Discov 16(5):315–337. https://doi.org/10.1038/nrd.2016.268
2. Bross PF, Beitz J, Chen G, Chen XH, Duffy E, Kieffer L, Roy S, Sridhara R, Rahman A, Williams G, Pazdur R (2001) Approval summary. Gemtuzumab ozogamicin in relapsed acute myeloid leukemia. Clin Cancer Res 7 (6):1490–1496
3. Junutula JR, Raab H, Clark S, Bhakta S, Leipold DD, Weir S, Chen Y, Simpson M, Tsai SP, Dennis MS, Lu Y, Meng YG, Ng C, Yang J, Lee CC, Duenas E, Gorrell J, Katta V, Kim A, McDorman K, Flagella K, Venook R, Ross S, Spencer SD, Lee Wong W, Lowman HB, Vandlen R, Sliwkowski MX, Scheller RH, Polakis P, Mallet W (2008) Site-specific conjugation of a cytotoxic drug to an antibody improves the therapeutic index. Nat Biotechnol 26:925. https://doi.org/10.1038/nbt.1480
4. Shen BQ, Xu K, Liu L, Raab H, Bhakta S, Kenrick M, Parsons-Reponte KL, Tien J, Yu SF, Mai E, Li D, Tibbitts J, Baudys J, Saad OM, Scales SJ, McDonald PJ, Hass PE, Eigenbrot C, Nguyen T, Solis WA, Fuji RN, Flagella KM, Patel D, Spencer SD, Khawli LA, Ebens A, Wong WL, Vandlen R, Kaur S, Sliwkowski MX, Scheller RH, Polakis P, Junutula JR (2012) Conjugation site modulates the *in vivo* stability and therapeutic activity of antibody-drug conjugates. Nat Biotechnol 30 (2):184–189. https://doi.org/10.1038/nbt.2108
5. Strop P, Liu SH, Dorywalska M, Delaria K, Dushin RG, Tran TT, Ho WH, Farias S, Casas MG, Abdiche Y, Zhou D, Chandrasekaran R, Samain C, Loo C, Rossi A, Rickert M, Krimm S, Wong T, Chin SM, Yu J, Dilley J, Chaparro-Riggers J, Filzen GF, O'Donnell CJ, Wang F, Myers JS, Pons J, Shelton DL, Rajpal A (2013) Location matters: site of conjugation modulates stability and pharmacokinetics of antibody drug conjugates. Chem Biol 20(2):161–167. https://doi.org/10.1016/j.chembiol.2013.01.010
6. Tumey LN, Charati M, He T, Sousa E, Ma D, Han X, Clark T, Casavant J, Loganzo F, Barletta F, Lucas J, Graziani EI (2014) Mild method for succinimide hydrolysis on ADCs: impact on ADC potency, stability, exposure, and efficacy. Bioconjug Chem 25 (10):1871–1880. https://doi.org/10.1021/bc500357n
7. Tumey LN, Li F, Rago B, Han X, Loganzo F, Musto S, Graziani EI, Puthenveetil S, Casavant J, Marquette K, Clark T, Bikker J, Bennett EM, Barletta F, Piche-Nicholas N, Tam A, O'Donnell CJ, Gerber HP, Tchistiakova L (2017) Site selection: a case study in the identification of optimal cysteine engineered antibody drug conjugates. AAPS J 19

(4):1123–1135. https://doi.org/10.1208/s12248-017-0083-7

8. Vollmar BS, Wei B, Ohri R, Zhou J, He J, Yu SF, Leipold D, Cosino E, Yee S, Fourie-O'Donohue A, Li G, Phillips GL, Kozak KR, Kamath A, Xu K, Lee G, Lazar GA, Erickson HK (2017) Attachment site cysteine Thiol pKa is a key driver for site-dependent stability of THIOMAB antibody-drug conjugates. Bioconjug Chem 28(10):2538–2548. https://doi.org/10.1021/acs.bioconjchem.7b00365
9. Agarwal P, Bertozzi CR (2015) Site-specific antibody-drug conjugates: the nexus of bioorthogonal chemistry, protein engineering, and drug development. Bioconjug Chem 26 (2):176–192. https://doi.org/10.1021/bc5004982
10. Hamann PR, Hinman LM, Hollander I, Beyer CF, Lindh D, Holcomb R, Hallett W, Tsou H-R, Upeslacis J, Shochat D, Mountain A, Flowers DA, Bernstein I (2002) Gemtuzumab ozogamicin, a potent and selective anti-CD33 antibody–calicheamicin conjugate for treatment of acute myeloid leukemia. Bioconjug Chem 13(1):47–58. https://doi.org/10.1021/bc010021y
11. Laguzza BC, Nichols CL, Briggs SL, Cullinan GJ, Johnson DA, Starling JJ, Baker AL, Bumol TF, Corvalan JRF (1989) New antitumor monoclonal antibody-vinca conjugates LY203725 and related compounds: design, preparation, and representative in vivo activity. J Med Chem 32(3):548–555. https://doi.org/10.1021/jm00123a007
12. Hinman LM, Hamann PR, Wallace R, Menendez AT, Durr FE, Upeslacis J (1993) Preparation and characterization of monoclonal antibody conjugates of the calicheamicins: a novel and potent family of antitumor antibiotics. Cancer Res 53(14):3336–3342
13. Zuberbühler K, Casi G, Bernardes GJL, Neri D (2012) Fucose-specific conjugation of hydrazide derivatives to a vascular-targeting monoclonal antibody in IgG format. Chem Commun 48(56):7100–7102. https://doi.org/10.1039/c2cc32412a
14. Senter PD (2009) Potent antibody drug conjugates for cancer therapy. Curr Opin Chem Biol 13(3):235–244. https://doi.org/10.1016/j.cbpa.2009.03.023
15. Kalia J, Raines RT (2008) Hydrolytic stability of hydrazones and oximes. Angew Chem Int Ed 47(39):7523–7526. https://doi.org/10.1002/anie.200802651
16. NIH: U.S. National Library of Medicine (2017) A dose-escalation study of ARX788, IV administered in subjects with advanced cancers with HER2 expression (Identifier: NCT03255070). https://clinicaltrials.gov/ct2/show/NCT03255070. Accessed 1 Feb 2019
17. LegoChem Biosciences, Inc. (2016) Pipeline. http://www.legochembio.com/m/eng/md/pipeline.asp. Accessed 1 Feb 2019
18. Dirksen A, Dawson PE (2008) Rapid oxime and hydrazone ligations with aromatic aldehydes for biomolecular labeling. Bioconjug Chem 19(12):2543–2548. https://doi.org/10.1021/bc800310p
19. Kölmel DK, Kool ET (2017) Oximes and hydrazones in bioconjugation: mechanism and catalysis. Chem Rev 117 (15):10358–10376. https://doi.org/10.1021/acs.chemrev.7b00090
20. Agarwal P, Kudirka R, Albers AE, Barfield RM, de Hart GW, Drake PM, Jones LC, Rabuka D (2013) Hydrazino-Pictet-Spengler ligation as a biocompatible method for the generation of stable protein conjugates. Bioconjug Chem 24(6):846–851. https://doi.org/10.1021/bc400042a
21. Drake PM, Albers AE, Baker J, Banas S, Barfield RM, Bhat AS, de Hart GW, Garofalo AW, Holder P, Jones LC, Kudirka R, McFarland J, Zmolek W, Rabuka D (2014) Aldehyde tag coupled with HIPS chemistry enables the production of ADCs conjugated site-specifically to different antibody regions with distinct in vivo efficacy and PK outcomes. Bioconjug Chem 25 (7):1331–1341. https://doi.org/10.1021/bc500189z
22. NIH: U.S. National Library of Medicine (2018) Study of TRPH-222 in patients with relapsed and/or refractory B-cell lymphoma (Identifier: NCT03682796). https://clinicaltrials.gov/ct2/show/NCT03682796. Accessed 1 Feb 2019
23. Kudirka R, Barfield Robyn M, McFarland J, Albers Aaron E, de Hart Gregory W, Drake Penelope M, Holder Patrick G, Banas S, Jones Lesley C, Garofalo Albert W, Rabuka D (2015) Generating site-specifically modified proteins via a versatile and stable nucleophilic carbon ligation. Chem Biol 22(2):293–298. https://doi.org/10.1016/j.chembiol.2014.11.019
24. Dilek O, Lei Z, Mukherjee K, Bane S (2015) Rapid formation of a stable boron-nitrogen heterocycle in dilute, neutral aqueous solution for bioorthogonal coupling reactions. Chem Commun 51(95):16992–16995. https://doi.org/10.1039/c5cc07453c
25. Schmidt P, Stress C, Gillingham D (2015) Boronic acids facilitate rapid oxime condensations at neutral pH. Chem Sci 6 (6):3329–3333. https://doi.org/10.1039/c5sc00921a

26. Stress CJ, Schmidt PJ, Gillingham DG (2016) Comparison of boron-assisted oxime and hydrazone formations leads to the discovery of a fluorogenic variant. Org Biomol Chem 14(24):5529–5533. https://doi.org/10.1039/c6ob00168h
27. Gillingham D (2016) The role of boronic acids in accelerating condensation reactions of alpha-effect amines with carbonyls. Org Biomol Chem 14(32):7606–7609. https://doi.org/10.1039/c6ob01193d
28. Gu H, Chio TI, Lei Z, Staples RJ, Hirschi JS, Bane S (2017) Formation of hydrazones and stabilized boron-nitrogen heterocycles in aqueous solution from carbohydrazides and *ortho*-formylphenylboronic acids. Org Biomol Chem 15(36):7543–7548. https://doi.org/10.1039/c7ob01708a
29. Chio TI, Gu H, Mukherjee K, Tumey LN, Bane S (2019) Site-specific bioconjugation and multi-bioorthogonal labeling via rapid formation of a boron-nitrogen heterocycle. Bioconjug Chem 30(5):1554–1564. https://doi.org/10.1021/acs.bioconjchem.9b00246
30. Pickens CJ, Johnson SN, Pressnall MM, Leon MA, Berkland CJ (2018) Practical considerations, challenges, and limitations of bioconjugation via Azide–alkyne cycloaddition. Bioconjug Chem 29(3):686–701. https://doi.org/10.1021/acs.bioconjchem.7b00633
31. Li X, Fang T, Boons G-J (2014) Preparation of well-defined antibody–drug conjugates through glycan remodeling and strain-promoted azide–alkyne cycloadditions. Angew Chem 126(28):7307–7310. https://doi.org/10.1002/ange.201402606
32. Zimmerman ES, Heibeck TH, Gill A, Li X, Murray CJ, Madlansacay MR, Tran C, Uter NT, Yin G, Rivers PJ, Yam AY, Wang WD, Steiner AR, Bajad SU, Penta K, Yang W, Hallam TJ, Thanos CD, Sato AK (2014) Production of site-specific antibody–drug conjugates using optimized non-natural amino acids in a cell-free expression system. Bioconjug Chem 25(2):351–361. https://doi.org/10.1021/bc400490z
33. Dennler P, Chiotellis A, Fischer E, Bregeon D, Belmant C, Gauthier L, Lhospice F, Romagne F, Schibli R (2014) Transglutaminase-based chemo-enzymatic conjugation approach yields homogeneous antibody-drug conjugates. Bioconjug Chem 25(3):569–578. https://doi.org/10.1021/bc400574z
34. van Geel R, Wijdeven MA, Heesbeen R, Verkade JMM, Wasiel AA, van Berkel SS, van Delft FL (2015) Chemoenzymatic conjugation of toxic payloads to the globally conserved N-glycan of native mAbs provides homogeneous and highly efficacious antibody–drug conjugates. Bioconjug Chem 26(11):2233–2242. https://doi.org/10.1021/acs.bioconjchem.5b00224
35. VanBrunt MP, Shanebeck K, Caldwell Z, Johnson J, Thompson P, Martin T, Dong H, Li G, Xu H, D'Hooge F, Masterson L, Bariola P, Tiberghien A, Ezeadi E, Williams DG, Hartley JA, Howard PW, Grabstein KH, Bowen MA, Marelli M (2015) Genetically encoded azide containing amino acid in mammalian cells enables site-specific antibody–drug conjugates using click cycloaddition chemistry. Bioconjug Chem 26(11):2249–2260. https://doi.org/10.1021/acs.bioconjchem.5b00359
36. Tang F, Yang Y, Tang Y, Tang S, Yang L, Sun B, Jiang B, Dong J, Liu H, Huang M, Geng M-Y, Huang W (2016) One-pot N-glycosylation remodeling of IgG with non-natural sialylglycopeptides enables glycosite-specific and dual-payload antibody–drug conjugates. Org Biomol Chem 14(40):9501–9518. https://doi.org/10.1039/c6ob01751g
37. Thompson P, Ezeadi E, Hutchinson I, Fleming R, Bezabeh B, Lin J, Mao S, Chen C, Masterson L, Zhong H, Toader D, Howard P, Wu H, Gao C, Dimasi N (2016) Straightforward glycoengineering approach to site-specific antibody–pyrrolobenzodiazepine conjugates. ACS Med Chem Lett 7(11):1005–1008. https://doi.org/10.1021/acsmedchemlett.6b00278
38. NIH: U.S. National Library of Medicine (2018) Study of STRO-001, an anti-CD74 antibody drug conjugate, in patients with advanced B-cell malignancies (Identifier: NCT03424603). https://clinicaltrials.gov/ct2/show/NCT03424603. Accessed 1 Feb 2019
39. NIH: U.S. National Library of Medicine (2018) Safety, tolerability, pharmacokinetics, and antitumor study of ADCT-601 to treat advanced solid tumors (Identifier: NCT03700294). https://clinicaltrials.gov/ct2/show/NCT03700294. Accessed 1 Feb 2019
40. Oliveira BL, Guo Z, Bernardes GJL (2017) Inverse electron demand Diels–Alder reactions in chemical biology. Chem Soc Rev 46(16):4895–4950. https://doi.org/10.1039/c7cs00184c
41. Oller-Salvia B, Kym G, Chin JW (2018) Rapid and efficient generation of stable antibody-drug conjugates via an encoded cyclopropene and an inverse-electron-demand Diels-Alder reaction. Angew Chem Int Ed 57(11):2831–2834. https://doi.org/10.1002/anie.201712370

42. Axup JY, Bajjuri KM, Ritland M, Hutchins BM, Kim CH, Kazane SA, Halder R, Forsyth JS, Santidrian AF, Stafin K, Lu Y, Tran H, Seller AJ, Biroc SL, Szydlik A, Pinkstaff JK, Tian F, Sinha SC, Felding-Habermann B, Smider VV, Schultz PG (2012) Synthesis of site-specific antibody-drug conjugates using unnatural amino acids. Proc Natl Acad Sci U S A 109 (40):16101–16106. https://doi.org/10.1073/pnas.1211023109
43. Tian F, Lu Y, Manibusan A, Sellers A, Tran H, Sun Y, Phuong T, Barnett R, Hehli B, Song F, DeGuzman MJ, Ensari S, Pinkstaff JK, Sullivan LM, Biroc SL, Cho H, Schultz PG, DiJoseph J, Dougher M, Ma D, Dushin R, Leal M, Tchistiakova L, Feyfant E, Gerber HP, Sapra P (2014) A general approach to site-specific antibody drug conjugates. Proc Natl Acad Sci U S A 111(5):1766–1771. https://doi.org/10.1073/pnas.1321237111
44. Zhou Q, Stefano JE, Manning C, Kyazike J, Chen B, Gianolio DA, Park A, Busch M, Bird J, Zheng X, Simonds-Mannes H, Kim J, Gregory RC, Miller RJ, Brondyk WH, Dhal PK, Pan CQ (2014) Site-specific antibody–drug conjugation through glycoengineering. Bioconjug Chem 25(3):510–520. https://doi.org/10.1021/bc400505q
45. Ramakrishnan B, Li J, Wang Y, Feng Y, Prabakaran P, Colantonio S, Dyba MA, Qasba PK, Dimitrov DS (2014) Site-specific antibody-drug conjugation through an engineered glycotransferase and a chemically reactive sugar AU - Zhu, Zhongyu. MAbs 6(5):1190–1200. https://doi.org/10.4161/mabs.29889
46. Thompson P, Bezabeh B, Fleming R, Pruitt M, Mao S, Strout P, Chen C, Cho S, Zhong H, Wu H, Gao C, Dimasi N (2015) Hydrolytically stable site-specific conjugation at the N-terminus of an engineered antibody. Bioconjug Chem 26(10):2085–2096. https://doi.org/10.1021/acs.bioconjchem.5b00355
47. J-j L, Choi H-J, Yun M, Kang Y, Jung J-E, Ryu Y, Kim TY, Y-j C, Cho H-S, Min J-J, Chung C-W, Kim H-S (2015) Enzymatic prenylation and oxime ligation for the synthesis of stable and homogeneous protein–drug conjugates for targeted therapy. Angew Chem Int Ed 54(41):12020–12024. https://doi.org/10.1002/anie.201505964
48. Kudirka RA, Barfield RM, McFarland JM, Drake PM, Carlson A, Banas S, Zmolek W, Garofalo AW, Rabuka D (2016) Site-specific tandem Knoevenagel condensation-Michael addition to generate antibody-drug conjugates. ACS Med Chem Lett 7(11):994–998. https://doi.org/10.1021/acsmedchemlett.6b00253
49. Xu Y, Jin S, Zhao W, Liu W, Ding D, Zhou J, Chen S (2017) A versatile chemo-enzymatic conjugation approach yields homogeneous and highly potent antibody-drug conjugates. Int J Mol Sci 18(11):2284
50. Kim Y, Park T, Woo S, Lee H, Kim S, Cho J, Jung D, Kim Y, Kwon H, Oh K, Chung Y, Park Y (2017) Antibody-active agent conjugates and methods of use. US Patent, 9,669,107, 6 Jun 2017
51. Saito F, Noda H, Bode JW (2015) Critical evaluation and rate constants of chemoselective ligation reactions for stoichiometric conjugations in water. ACS Chem Biol 10 (4):1026–1033. https://doi.org/10.1021/cb5006728
52. Dirksen A, Hackeng TM, Dawson PE (2006) Nucleophilic catalysis of oxime ligation. Angew Chem Int Ed 45(45):7581–7584. https://doi.org/10.1002/anie.200602877
53. Kumar A, Kinneer K, Masterson L, Ezeadi E, Howard P, Wu H, Gao C, Dimasi N (2018) Synthesis of a heterotrifunctional linker for the site-specific preparation of antibody-drug conjugates with two distinct warheads. Bioorg Med Chem Lett 28(23):3617–3621. https://doi.org/10.1016/j.bmcl.2018.10.043
54. Kumar A, Kinneer K, Masterson L, Ezeadi E, Howard P, Wu H, Gao C, Dimasi N (2018) Characterization and in vitro data of antibody drug conjugates (ADCs) derived from heterotrifunctional linker designed for the site-specific preparation of dual ADCs. Data Brief 21:2208–2220. https://doi.org/10.1016/j.dib.2018.11.005
55. Blanden AR, Mukherjee K, Dilek O, Loew M, Bane SL (2011) 4-Aminophenylalanine as a biocompatible nucleophilic catalyst for hydrazone ligations at low temperature and neutral pH. Bioconjug Chem 22(10):1954–1961. https://doi.org/10.1021/bc2001566
56. Davis DL, Price EK, Aderibigbe SO, Larkin MXH, Barlow ED, Chen R, Ford LC, Gray ZT, Gren SH, Jin Y, Keddington KS, Kent AD, Kim D, Lewis A, Marrouche RS, O'Dair MK, Powell DR, Scadden MHC, Session CB, Tao J, Trieu J, Whiteford KN, Yuan Z, Yun G, Zhu J, Heemstra JM (2016) Effect of buffer conditions and organic cosolvents on the rate of strain-promoted azide–alkyne cycloaddition. J Org Chem 81(15):6816–6819. https://doi.org/10.1021/acs.joc.6b01112

Chapter 7

Utilizing Solid-Phase to Enable High-Throughput, Site-Specific Conjugation and Dual-Labeled Antibody and Fab Conjugates

Sujiet Puthenveetil

Abstract

For therapeutic and diagnostic applications, site-specific antibody conjugates have proven superior for both the ease of characterization as well as for optimal biophysical and therapeutic properties. Screening multiple antibodies on multiple sites with multiple linker-drugs can become very tedious and time-consuming. As solid-phase reactions are best suited to simplify multistep reactions, readily available protein A/L agarose beads can be utilized to generate site-specific, antibody –drug conjugates on engineered cysteines. Multiple site-specific labels on an antibody with either fluorophore or other-linker drugs is highly desired to evaluate antibody trafficking or payload-synergy for therapeutics. Utilizing solid-phase conjugation, a simple method to generate dual-labeled, site-specific antibody and Fab conjugates from antibody with engineered cysteine is also been described.

Key words Solid-phase conjugation, Site-specific conjugation, On-bead conjugation, Antibody–drug conjugate, Fab conjugate, Dual-label

1 Introduction

Any multistep chemical reaction can be simplified by the use of solid-phase tethering of the reactants because it eliminates the time-consuming intermediate purification steps. One key requisite for such a reaction is a straightforward method to covalently or non-covalently bind the reactant to the solid-phase and a simple elution methodology. Antibodies and Fab fragments are uniquely suited to this kind of binding and elution, as an affinity capture step is typically employed during their purification from the media. With the advent of multiple therapeutic antibody–drug conjugates (ADCs) in the clinic and several more in preclinical space [1], the use of high-throughput, solid-phase mediated antibody conjugation could greatly facilitate early-research efforts.

Early ADCs have been generated by conjugating linker-drugs to the lysines present on the surface of the antibody. As there are

L. Nathan Tumey (ed.), *Antibody-Drug Conjugates: Methods and Protocols*, Methods in Molecular Biology, vol. 2078, https://doi.org/10.1007/978-1-4939-9929-3_7,

over 70 lysines on an antibody, this methodology generates a very heterogeneous mixture of drug conjugate. Hence, despite utilizing lysine conjugation for generating early marketed ADCs like KADCYLA and MYLOTARG, the field has moved on to more homogeneous conjugates, due to ease of analytical characterization and improved ADC properties [2]. The second-generation ADCs like ADCETRIS have targeted interchain disulfide bonds of the antibody for conjugating linker-drugs to endogenous cysteines, to generate a more homogeneous conjugate [3]. For example, the eight interchain disulfides on a human IgG1 can be selectively reduced and partial reduction of these disulfide bonds allows for a more homogeneous mixture compared to the lysine conjugation. Despite lower heterogeneity with respect to the hinge-cysteine conjugation, the conjugation of linker-drugs is still restricted to the hinge region, which may not be ideal for overall ADC properties. For example, conjugation of multiple, hydrophobic linker-drugs all to the same region of the antibody may lead to increased aggregation or poor exposure in vivo [4].

The shift to third-generation, site-specific conjugation has been instrumental in overcoming these limitations [5]. By selecting the site of conjugation, it is easy to modulate the accessibility of protease susceptible linker-drugs, thus in turn, modulating their stability in vivo [6, 7]. It is also been shown that by distributing the linker-drugs to well-defined sites farther away from each other, a more stable ADC with higher drug-to-antibody ratio (DAR) can be achieved [4]. There are over a dozen site-specific ADCs in the clinic, highlighting the promise of the third generation of well-defined, site-specific ADCs [8]. At the early discovery stage, it is crucial to select the optimal linker-drug, site of conjugation and an optimal clone of the antibody for target of interest. As one can imagine, this combination of variables can lead to the generation of large sets of ADCs for screening, thus, necessitating a method to generate and purify ADCs in a high-throughput fashion. Previously, solid-phase bound antibody conjugations to the hinge-cysteines have been reported [9, 10]. Here, we describe the methods of generating site-specific antibody and Fab drug conjugates on solid-phase support, utilizing readily available protein-A/G/L agarose beads [11]. Furthermore, the ADC field has also been exploring the conjugation of multiple linker-drugs to potentially reduce the toxicity or improve efficacy of the ADCs by the synergistic effects of the combination of linker-drugs [12–14]. Sequential conjugation of multiple linker-drugs to different sites adds more reaction and purification steps towards the generation of dual-labeled-ADCs. Therefore, the solid-phase conjugation method described here is uniquely suited for such multistep labeling protocols.

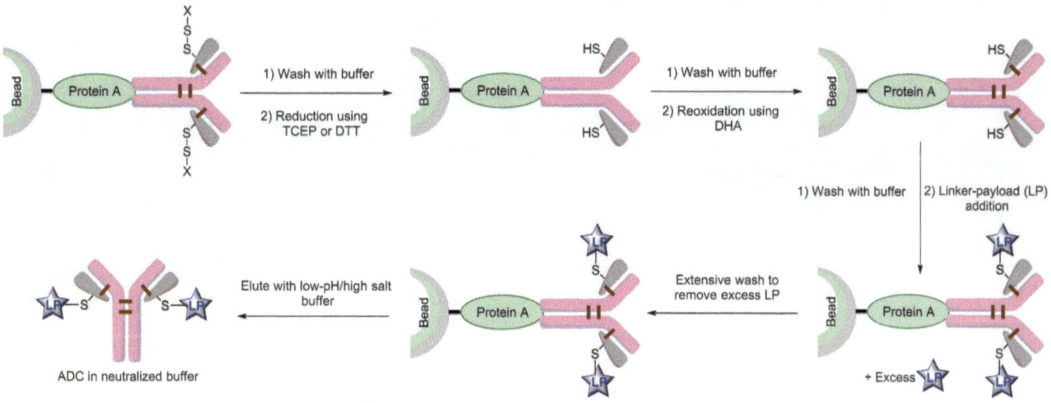

Fig. 1 Schematic representation for generation of site-specific ADCs using protein-A agarose beads. (Reprinted with permission from "Development of Solid-Phase Site-Specific Conjugation and Its Application toward Generation of Dual Labeled Antibody and Fab Drug Conjugates" by Puthenveetil S, Musto S, Loganzo F, Tumey LN, O'Donnell CJ, Graziani E. Bioconjug Chem. 2016;27(4):1030–9. Copyright 2016 American Chemical Society)

1.1 High-Throughput, Solid-Phase Site-Specific Conjugation of Engineered Cysteines on Antibody

A brief outline of the conjugation is as follows; first, an appropriate binding medium is chosen based on the type of antibody selected for the conjugation. For example, the method below describes the conjugation and purification of human IgG1 ADCs on protein-A agarose beads (Fig. 1). Based on the binding capacity of the solid-phase agarose beads, appropriate amount of antibody is bound, following which the solvent medium is changed to an appropriate reaction buffer. For a site-specific cysteine conjugation, the antibody is engineered to have surface cysteines on selected sites. The extra-engineered cysteine on the antibody is often unavailable for conjugation due to formation of disulfide bond with free cellular cysteine or glutathione. As it is difficult to selectively reduce the surface cysteines, both the interchain disulfides and the surface-engineered cysteines of the solid-phase bound antibody are reduced with excess reducing agent, like tris (2-carboxyethyl) phosphine hydrochloride (TCEP). After the reduction is complete, the reducing agent and any reduced free cysteine or glutathione is removed by washing the beads with an appropriate buffer. To re-form the interchain disulfide, the bound antibody is treated with an oxidizing reagent like dehydroascorbic acid (DHA), thereby selectively rendering the engineered cysteine available for site-specific conjugation. Once the excess oxidizing reagent is washed off the beads, a cysteine reactive linker-drug is added to the solid-phase bound antibody. After incubation for an appropriate time, the excess linker-drug is washed and subsequently the ADC is eluted using an appropriate elution buffer.

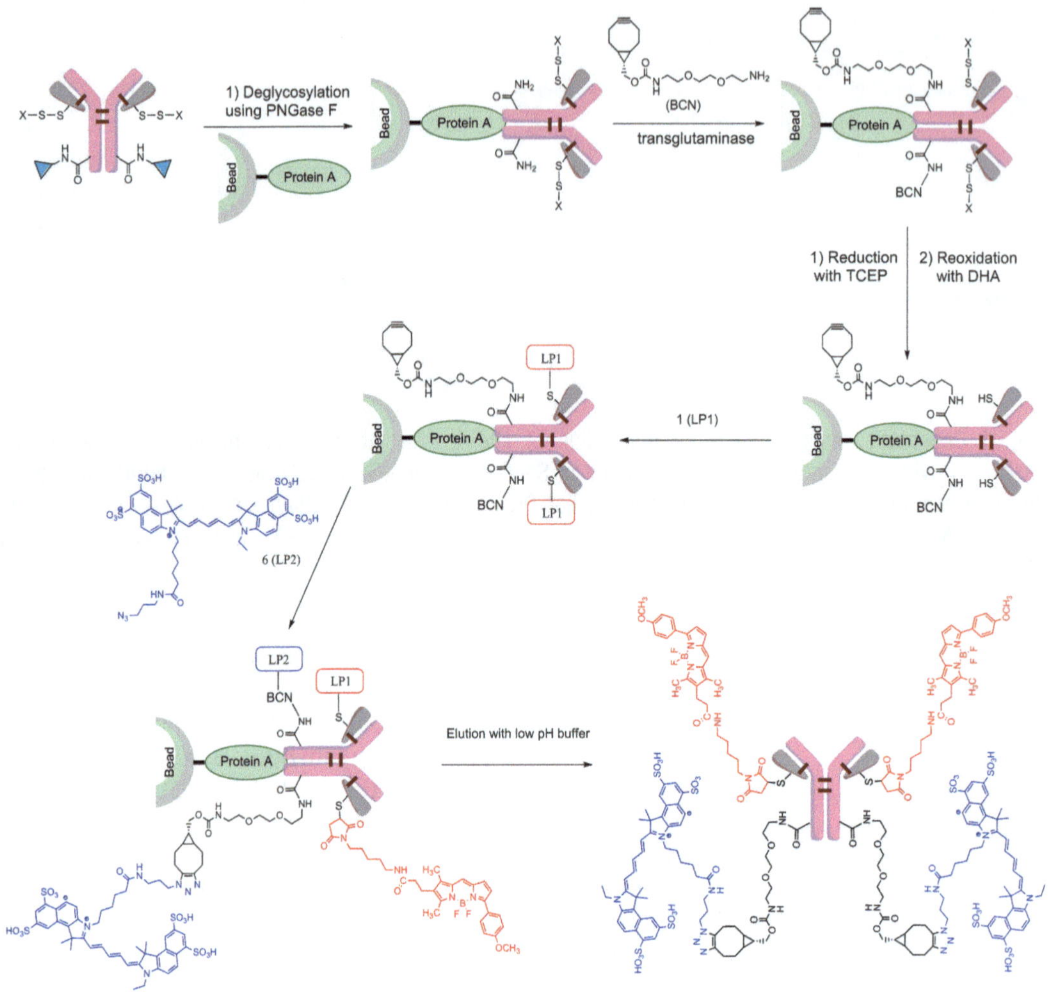

Fig. 2 Schematic representation for generation of dual-payload labeled, site-specific antibody conjugates on solid-phase. (Reprinted with permission from "Development of Solid-Phase Site-Specific Conjugation and Its Application toward Generation of Dual Labeled Antibody and Fab Drug Conjugates" by Puthenveetil S, Musto S, Loganzo F, Tumey LN, O'Donnell CJ, Graziani E. Bioconjug Chem. 2016;27(4):1030–9. Copyright 2016 American Chemical Society)

1.2 Generation of Dual-Labeled Site-Specific ADC on Solid-Phase Support

To site-specifically conjugate multiple linker-drugs, an appropriate complimentary conjugation methodology can be employed along with the engineered cysteine conjugation. Here we describe an enzymatic conjugation using microbial transglutaminase as a complimentary site-specific conjugation methodology to engineered cysteine conjugation (Fig. 2). In the method described below, for dual linker-drug conjugation to an IgG1 with extra-engineered cysteines, the antibody was first deglycosylated in order to render the vicinal glutamine-295 available for enzymatic conjugation. The deglycosylated antibody was then bound to protein-A agarose beads, followed by an on-bead bio-conjugation of N-[(1R,8S,9s)-bicyclo[6.1.0]non4-yn-9-ylmethyloxycarbonyl]-1,8-diamino-3,6-

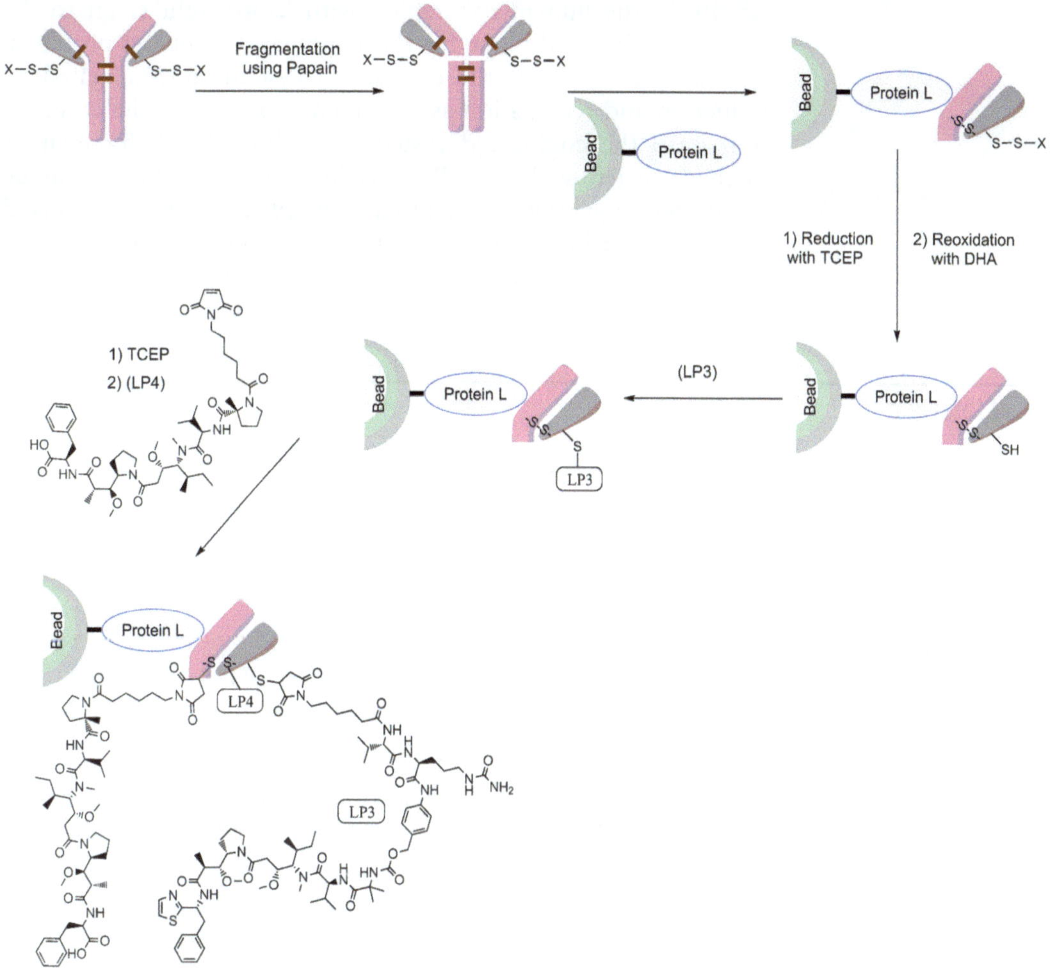

Fig. 3 Schematic representation for generation of dual-labeled Fab conjugate. (Reprinted with permission from "Development of Solid-Phase Site-Specific Conjugation and Its Application toward Generation of Dual Labeled Antibody and Fab Drug Conjugates" by Puthenveetil S, Musto S, Loganzo F, Tumey LN, O'Donnell CJ, Graziani E. Bioconjug Chem. 2016;27(4):1030–9. Copyright 2016 American Chemical Society)

dioxaoctane (BCN) to the 295Q using transglutaminase enzyme. The excess enzyme and the linker-drug were removed by washing the beads. Following the conjugation of BCN, the second cysteine reactive linker-drug was site-specifically conjugated as mentioned above. Any azide carrying payload can be then coupled to BCN via strain-promoted 1,3 dipolar cycloaddition reaction for dual-labeled antibody conjugate [15].

1.3 Generation of Dual-Labeled Fab Conjugate on Solid-Phase Support

Lastly, a simple way to generate dual-labeled Fab–drug conjugate is also described (Fig. 3). If a cysteine-engineered Fab fragment is not available, an antibody with an engineered cysteine on the Fab region can be digested to obtain Fab fragment with one interchain disulfide and one engineered cysteine for conjugation. Due to the affinity of the human Fab region with kappa light chain to the protein-L, the solid-phase for this conjugation employs protein-L agarose beads. Firstly, the engineered cysteine is conjugated by reduction and reoxidation as described above. After the conjugation onto the engineered cysteine, the bound Fab fragment is further treated with TCEP to reduce the interchain disulfide bond. Subsequently, the endogenous cysteines are conjugated with a second linker-drug to obtain dual-labeled Fab conjugate. Multiple-engineered cysteines can be introduced onto the antibody/Fab to obtain different ratios of the linker-drugs.

2 Materials

2.1 High-Throughput, Solid-Phase Site-Specific Conjugation of Engineered Cysteines on Antibody

1. Dulbecco's Phosphate Buffered Saline (DPBS, 1×, 9.5 mM PO_4 without Calcium or Magnesium), pH 7.4.
2. 100 mM Tris buffer pH 8.0.
3. Dimethyl sulfoxide (DMSO).
4. Dimethylacetamide (DMA).
5. Human IgG1 with engineered cysteines (1–10 mg/mL).
6. 0.5 M 2,2′,2″,2‴-(ethane-1,2-diyldinitrilo)tetraacetic acid (EDTA) solution pH 7.5 (Teknova).
7. 1 mL Protein-A agarose beads (such as Pierce™ Protein A Plus Agarose beads or GE MabSelect™ SuRe™ antibody purification resin).
8. Micro-spin columns (Pierce™ # 89879) for single conjugation or 96-well deep well hydrophilic filter plates (such as Millipore MDRLN0410 Multiscreen deep-well solvinert, 0.45 μm pore size, Hydrophilic Polytetrafluoroethylene (PTFE), volume 1.9 mL) for high-throughput conjugation.
9. MultiScreen®HTS Vacuum Manifold (Millipore #MSVMHTS00) is required for vacuum filtering the 96-well plates. A table-top microcentrifuge can be used to filter micro-spin columns as per manufacturer's instruction.
10. 96-well deep-well collection plates (Millipore # MDCPN2M50) for collecting eluted antibody and washing eluents.
11. Orbital shaker (optional: temperature controlled).
12. 0.5 M tris (2-carboxyethyl) phosphine hydrochloride (TCEP) solution, pH 7.0 (sigma # 646547)
13. 50 mM (L)-Dehydroascorbic acid (DHA) (in 1:4:5, DMSO: DPBS: Ethanol).
14. Thiol reactive (such as maleimide or haloacetamide) payload stored at 5 mM in DMSO or DMA at −80 °C.

15. Antibody elution buffer (0.1 M Glycine.HCl pH 3.0 or Pierce elution buffer #21004).
16. Neutralization buffer (1 M Tris buffer, pH 8.0).
17. Nanodrop UV-Vis spectrophotometer.
18. Optional: Multichannel pipette (10–100 μL and 100–1000 μL).

2.2 Additional Material for Dual-Labeled Site-Specific ADC

1. PNGase F enzyme for deglycosylation ((NEB# P0704L).
2. (a) 30 mM N-[(1R,8S,9s)-bicyclo[6.1.0]non4-yn-9-ylmethyloxycarbonyl]-1,8-diamino-3,6-dioxaoctane (BCN-amine, Sigma-Aldrich # 745073) in DMA and 10 mM payload with an azide handle for two-step click reaction.

   (b) 30 mM Linker-Drug in DMA with alkyl-amine (5-aminopentyl) reactive handle as a direct transglutaminase substrate.
3. Bacterial transglutaminase enzyme (Ajinomoto, Activa TI).
4. Optional: human IgG1 with N297A or LLQG [16] tag in addition to the engineered cysteine.

2.3 Additional Material for Dual-Labeled Fab Conjugate

1. Pierce protein-L plus agarose beads (Thermo Fisher Scientific # 20520).
2. Optional: Pierce™ Fab Preparation Kit papain (Thermo Fisher Scientific # 44985).

3 Method

3.1 High-Throughput, Solid-Phase Site-Specific Conjugation of Engineered Cysteines on Antibody

1. Equilibrate all the buffers and agarose beads to room temperature.
2. Pipette into each well of Millipore 96-well filter plates, 100 μL suspension of protein-A beads (Pierce™ Protein A Plus Agarose beads has a binding capacity of up to 35 mg IgG1/mL beads) (*see* **Notes 1** and **2**).
3. Place a 96-well collection plate in MultiScreen®HTS Vacuum Manifold (Millipore #MSVMHTS00) and filter out the solution from Protein-A suspension at a vacuum of −20 kPa to −50 kPa. Discard the flow-through (*see* **Note 3**).
4. Rinse the protein-A beads by resuspending the beads with 300 μL DPBS and using vacuum manifold to remove the flow-through in 96-well filter plate, as described above. Repeat the wash twice more for a total of three washes.
5. *Antibody binding steps:* Switch off the vacuum and then add 1 mg of human IgG1 antibody with extra-engineered cysteines in DPBS to the rinsed beads, while resuspending them (*see* **Notes 4** and **5**).

6. Place the filter plate on top of the collection plate and incubate for 15 min at room temperature while gently rocking on an orbital shaker at 50–150 rpm. If the volume is more than 300 μL resuspend the beads at half-way time point (*see* **Note 6**).
7. After the antibody is bound to the protein A beads, rinse the beads with 300 μL of fresh DPBS using the vacuum manifold as described above. Discard the flow-through. Repeat the wash once more for a total of two washes (*see* **Note 7**).
8. *Antibody reduction steps:* Make fresh reducing buffer by adding TCEP and EDTA to DPBS to make 2.22 mM TCEP (100 equivalents), 5 mM EDTA, DPBS (*see* **Note 8**).
9. Add 300 μL of this fresh reducing buffer to the antibody bound on the beads and incubate for 1 h at room temperature while gently rocking on an orbital shaker at 50–150 rpm as was performed for antibody binding step.
10. After the antibody is reduced with excess TCEP, use the vacuum manifold to remove the reducing buffer. Discard the flow-through. Rinse the beads with 300 μL of DPBS, 5 mM EDTA. Repeat the wash twice more for a total of three washes. Discard the flow-through (*see* **Note 9**).
11. *Antibody reoxidation steps:* Make fresh reoxidation buffer by adding DHA solution in DPBS to obtain a final concentration of 0.85 mM DHA (40 equivalents), DPBS (*see* **Note 8**).
12. Add 300 μL of this fresh reoxidation buffer to the antibody bound on the beads and incubate for 1 h at room temperature while gently rocking on an orbital shaker at 50–150 rpm as was performed for previous steps.
13. After the antibody is reoxidized, use the vacuum manifold to remove the reoxidation buffer. Discard the flow-through. Rinse the beads with 300 μL of DPBS, 5 mM EDTA. Repeat the wash twice more for a total of three washes. Discard the flow-through.
14. *Site-specific cysteine conjugation step*: Mix 10 μL of 5 mM maleimide linker-drug (6 equivalents) solution to 290 μL of DPBS, 5 mM EDTA pH 7.4. Add up to 20 μL more of DMA/DMSO if the solution turns cloudy due to incomplete solubility (*see* **Notes 8** and **10**).
15. Add this linker-drug solution to the reoxidized antibody bound to the agarose and incubate for 2 h at room temperature while gently rocking on an orbital shaker at 50–150 rpm, as was performed for previous steps (*see* **Note 11**).
16. *Linker-drug washing steps*: After the conjugation step, use the vacuum manifold to remove the linker-drug. As it is critical to remove all traces of linker-drug, rinse the bead-bound ADCs

with 500 μL 10% DMSO in DPBS for seven times using the vacuum manifold (*see* **Note 12**).

17. Perform three additional washes with 300 μL of DPBS. Discard all flow-through.
18. *Elution of ADC*: Add 75 μL (1/10th the volume of elution buffer) of neutralization buffer (1 M Tris pH 8.0) to the 96-well collection plate.
19. Add 250 μL of the elution buffer to each well of the 96-well filter plate containing ADC bound to agarose beads. Using the vacuum manifold, collect the flow-through containing ADCs, into the neutralization buffer containing 96-well collection plate. Repeat the elution times two more times by adding 250 μL to the same well and collecting to the same collection plate (*see* **Notes 13–15**).
20. Mix the neutralized ADC solution using a multichannel pipette and measure the absorbance at 280 nm to obtain their concentration.
21. Drug-to-antibody ratio (DAR) can be calculated using an appropriate liquid chromatography–mass spectrometry (LC-MS) method.

3.2 Solid-Phase Dual-Labeled Site-Specific ADC

1. Mix 0.2 μL of PNGase F to 1 mg of human IgG1 antibody engineered with selected extra cysteine (2–10 mg/mL) and incubate the mixture for 37 °C overnight.
2. Incubate the reaction mixture with protein-A agarose beads as described in Subheading 3.1. Follow the steps from Subheading 3.1, **steps 1–7**.
3. Make a transglutaminase reaction mix with 0.555 mM BCN-amine or other transglutaminase substrate (5.55 μL of 30 mM BCN amine in 300 μL PBS). To this solution, mix 20 mg of transglutaminase/maltodextrin powder.
4. Add 300 μL of this TG (Transglutaminase) reaction mix to the antibody bound on the beads and incubate for 24–48 h at 37 °C while gently rocking on an orbital shaker at 50–150 rpm as was performed for antibody-binding step (*see* **Notes 16–18**).
5. After the antibody is enzymatically conjugated, use the vacuum manifold to remove the transglutaminase reaction mix. Discard the flow through. Rinse the beads with 300 μL of DPBS, 5 mM EDTA. Repeat the wash twice more for a total of three washes. Discard the flow-through.
6. To conjugate the cysteine-engineered antibody with second linker-drug, follow steps from Subheading 3.1, **steps 8–17**.

7. If in Subheading 3.2, **step 3** the desired final transglutaminase substrate was enzymatically conjugated, then follow antibody elution Subheading 3.1, **steps 18–21**.
8. If BCN-amine was conjugated in Subheading 3.2, **step 3**, the strained alkyne on BCN is coupled to azide carrying linker-drug using copper-free click chemistry. Mix 0.133 mM azido-linker-drug (6 equivalents) with up to 10% DMSO in DPBS (4 μL of 10 mM azido linker-drug and 20 μL DMSO in 300 μL DMSO).
9. Add this solution to agarose-bound antibody from Subheading 3.2, **step 7** and incubate for 4 h at room temperature while gently rocking on an orbital shaker at 50–150 rpm as was performed for antibody binding step (*see* **Note 19**).
10. Follow linker-drug washing and antibody elution step as described in Subheading 3.1, **steps 16–21**.

3.3 Dual-Labeled Fab Conjugation on Solid-Phase

1. Bind 1 mg of cysteine-engineered human Fab fragment to 200 μL Pierce protein-L plus agarose beads following binding and washing procedure as described in Subheading 3.1, **steps 1–4** (*see* **Note 20**).
2. Following the procedure described in Subheading 3.1, **steps 5–17**, site specifically conjugate the first linker-drug to the engineered cysteine.
3. To reduce the interchain disulfide bond, make fresh reducing buffer by adding TCEP and EDTA to a final concentration of 0.444 mM TCEP (20 equivalents), 5 mM EDTA to DPBS.
4. Add 300 μL of this fresh reducing buffer to the antibody bound on the beads and incubate for 1 h at room temperature while gently rocking on an orbital shaker at 50–150 rpm as was performed for antibody binding step.
5. After the antibody is reduced with excess TCEP, use the vacuum manifold to remove the reducing buffer. Discard the flow-through. Rinse the beads with 300 μL of DPBS, 5 mM EDTA. Repeat the wash twice more for a total of three washes. Discard the flow-through.
6. Follow **steps 14–21** of Subheading 3.1 to conjugate the second linker-drug to the reduced endogenous cysteines and elute the Fab dual-drug conjugate.

4 Notes

1. Mix the agarose beads by inverting or gently shaking the bottle. Cut the pipette tip for uniform agarose suspension dispensing.

2. When not all of the wells of the 96-well filter plates are being used, sealing the unused wells with a tape helps with obtaining an efficient vacuum in the vacuum manifold.
3. Any other suitable multiwell plate vacuum manifold such as (PALL# 5017) or centrifuge with plate adaptors can be used to filter the solution out of Protein-A agarose beads.
4. If the antibody is in a different buffer, add 10× DPBS buffer and double the volume by adding equal amount of distilled water to bring the final antibody solution to 1× DPBS.
5. While adding buffers or reagents, do not resuspend the agarose using the pipette to avoid loss of agarose sticking to the tips. Pipet the solutions over the beads such that the beads get resuspended without spilling outside.
6. If using the micro-spin column for individual conjugation reaction, incubate the beads while mixing end over end.
7. To measure if the antibody is efficiently bound to agarose beads, measure the relative absorption of the flow-through at 280 nm.
8. Amount of reducing agent (100 equivalents), reoxidizing agent (40 equivalents), and maleimide linker-drug (6 equivalents), were added with the assumption that the antibody binding to agarose beads is quantitative.
9. If some engineered cysteine sites do not get completely reduced on solid-phase, reduce the antibody in solution overnight followed by binding the mixture to protein-A agarose beads as described in the antibody-binding step.
10. If using haloacetamide linker-drugs instead of maleimides, the reaction is more efficient in 100 mM Tris pH 8.0, longer reaction time to 6 h to overnight, and incubating the reaction mixture at 37 °C in the orbital shaker.
11. Some linker-drugs are slower to react, therefore, optimization of conditions using an increased reaction time and temperature to 37 °C could facilitate better conjugation efficiency.
12. Occasionally, some of the wells of the filter well plates show reduced flow under vacuum. This could be due to clogged filter or manufacturing defects. Under these circumstances it is best to resuspend the agarose in the buffer being used and transfer it to a fresh well. The loss of sample during transfer is very marginal.
13. Typical ADC yield eluted from the protein A agarose beads is 55–70%. To obtain a more concentrated ADC solution, the antibody can be eluted with lower amount of elution buffer. Two times with 150 μL instead of three times with 250 μL of elution buffer. About 10–20% further loss of yield could result.

14. Cytotoxic ADCs generated for oncology using this method did not show a difference in the in vitro activity regardless of whether the neutralized buffer was further buffer exchanged into DPBS. Further buffer exchange can be achieved using 96-well desalting plates such as GE PD MultiTrap G-25 (GE # 28918006) or 96-well dialysis plate such as Pierce™ 96-well Microdialysis Plate, 10 K MWCO (ThermoFisher Scientific #88260).
15. If the linker-drug is sensitive to low pH of elution buffer, high salt Pierce™ Gentle Ag/Ab Elution Buffer, pH 6.6 (# 21027) can be used, followed by buffer exchange as described above. Gentle Ag/Ab Binding Buffer: pH 8.0; phosphate-free rinse of the agarose beads is recommended prior to high-salt elution.
16. Transglutaminase conjugation on antibodies with an engineered transglutaminase tag is more efficient than with the deglycosylated antibody. If the conjugation efficiency is lower for certain transglutaminase substrates, an insertion of transglutaminase tag LLQG to selected sites is recommended [16]. Alternatively, transglutaminase conjugation on deglycosylated antibody can be performed in solution and then the conjugated antibody mixture can be bound to protein-A agarose beads for subsequent purification and conjugation.
17. 20 μL of antibody bound to protein-A agarose beads can be removed and eluted using elution buffer using a micro-spin column. A LC-MS analysis of this ADC can be performed to calculate DAR. If the transglutaminase conjugation of deglycosylated human IgG1on the solid-phase is not very efficient, the reaction can be repeated two more times with fresh transglutaminase and linker-drug solution as described in Subheading 3.2, **steps 3** and **4**, after removing the previous transglutaminase reaction mix. Changing the reaction buffer from PBS to 50 mM Tris, 150 mM NaCl, pH 8.0 is also beneficial for some linker-drug transglutaminase conjugation.
18. The transglutaminase conjugation to deglycosylated antibody bound to solid-phase was carried out using 20 mg transglutaminase powder/mg of antibody, assuming quantitative binding of antibody to agarose beads. 25 equivalents of the transglutaminase linker-drug was used. Optimization of the transglutaminase reaction includes reducing or increasing the amount of transglutaminase powder from 1 to 30 mg.
19. Copper-free click chemistry on agarose beads can be optimized further by increasing the reaction temperature to 37 °C and increasing the reaction time.
20. Dual-labeled Fab conjugate can also be readily generated using IgG1 with engineered cysteines on the Fab region. A Fab-generation kit which uses immobilized papain (Thermo

Fisher Scientific # 20341) can be used to generate Fab and can be utilized for conjugation described in Subheading 3.3. To remove the nonfragmented antibody Ni-NTA agarose beads is recommended over protein-A agarose beads for better yield.

References

1. Jackson D, Stover D (2015) Using the lessons learned from the clinic to improve the preclinical development of antibody drug conjugates. Pharm Res 32(11):3458–3469. https://doi.org/10.1007/s11095-014-1536-7
2. Kim EG, Kim KM (2015) Strategies and advancement in antibody-drug conjugate optimization for targeted cancer therapeutics. Biomol Ther (Seoul) 23(6):493–509. https://doi.org/10.4062/biomolther.2015.116
3. Francisco JA, Cerveny CG, Meyer DL, Mixan BJ, Klussman K, Chace DF, Rejniak SX, Gordon KA, DeBlanc R, Toki BE, Law CL, Doronina SO, Siegall CB, Senter PD, Wahl AF (2003) cAC10-vcMMAE, an anti-CD30-monomethyl auristatin E conjugate with potent and selective antitumor activity. Blood 102(4):1458–1465. https://doi.org/10.1182/blood-2003-01-0039
4. Strop P, Delaria K, Foletti D, Witt JM, Hasa-Moreno A, Poulsen K, Casas MG, Dorywalska M, Farias S, Pios A, Lui V, Dushin R, Zhou D, Navaratnain T, Trani TT, Sutton J, Lindquist KC, Han B, Litt SH, Shelton DL, Pons J, Rajpal A (2015) Site-specific conjugation improves therapeutic index of antibody drug conjugates with high drug loading. Nat Biotechnol 33(7):694–696. https://doi.org/10.1038/nbt.3274
5. Panowksi S, Bhakta S, Raab H, Polakis P, Junutula Jagath R (2014) Site-specific antibody drug conjugates for cancer therapy. MAbs 6 (1):34–45
6. Tumey LN, Leverett CA, Vetelino B, Li F, Rago B, Han X, Loganzo F, Musto S, Bai G, Sukuru SCK, Graziani EI, Puthenveetil S, Casavant J, Ratnayake A, Marquette K, Hudson S, Doppalapudi VR, Stock J, Tchistiakova L, Bessire AJ, Clark T, Lucas J, Hosselet C, O'Donnell CJ, Subramanyam C (2016) Optimization of Tubulysin antibody--drug conjugates: a case study in addressing ADC metabolism. ACS Med Chem Lett 7 (11):977–982
7. Strop P, Liu S-H, Dorywalska M, Delaria K, Dushin RG, Tran T-T, Ho W-H, Farias S, Casas MG, Abdiche Y, Zhou D, Chandrasekaran R, Samain C, Loo C, Rossi A, Rickert M, Krimm S, Wong T, Chin SM, Yu J, Dilley J, Chaparro-Riggers J, Filzen GF, O'Donnell CJ, Wang F, Myers JS, Pons J, Shelton DL, Rajpal A (2013) Location matters: site of conjugation modulates stability and pharmacokinetics of antibody drug conjugates. Chem Biol 20(2):161–167. https://doi.org/10.1016/j.chembiol.2013.01.010
8. van Berkel SS, van Delft FL (2018) Enzymatic strategies for (near) clinical development of antibody-drug conjugates. Drug Discov Today Technol 30:3–10. https://doi.org/10.1016/j.ddtec.2018.09.005
9. Nath N, Godat B, Benink H, Urh M (2015) On-bead antibody-small molecule conjugation using high-capacity magnetic beads. J Immunol Methods 426:95–103. https://doi.org/10.1016/j.jim.2015.08.008
10. Lyon RP, Meyer DL, Setter JR, Senter PD (2012) Conjugation of anticancer drugs through endogenous monoclonal antibody cysteine residues. Methods Enzymol 502(Protein Engineering for Therapeutics, Part A):123–138. https://doi.org/10.1016/b978-0-12-416039-2.00006-9
11. Puthenveetil S, Musto S, Loganzo F, Tumey LN, O'Donnell CJ, Graziani E (2016) Development of solid-phase site-specific conjugation and its application toward generation of dual labeled antibody and fab drug conjugates. Bioconjug Chem 27(4):1030–1039. https://doi.org/10.1021/acs.bioconjchem.6b00054
12. Hallam T (2013) Producing homogeneous ADCs with combination warheads. In: World ADC Summit, San Francisco, California, USA, 14–17 Oct 2013
13. Li X, Patterson JT, Sarkar M, Pedzisa L, Kodadek T, Roush WR, Rader C (2015) Site-specific dual antibody conjugation via engineered cysteine and selenocysteine residues. Bioconjug Chem 26:2243–2248. https://doi.org/10.1021/acs.bioconjchem.5b00244
14. Maruani A, Smith ME, Miranda E, Chester KA, Chudasama V, Caddick S (2015) A plug-and-play approach to antibody-based therapeutics via a chemoselective dual click strategy. Nat Commun 6:6645. https://doi.org/10.1038/ncomms7645
15. Pickens CJ, Johnson SN, Pressnall MM, Leon MA, Berkland CJ (2018) Practical

considerations, challenges, and limitations of bioconjugation via azide-alkyne cycloaddition. Bioconjug Chem 29(3):686–701. https://doi.org/10.1021/acs.bioconjchem.7b00633

16. Strop P, Dorywalska MG, Rajpal A, Shelton D, Liu S-H, Pons J, Dushin R (2012) Engineered polypeptide conjugates and methods for making thereof using transglutaminase. Application: WO. WO Patent 2011-IB54899, 2012059882

Chapter 8

Bridged Cysteine Conjugations

Matthew Bird, Joao Nunes, and Mark Frigerio

Abstract

Preparation of antibody–drug conjugates (ADCs) with a highly homogeneous drug loading in general requires site-selective conjugation of a cytotoxic payload. Typically, functionality utilized for attachment of the payload is achieved through engineering of suitable chemical handles or by enzymatic modification of the antibody. Relatively few methods to produce ADCs with homogeneous drug loading via endogenous amino acid conjugation have been developed. Herein we describe a robust method for the conjugation of antibodies using a cysteine rebridging approach to produce ADCs with highly homogeneous drug-to-antibody ratios (DAR) at the native interchain disulfides, called ThioBridge®. The process described relies upon an elegant cascade of addition–elimination reactions carried out under mild aqueous conditions that can be readily applied to wild-type antibodies without the need for prior modification via recombinant or enzymatic means. Using this method, conversions to a conserved DAR ADC are typically in the range of 70–95% and overall process yields of >70% are readily achieved.

Key words Interchain disulfide, Cysteine rebridging, Michael addition, Homogeneous drug loading, ThioBridge® conjugation

1 Introduction

Early methods for chemical conjugation of cytotoxic drugs to antibodies focused on attachment at native lysine and cysteine residues. These methods typically resulted in the first-generation ADCs being composed of mixtures of positional isomers [1, 2]. Lysine conjugation, often performed using NHS ester-based reagents, targets the ε-amino group in solvent accessible lysines, which can number at least 40–60 residues in a typical IgG1 antibody [3], resulting in highly heterogeneous mixtures [1, 4, 5].

Cysteine conjugation often uses maleimide-based reagents to target sulfhydryl residues, made available through reduction of the interchain disulfide bonds present in the antibody structure, and despite fewer sites being available for conjugation when compared to lysine modification, this strategy also results in a heterogeneous mixture of ADC species [2, 6]. The loss of structural integrity resulting from disulfide reduction can also contribute to an

L. Nathan Tumey (ed.), *Antibody-Drug Conjugates: Methods and Protocols*, Methods in Molecular Biology, vol. 2078,
https://doi.org/10.1007/978-1-4939-9929-3_8,

increased physicochemical instability to stress conditions [7, 8]. A known limitation of maleimide conjugation is the susceptibility to cross-conjugation to protein thiols and also to deconjugation via a retro-Michael reaction, compromising the pharmacokinetic (PK) profile [9–11]. Deconjugation can be modulated by hydrolysis of the succinimide ring to the maleamic acid by incorporation of an amine group on the *N*-alkyl spacer [12] or by use of an *N*-aryl spacer [13], resulting in improved PK and in vivo efficacy [9, 12, 14]. These strategies however do not address the general problem of heterogeneity resulting from poor control of conjugation site location leading to variations in drug loading. Heterogeneous lysine and maleimide-based ADCs therefore consist of both less-potent low drug-loaded species and high drug-loaded species subject to increased clearance rates, resulting in suboptimal therapeutic indexes [5, 7, 10, 15–18].

Disulfide rebridging strategies can address the issues of site-selectivity and homogeneity and offer several key advantages over the more stochastic conjugation methods, including homogeneous drug loading and controlling the site of conjugation at the interchain disulfides. The specific chemistry and dual points of attachment per conjugation site may deliver improved stability and rebridging can improve the antibody structural stability which is affected in maleimide ADCs. Finally, antibody engineering through site-directed mutagenesis is avoided, enabling disulfide rebridging to be readily applicable to commercial and off-the-shelf antibodies.

Disulfide rebridging methods for ADC production includes Abzena's ThioBridge® technology and typically involves a two-step sequence (Fig. 1). The first step is the reduction of the interchain disulfide bonds to release sulfhydryl residues for conjugation, typically achieved using either phosphine-based reductants such as tris(2-carboxyethyl)phosphine (TCEP) or by thiol-based reductants such as dithiothreitol (DTT). TCEP offers the advantages of being highly reactive, is odorless, relatively stable in aqueous conditions, and leads to an irreversible reduction with fewer equivalents of reducing agent used when compared to DTT [19]. There is also the added advantage of not requiring the removal of TCEP from the reduction step prior to conjugation. The use of EDTA as a metal scavenger in the reaction buffer during conjugation is a standard procedure employed to avoid any disulfide bond reoxidation processes that can take place due to trace metal catalysis. Thus, for a typical human IgG1, four reduced disulfide bonds yield eight free sulfhydryl residues. The second step involves conjugation of a bis-functional electrophilic reagent capable of reacting with a pair of sulfhydryl residues to covalently rebridge the disulfide bonds. A small amount of water miscible organic solvent may be required to solubilize the reagent for conjugation, and the buffer is typically at neutral or mildly basic pH to generate the sulfhydryl thiolate anion as the reactive species. Once

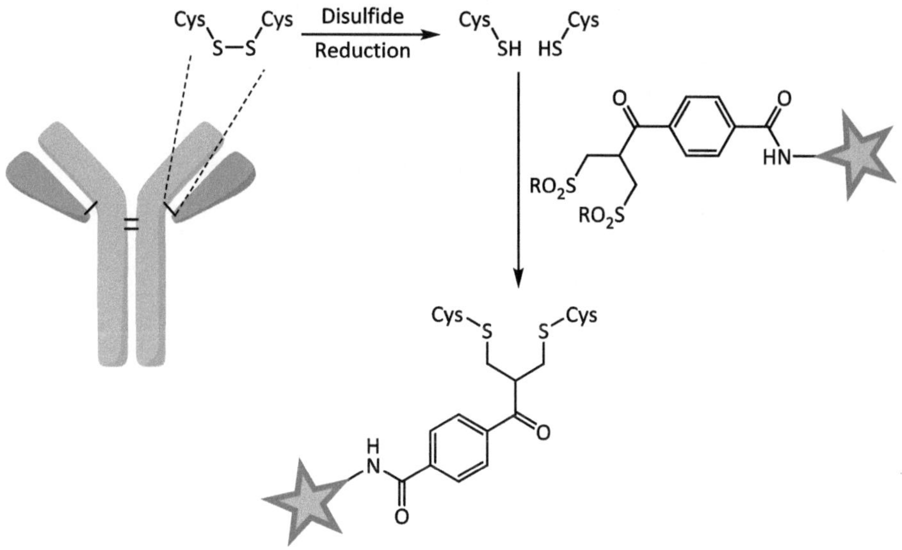

Fig. 1 Disulfide rebridging conjugation. Interchain disulfide of IgG1 bonds are reduced to produce four pairs of cysteine residues, each containing a reactive thiol side chain. Four reagent molecules conjugate at the reduced disulfides, linking the cysteine residues via a three-carbon bridge

fully rebridged, the resulting ADC will bear exactly one conjugating linker per disulfide bond.

Reaction monitoring can be carried out by hydrophobic interaction chromatography (HIC), and SDS-PAGE, and LC-MS to confirm antibody reduction as well as progress of conjugation. Purification and/or polishing of the final ADC is typically carried out by preparative HIC, ceramic hydroxyapatite, ion-exchange, or by TFF/buffer exchange. Final characterization is typically performed by analytical HIC, MS, or UV for DAR determination, analytical SEC for monomeric purity, UV absorbance for content determination, SDS-PAGE and LC-MS for conjugate rebridging confirmation.

There are other approaches for antibody disulfide rebridging in addition to Abzena's ThioBridge® bis-sulfones, which include Thiologics' dibromo maleimides and pyridazinediones [20–26], Concortis Biotherapeutics' bis-halo C-Lock™ [27], and divinylpyrimidine linkers [28].

Abzena's ThioBridge® platform uses a reagent composed of a bis-sulfone bis-alkylating conjugation unit, a spacer containing a polymeric chain (typically PEG or cyclodextrin), a self immolative release linker (e.g. valine-citrulline-*p*-aminobenzyloxycarbonyl, val-cit-PAB), and a payload (drug or reporter molecule). Reduction and conjugation is typically achieved with modest and efficient amounts of reagent at 1.3–1.6 equivalents per disulfide bond. Elimination of one sulfinic acid leaving group in aqueous conditions at neutral or mildly basic pH generates one reactive

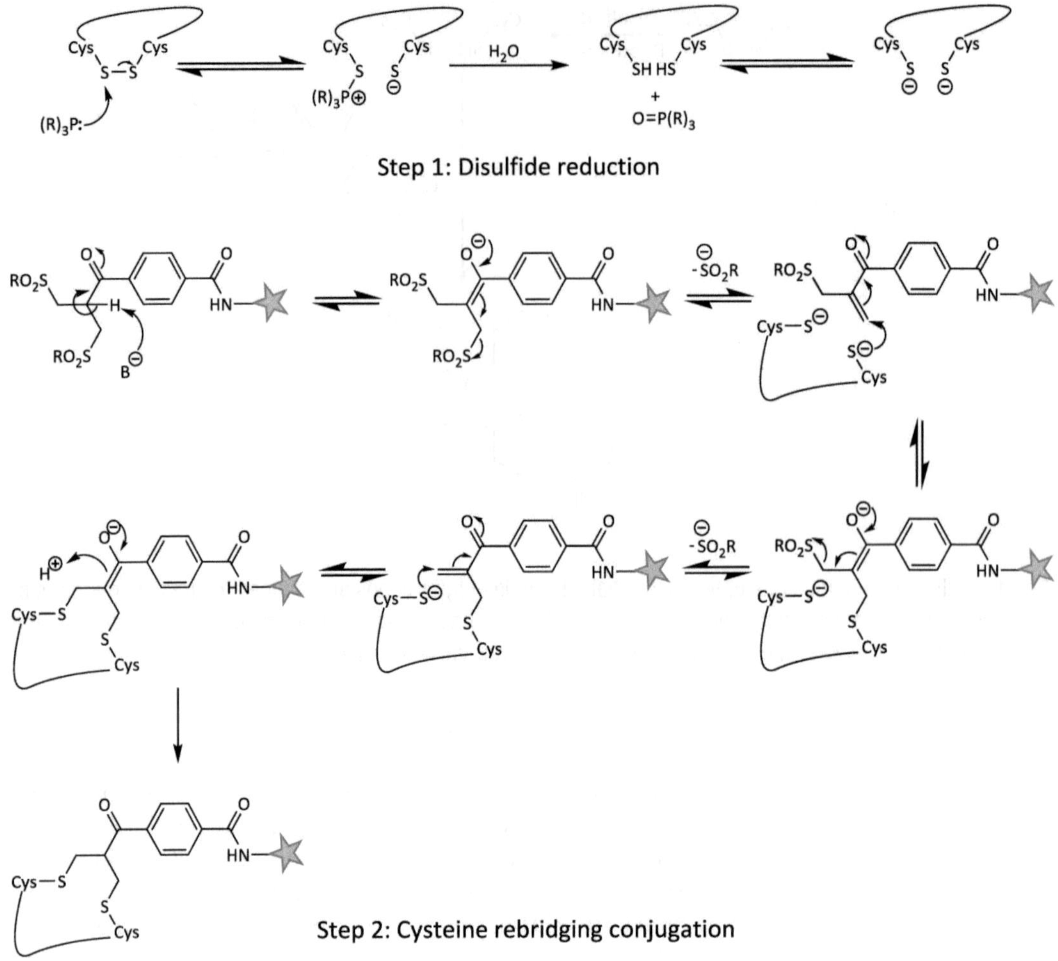

Fig. 2 Reaction mechanism for cysteine rebridging conjugation. Step 1. Disulfide reduction using TCEP produces two free thiols (thiolates); Step 2. β-elimination of sulfone leaving group to generate a reactive α,β-unsaturated ketone followed by sequential Michael addition reactions of the free cysteine thiolates to rebridge the disulfide via a three-carbon linkage

α,β-unsaturated group that is amenable to 1,4-addition of a sulfhydryl residue to generate a thioether bond. Repeat of this elimination–addition mechanism leads to a rebridging of the two sulfhydryl residues with a three-carbon bridge (Fig. 2).

An advantage of ThioBridge® over other rebridging approaches is that ThioBridge® is tolerant of TCEP during the conjugation, avoiding the need to perform a TCEP removal step, which is the case for dibromomaleimides. In addition, ThioBridge® does not require a hydrolysis step to confer stability, as it is resistant to deconjugation and cross conjugation; however, hydrolysis of dibromomaleimde conjugates is required to stabilize the linker. Finally, ThioBridge® reacts in an extremely efficient manner, with only slight stoichiometric excesses required, rather than the large reagent excess typically required for divinylpyrimidines (up to 10 eq. per disulfide) and the bis-halo linkers (2.5 eq. per disulfide).

The ThioBridge® platform is compatible with a wide variety of cytotoxic drugs, fluorescent labels, metal chelators, peptides, binding agents, and oligonucleotides. For example, it has been used to conjugate monomethyl auristatin E (MMAE) to trastuzumab [29, 30] and brentuximab [31], affording 70–95% conversion to DAR 4 ADCs, free from any unconjugated antibody. Preparative HIC polishing raises the DAR 4 ADC purity to >95%. Analogous conjugation applied to Fab fragments afford Fab ThioBridge® MMAE fragment–drug conjugates (FDCs) with a drug-to-fragment ratio (DFR) of 1 [29].

ThioBridge® DAR 4 ADCs demonstrate excellent stability against retro-Michael deconjugation, retention of antigen binding potency identical to the native mAb, and antigen-selective in vitro and in vivo potency comparable to that of the parent drug. Good in vivo tolerability and superior efficacy of a ThioBridge® trastuzumab DAR 4 ADC was also demonstrated when compared to trastuzumab-DM1 (Kadcyla®) in a mouse xenograft study [29, 30, 32]. The evaluation of several spacer designs such as incorporation of a spacer PEG polymer versus a PEG polymer attached via a glutamic acid branching point, a cyclic (i.e. macrocyclic) PEG polymer [33], and cyclodextrins [34] has also been carried out to investigate optimal ADC design space. Incorporation of two branching points within the ThioBridge® architecture optionally positions two drugs per reagent, resulting in a DAR 8 ADC that has demonstrated high efficacy in vivo [31].

Herein we present a detailed protocol that illustrates the application of disulfide rebridging using a ThioBridge® reagent for the purposes of preparing a human IgG1 antibody–drug conjugate with a DAR of 4.

2 Materials

Prepare all preparative-grade buffers and solutions using endotoxin-free deionized water. Prepare analytical-grade buffers with ultrapure water. Store all buffers at 2–8 °C unless otherwise stated. Use buffers after pre-equilibration at ambient temperature. Store cytotoxic reagents for antibody–drug conjugation at −20 °C and warm to room temperature prior to use.

2.1 Preparation of hIgG1 Antibody

1. Antibody solution preferably at >8 mg/mL. Where antibodies are <8 mg/mL, concentration can be performed using a Vivaspin centrifugal concentrator (30 kDa molecular weight cut-off (MWCO) poly(ether sulfone) (PES) membranes) or equivalent.

2. Reaction Buffer: 20 mM sodium phosphate buffer, pH 7.5 containing 150 mM NaCl and 20 mM EDTA. To a 1 L graduated measuring cylinder or beaker add monosodium dihydrogen phosphate dihydrate (0.59 g), disodium monohydrogen phosphate dodecahydrate (5.82 g), sodium chloride (8.77 g) and disodium ethylenediaminetetraacetic acid (EDTA) dihydrate (7.44 g). Add water (ca. 950 mL) and stir until complete dissolution has been achieved. Adjust pH to 7.5 by the addition of 2 M NaOH, add water to the 1 L graduation and then mix thoroughly. Filter the buffer into a sterile container using a 0.22 μm PES filter.
3. PD-10 desalting column.

2.2 Interchain Disulfide Reduction

1. Preparation of 5 mM tris(carboxyethyl)phosphine (TCEP) solution: Open a fresh 1 mL ampule of 0.5 M TCEP. To two clean 1.5 mL tubes add water (900 μL). Add 0.5 M TCEP (100 μL) to a tube containing water to prepare a 50 mM TCEP solution. Seal the tube, mix thoroughly using a vortexer and centrifuge the tube. Add 50 mM TCEP (100 μL) to the second tube containing water to prepare a 5 mM TCEP solution. Seal the tube, mix thoroughly using a vortexer and centrifuge the tube.
2. Eppendorf thermoblock.

2.3 Cysteine Rebridging Conjugation

1. Organic solvents for reagent dissolution, e.g. acetonitrile, *N*,*N*-dimethylformamide (DMF), 1,2-propandiol.
2. Cysteine rebridging reagent, (structure 1 Fig. 3).

2.4 Preparative Hydrophobic Interaction Chromatography (HIC) Purification

1. ÄKTA prime plus.
2. ToyoPearl Phenyl-650S column (1 mL).
3. HIC loading buffer: 50 mM sodium phosphate buffer, pH 7.0 containing 4 M NaCl. To a 250 mL graduated measuring cylinder or beaker add monosodium dihydrogen phosphate dihydrate (0.82 g), disodium monohydrogen phosphate dodecahydrate (2.58 g) and sodium chloride (58.4 g). Add water (ca. 230 mL) and stir until complete dissolution is achieved. Adjust pH to 7.0 by the addition of 2 M NaOH, add water to the 250 mL graduation and mix thoroughly. Filter the buffer into a sterile container using a 0.22 μm PES filter. Store HIC loading buffer at room temperature (*see* **Note 1**).
4. HIC buffer A: 50 mM sodium phosphate buffer, pH 7.0 containing 2 M NaCl. To a 1 L graduated measuring cylinder or beaker add monosodium dihydrogen phosphate dihydrate (3.30 g), disodium monohydrogen phosphate dodecahydrate (10.3 g) and sodium chloride (116.9 g). Add water (ca. 950 mL) and stir until complete dissolution is achieved.

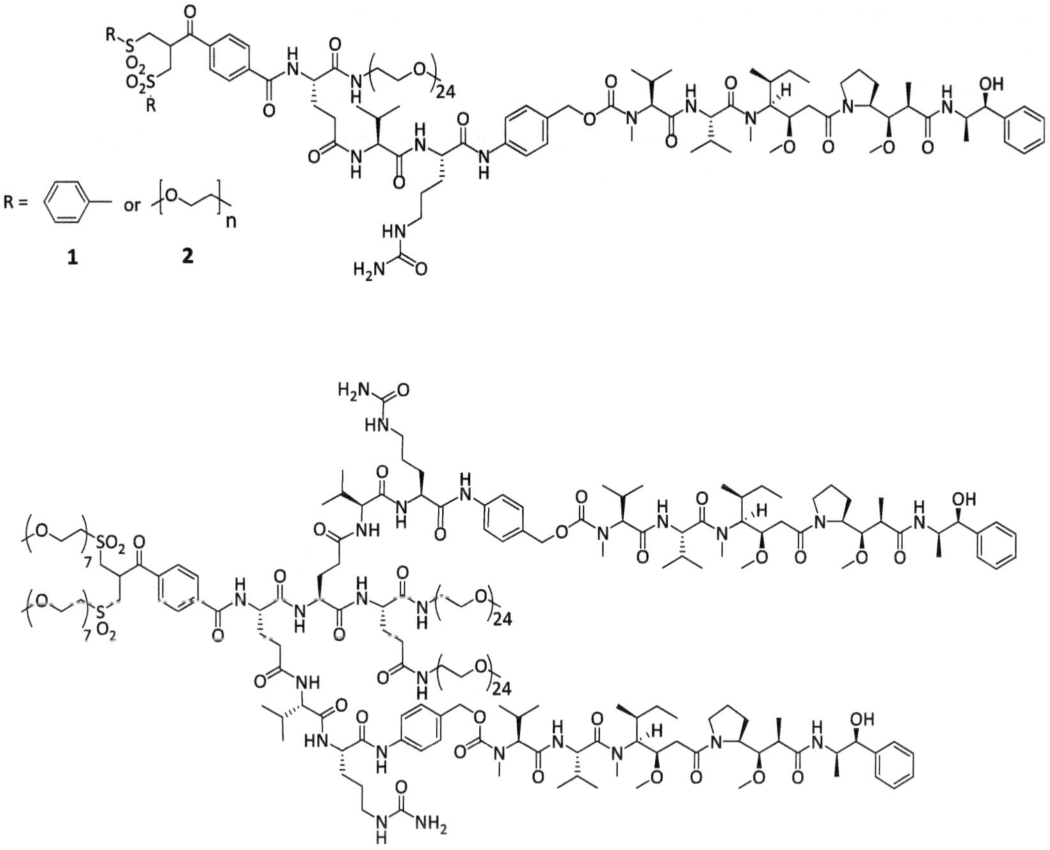

1 2

3

Fig. 3 Molecular structures of mono- and di-drug (MMAE)-loaded cysteine rebridging reagents

Adjust pH to 7.0 by the addition of 2 M NaOH, add water to the 1 L graduation and mix thoroughly. Filter the buffer into a sterile container using a 0.22 μm PES filter. Store HIC buffer A at room temperature.

5. HIC buffer B: 50 mM sodium phosphate buffer, pH 7.0 containing 20% v/v 2-propanol. To a 1 L graduated measuring cylinder or beaker add monosodium dihydrogen phosphate dihydrate (3.30 g) and disodium monohydrogen phosphate dodecahydrate (10.3 g). Add water (ca. 750 mL) and stir until complete dissolution is achieved. To the buffer add 2-propanol (200 mL) and adjust the pH to 7.0 with 2 M NaOH. Add water to the 1 L graduation and mix thoroughly. Filter the buffer into a sterile container using a 0.22 μm PES filter.
6. Luer lock syringe.
7. Blunt-end needle.
8. 15 mL Falcon tubes.

2.5 Buffer Exchange and Sample Sterilization

1. Endotoxin-free deionized water.
2. 70% ethanol.
3. Dulbecco's phosphate buffer saline (DPBS).
4. Vivaspin20 centrifugal concentrator (30 kDa MWCO PES membranes).
5. PD-10 desalting column.
6. Luer lock syringe.
7. Blunt-end needle.
8. 0.22 μm PVDF sterile filter.

2.6 In-Process Analytics (UV-A280)

1. Nanodrop spectrophotometer.
2. Diluent: Reaction buffer (*see* Subheading 2.1) and DPBS.

2.7 In-Process Analytics (SDS-PAGE)

1. 200 mM ammonium bicarbonate buffer, pH 8.0. To a 50 mL graduated measuring cylinder add ammonium bicarbonate (0.79 g). Add water (ca. 45 mL) and stir until complete dissolution is achieved. Adjust pH to 8.0 by the addition of 2 M HCl, add water to the 50 mL graduation and mix thoroughly. Filter the solution using a 0.22 μm PVDF syringe filter.
2. 375 mM Iodoacetamide solution: Add 200 mM ammonium bicarbonate buffer, pH 8.0 (132 μL) to an aliquot of iodoacetamide (9.3 mg). Mix the solution and store at room temperature protected from light (*see* **Note 2**).
3. Sodium dodecyl sulfate 20% w/v in water (*see* **Note 3**).
4. NuPAGE LDS sample buffer (4×).
5. Novex sharp pre-stained protein standard.
6. NuPAGE 4–12% Bis-Tris protein gels, 1.0 mm, 10-well.
7. MES running buffer: To a 1 L graduated measuring cylinder add water (950 mL) and 20× MES running buffer (50 mL). Mix the solution and transfer to a 1 L bottle. To the solution add NuPAGE antioxidant (75 μL) and mix.
8. XCell Surelock mini-cell electrophoresis system.
9. Variable power supply.
10. InstantBlue™ protein stain.
11. Plastic container.

2.8 In-Process Analytics (Analytical HIC)

1. TOSOH TSKgel Butyl-NPR column (3.5 cm × 4.6 mm).
2. Analytical HIC loading buffer: 50 mM sodium phosphate buffer, pH 7.0 containing 3 M ammonium sulfate. To a 250 mL graduated measuring cylinder or beaker add monosodium dihydrogen phosphate dihydrate (0.82 g), disodium monohydrogen phosphate dodecahydrate (2.58 g) and

ammonium sulfate (99.1 g). Add water (ca. 230 mL) and stir until complete dissolution is achieved. Adjust pH to 7.0 by the addition of 2 M NaOH, add water to the 250 mL graduation and mix thoroughly. Filter the buffer into a sterile container using a 0.22 μm PES filter. Store analytical HIC loading buffer at room temperature.

3. Analytical HIC buffer A: 50 mM sodium phosphate buffer, pH 7.0 containing 1.5 M ammonium sulfate. To a 2 L graduated measuring cylinder or beaker add monosodium dihydrogen phosphate dihydrate (6.60 g), disodium monohydrogen phosphate dodecahydrate (20.7 g) and ammonium sulfate (396.4 g). Add water (ca. 1.9 L) and stir until complete dissolution is achieved. Adjust pH to 7.0 by the addition of 2 M NaOH, add water to the 2 L graduation and mix thoroughly. Filter the buffer into a sterile container using a 0.22 μm PES filter. Store analytical HIC buffer A at room temperature.
4. Analytical HIC buffer B: 50 mM sodium phosphate buffer, pH 7.0 containing 20% v/v 2-propanol. To a 2 L graduated measuring cylinder or beaker add monosodium dihydrogen phosphate dihydrate (6.60 g) and disodium monohydrogen phosphate dodecahydrate (20.7 g). Add water (ca. 1.5 L) and stir until complete dissolution is achieved. To the buffer add 2-propanol (400 mL) and adjust the pH to 7.0 with 2 M NaOH. Add water to the 2 L graduation and mix thoroughly. Filter the buffer into a sterile container using a 0.22 μm PES filter.

3 Methods

3.1 Preparation of Antibody

1. Equilibrate a PD-10 column with Reaction Buffer (≥25 mL). To the column add the antibody solution (2.5 mL) and allow it to pass into the bed. Elute the antibody by the addition of Reaction Buffer (3.5 mL) to the column, collecting the eluate into a clean tube. Mix the solution and then centrifuge (*see* **Note 4**).
2. Measure the antibody content by UV A280 using the extinction coefficient, $\varepsilon_{0.1\%}$ to convert absorbance values into concentration in mg/mL units (*see* Subheading 3.6).
3. Dilute the antibody solution to 5.2 mg/mL using Reaction Buffer.
4. Transfer the antibody (5.1 mg, 981 μL) to a clean tube via pipette and incubate the solution for 15 min in a preheated heating block set at 40 °C.

3.2 Interchain Disulfide Reduction

1. To the antibody solution add 5 mM TCEP (40.8 μL, 6.0 eq.) and mix the solution using a vortexer.
2. Incubate the reduction mixture at 40 °C for 1 h.
3. Cool the reduced antibody solution to 22 °C allowing a 15 min cooling period.
4. Prior to opening, centrifuge the tube. Remove 2 × 10 μL aliquots of antibody solution and place into clean tubes, freeze the one aliquot at −80 °C and alkylate the second aliquot with iodoacetamide prior to SDS-PAGE analysis (*see* Subheading 3.7).

3.3 Cysteine Rebridging Conjugation (See Note 5)

1. To an aliquot of reagent (0.256 μmol) add acetonitrile (85.7 μL) to prepare a 3.0 mM reagent solution. Vortex the vial until complete dissolution is achieved. Centrifuge the reagent solution.
2. To the reduced antibody solution (5.0 mg) add Reaction buffer (188 μL) followed by reagent solution (62.5 μL, 5.6 eq. per antibody). Mix the conjugation reaction using a vortexer and then incubate at 22 °C overnight.
3. Sample the crude reaction from 16 h and analyze the progress of the reaction by analytical HIC (*see* **Note 6** and Subheading 3.8).

3.4 Preparative HIC Purification

1. Prior to purification of the ADC, mount a ToyoPearl Phenyl-650S column to an ÄKTA prime and wash the system (*see* **Note 7**) with 0.2 M NaOH followed endotoxin-free deionized water (*see* **Note 8**).
2. Purge the system with HIC buffer B followed by HIC buffer A (*see* **Note** 7). Once all wash steps are complete terminate the wash run prior to initiation of the purification run.
3. Load the fraction collection carousel with 15 mL Falcon tubes.
4. Mix the crude ADC in 1:1 v/v ratio with HIC load buffer. Centrifuge the vial and fill a syringe with the solution via a blunt-end needle.
5. Load the sample into the injection loop.
6. Once the sample injection is complete, initiate elution of the ADC by setting flow at 1 mL/min and a linear gradient of 0–100% B. Collect fractions of appropriate volume.
7. Wash the ÄKTA system at 100% B until the conductivity and UV measurements reach a steady state and end the run.
8. Analyze eluate fractions by analytical HIC to determine fractions containing DAR 4 ADC (*see* Subheading 3.8).

3.5 Sample Processing

1. Pool fractions containing DAR 4 ADC.
2. Wash a Vivaspin20 centrifugal concentrator (30 kDa MWCO PES membranes) with endotoxin-free deionized water, 70% ethanol and DPBS using a centrifuge (3000 × *g*) prior to use.
3. Add the DAR 4 ADC pool to the centrifugal concentrator and concentrate the sample to ca. 2 mL.
4. Remove the ADC from the concentrator using a pipette and add it to a clean vial. Wash the centrifugal concentrator with DPBS (ca. 0.5 mL) and add the washings to the ADC to give a final solution volume of 2.5 mL.
5. Equilibrate a PD-10 column with DPBS (≥25 mL). To the column add the ADC (2.5 mL) and allow it to pass into the bed. Elute the antibody by the addition of DPBS (3.5 mL) to the column, collecting the eluate into a clean tube. Mix the solution and then centrifuge.
6. Fill a luer lock syringe with the ADC using a blunt-end needle and sterile filter the ADC solution through a 0.22 μm PVDF syringe filter (*see* **Note 9**).

3.6 In-Process Analytics (UV-A280)

Initial antibody and final ADC concentrations are measured by UV A280 and may be performed using a Nanodrop spectrophotometer.

1. For Nanodrop measurements of antibody and ADC samples, blank the instrument with the sample buffer (Reaction buffer and DPBS respectively) and analyze samples in triplicate without further dilution (*see* **Note 10**).

3.7 In-Process Analytics (SDS-PAGE)

To assess the efficiency of disulfide reduction SDS-PAGE can be performed (*see* **Note 11**) (Fig. 4).

1. To the TCEP reduced antibody aliquot (10 μL, Subheading 3.2, **step 4**) add 200 mM ammonium bicarbonate buffer, pH 8.0 (40 μL) and mix. Next, add 375 mM iodoacetamide solution (1.00 μL) to the diluted TCEP reduced antibody and fully reduced antibody control, mix and incubate the samples at room temperature for 30 min in the dark (*see* **Note 2**).
2. Thaw the second TCEP reduced antibody (10 μL) at 2–8 °C and analyze without iodoacetamide treatment.
3. Dilute antibody, and the reduced antibody samples to 0.5 mg/mL with DPBS. To the samples (10 μL), add 20% SDS (10 μL), mix using a vortexer and incubate at 40 °C for 1 h. Next add NuPAGE sample buffer (6.67 μL) to the samples and mix using a vortexer.
4. Insert a 10-well 4–12% Bis-Tris SDS-PAGE gel and a blank cassette into a XCell Surelock mini-cell and close the lock. Fill

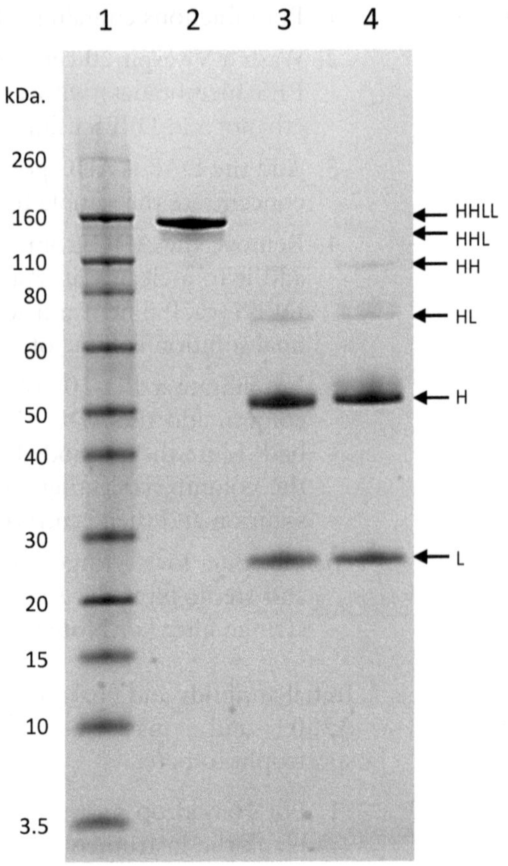

Fig. 4 SDS-PAGE analysis of lane 1. Novex Markers; lane 2. IgG1; lane 3. disulfide reduced IgG1 (0.2 mM TCEP, 1 h 40 °C); lane 4 disulfide reduced-alkylated IgG1 (0.2 mM TCEP, 1 h, 40 °C; 7.4 mM iodoacetamide, 30 min, RT)

the upper (ca. 200 mL) and lower (ca. 600 mL) chambers with MES running buffer.

5. Load the Novex sharp pre-stained protein standard (3–5 μL) and the antibody samples (1 μg, 5.33 μL) onto the gel. Place the lid onto the cell ensuring the electrical connectors are correctly in place. Attach the connector cables into the variable power supply and then turn the power supply on. Set the system to run at 200 V for 35 min with the current set to maximum ampage.
6. Remove the lid from the tank and unlock the gel. Remove the gel from the tank and pry open the cassette using a gel knife. Place the gel into a plastic container and wash with water (100 mL) for 10 min. Decant the water and then stain the gel with InstantBlue™ gel stain (20 mL) at room temperature for 1 h. De-stain the gel with water for 1 h (2 × 100 mL), changing water after 30 min.

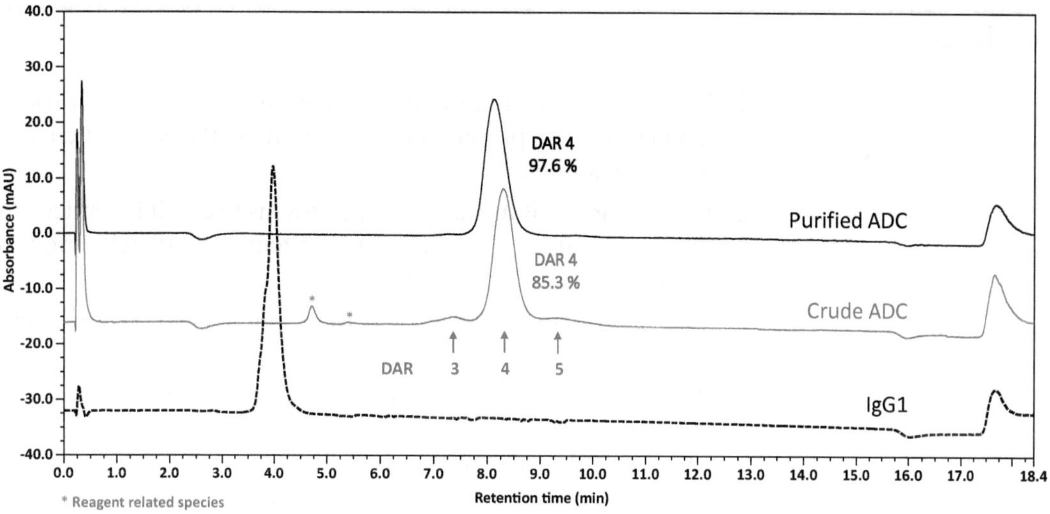

Fig. 5 Hydrophobic Interaction Chromatography of (1) IgG1; (2) crude cysteine-rebridged IgG1-MMAE ADC; (3) purified cysteine-rebridged IgG1-MMAE ADC

7. Image the gel using an imaging system (e.g. IMAGEQUANT™ LAS 4010 or Chemidoc™) and measure band densities to determine reduction efficiency.

3.8 In-Process Analytics (Analytical HIC)

Hydrophobic interaction chromatography is used to analyze crude reaction mixtures, preparative HIC fractions, and the purified ADC (Fig. 5).

1. Antibody and conjugate samples are prepared for analysis by diluting the sample to 0.15 mg/mL with DPBS (80 μL final sample volume) in a HPLC vial (*see* **Note 12**). To the diluted sample (80 μL), add analytical HIC load buffer (40 μL), cap the vial and vortex to mix.
2. Where sample concentration is unknown (e.g. preparative HIC fractions) prepare the sample as above without prior dilution with DPBS.
3. Attach a TOSOH TSKgel Butyl-NPR column to a HPLC and prime the system with analytical HIC buffer A and B (*see* **Note 13**).
4. Inject the samples onto the system in analytical buffer A and elute with a gradient of analytical HIC buffer B (*see* **Note 14**).
5. Integrate chromatograms and assign DAR values by retention time (and absorbance ratios). Use integrals to determine conjugation conversion, fraction purity, and final ADC purity.

4 Notes

1. Buffers containing high salt concentrations are stored at room temperature to prevent crystallization of the salt which can occur on cooling.
2. Iodoacetamide is unstable and photosensitive so it is prudent to prepare solutions of the alkylating agent immediately prior to use and to protect from light using foil.
3. Store SDS solutions at ≥25 °C to prevent crystallization of the surfactant.
4. Prior to opening vials containing liquid, centrifugation of the vial draws liquid that may have collected in the cap or that is adhered to the sides of the vial into a single pool at the bottom of the vial aiding its recovery via pipette.
5. When handling cytotoxic materials appropriate personnel protective equipment must be used. Typically, this includes lab coat, safety glasses, and gloves. Handle cytotoxics under suitable local exhaust ventilation (LEV) such as an isolator, reverse laminar flow cabinet, or vented fume hood. Generally, LEV systems should be fitted with double high-efficiency particulate air (HEPA) filters.
6. Conjugation reaction rates vary; typically 16–22 h is sufficient to attain high conversion to DAR 4 ADC under the reaction conditions described.
7. When cleaning the ÄKTA system ensure both buffer lines, the injection loop and the outlet tube to the fraction collector, are all washed to remove contaminants prior to application of the sample to the column.
8. Online conductivity measurements can be used to determine when the system has been equilibrated with the various washing solutions and running buffers.
9. Sterile filtration must be carried out under a category II biosafety cabinet using standard aseptic handling techniques.
10. We perform Nanodrop measurements using a Nanodrop 2000 instrument with a 3 μL sample volume. Several other Nanodrop type instruments are available and may be used to produce equivalent results.
11. Other non-native analytical techniques such as CE-SDS, denaturing SEC, RP-HPLC, or LC-MS can also be used to quantitatively or qualitatively analyze reduced antibody samples.
12. For HIC analysis, use skirted HPLC vials with snap caps.
13. Prior to sample injection it is advisable to inject blank samples onto the system until a stable baseline is achieved.

14. The resolution of ADC DAR variants varies greatly with the linker-payload conjugated. The gradient applied for optimal separation requires development on a case-to-case basis.

Acknowledgement

The authors would like to thank the past and present colleagues at Abzena for their contributions to this work.

References

1. Wakankar AA, Feeney MB, Rivera J, Chen Y, Kim M, Sharma VK, Wang YJ (2010) Physicochemical stability of the antibody-drug conjugate Trastuzumab-DM1: changes due to modification and conjugation processes. Bioconjug Chem 21:1588–1595. https://doi.org/10.1021/bc900434c
2. Doronina SO, Toki BE, Torgov MY, Mendelsohn BA, Cerveny CG, Chace DF, DeBlanc RL, Gearing RP, Bovee TD, Siegall CB, Francisco JA, Wahl AF, Meyer DL, Senter PD (2003) Development of potent monoclonal antibody auristatin conjugates for cancer therapy. Nat Biotechnol 21:778–784. https://doi.org/10.1038/nbt832
3. Wang L, Amphlett G, Blättler WA, Lambert JM, Zhang W (2005) Structural characterization of the maytansinoid-monoclonal antibody immunoconjugate, huN901-DM1, by mass spectrometry. Protein Sci 14:2436–2446. https://doi.org/10.1110/ps.051478705
4. Sun X, Ponte JF, Yoder NC, Laleau R, Coccia J, Lanieri L, Qiu Q, Wu R, Hong E, Bogalhas M, Wang L, Dong L, Setiady Y, Maloney EK, Ab O, Zhang X, Pinkas J, Keating TA, Chari R, Erickson HK, Lambert JM (2017) Effects of drug–antibody ratio on pharmacokinetics, biodistribution, efficacy, and tolerability of antibody–maytansinoid conjugates. Bioconjug Chem 28:1371–1381. https://doi.org/10.1021/acs.bioconjchem.7b00062
5. Junutula JR, Flagella KM, Graham RA, Parsons KL, Ha E, Raab H, Bhakta S, Nguyen T, Dugger DL, Li G, Mai E, Lewis Phillips GD, Hiraragi H, Fuji RN, Tibbitts J, Vandlen R, Spencer SD, Scheller RH, Polakis P, Sliwkowski MX (2010) Engineered thio-trastuzumab-DM1 conjugate with an improved therapeutic index to target human epidermal growth factor receptor 2-positive breast cancer. Clin Cancer Res 16:4769–4778. https://doi.org/10.1158/1078-0432.CCR-10-0987
6. Francisco JA, Cerveny CG, Meyer DL, Mixan BJ, Klussman K, Chace DF, Rejniak SX, Gordon KA, DeBlanc R, Toki BE, Law C-L, Doronina SO, Siegall CB, Senter PD, Wahl AF (2003) cAC10-vcMMAE, an anti-CD30-monomethyl auristatin E conjugate with potent and selective antitumor activity. Blood 102:1458–1465. https://doi.org/10.1182/blood-2003-01-0039
7. Adem YT, Schwarz KA, Duenas E, Patapoff TW, Galush WJ, Esue O (2014) Auristatin antibody drug conjugate physical instability and the role of drug payload. Bioconjug Chem 25:656–664. https://doi.org/10.1021/bc400439x
8. Beckley NS, Lazzareschi KP, Chih H-W, Sharma VK, Flores HL (2013) Investigation into temperature-induced aggregation of an antibody drug conjugate. Bioconjug Chem 24:1674–1683. https://doi.org/10.1021/bc400182x
9. Shen B-Q, Xu K, Liu L, Raab H, Bhakta S, Kenrick M, Parsons-Reponte KL, Tien J, Yu S-F, Mai E, Li D, Tibbitts J, Baudys J, Saad OM, Scales SJ, McDonald PJ, Hass PE, Eigenbrot C, Nguyen T, Solis WA, Fuji RN, Flagella KM, Patel D, Spencer SD, Khawli LA, Ebens A, Wong WL, Vandlen R, Kaur S, Sliwkowski MX, Scheller RH, Polakis P, Junutula JR (2012) Conjugation site modulates the in vivo stability and therapeutic activity of antibody-drug conjugates. Nat Biotechnol 30:184–189. https://doi.org/10.1038/nbt.2108
10. Jackson D, Atkinson J, Guevara CI, Zhang C, Kery V, Moon S-J, Virata C, Yang P, Lowe C, Pinkstaff J, Cho H, Knudsen N, Manibusan A, Tian F, Sun Y, Lu Y, Sellers A, Jia X-C, Joseph I, Anand B, Morrison K, Pereira DS, Stover D (2014) In vitro and in vivo evaluation of cysteine and site specific conjugated herceptin antibody-drug conjugates. PLoS One 9:

e83865. https://doi.org/10.1371/journal.pone.0083865

11. Alley SC, Benjamin DR, Jeffrey SC, Okeley NM, Meyer DL, Sanderson RJ, Senter PD (2008) Contribution of linker stability to the activities of anticancer immunoconjugates. Bioconjug Chem 19:759–765. https://doi.org/10.1021/bc7004329
12. Lyon RP, Setter JR, Bovee TD, Doronina SO, Hunter JH, Anderson ME, Balasubramanian CL, Duniho SM, Leiske CI, Li F, Senter PD (2014) Self-hydrolyzing maleimides improve the stability and pharmacological properties of antibody-drug conjugates. Nat Biotechnol 32:1059–1065. https://doi.org/10.1038/nbt.2968
13. Christie RJ, Fleming R, Bezabeh B, Woods R, Mao S, Harper J, Joseph A, Wang Q, Xu ZQ, Wu H, Gao C, Dimasi N (2015) Stabilization of cysteine-linked antibody drug conjugates with N-aryl maleimides. J Control Release 220:660–670. https://doi.org/10.1016/j.jconrel.2015.09.032
14. Tumey LN, Charati M, He T, Sousa E, Ma D, Han X, Clark T, Casavant J, Loganzo F, Barletta F, Lucas J, Graziani EI (2014) Mild method for succinimide hydrolysis on ADCs: impact on ADC potency, stability, exposure, and efficacy. Bioconjug Chem 25:1871–1880. https://doi.org/10.1021/bc500357n
15. Junutula JR, Raab H, Clark S, Bhakta S, Leipold DD, Weir S, Chen Y, Simpson M, Tsai SP, Dennis MS, Lu Y, Meng YG, Ng C, Yang J, Lee CC, Duenas E, Gorrell J, Katta V, Kim A, McDorman K, Flagella K, Venook R, Ross S, Spencer SD, Lee Wong W, Lowman HB, Vandlen R, Sliwkowski MX, Scheller RH, Polakis P, Mallet W (2008) Site-specific conjugation of a cytotoxic drug to an antibody improves the therapeutic index. Nat Biotechnol 26:925–932. https://doi.org/10.1038/nbt.1480
16. Hamblett KJ, Senter PD, Chace DF, Sun MMC, Lenox J, Cerveny CG, Kissler KM, Bernhardt SX, Kopcha AK, Zabinski RF, Meyer DL, Francisco JA (2004) Effects of drug loading on the antitumor activity of a monoclonal antibody drug conjugate. Clin Cancer Res 10:7063–7070. https://doi.org/10.1158/1078-0432.CCR-04-0789
17. Boswell CA, Mundo EE, Zhang C, Bumbaca D, Valle NR, Kozak KR, Fourie A, Chuh J, Koppada N, Saad O, Gill H, Shen B-Q, Rubinfeld B, Tibbitts J, Kaur S, Theil F-P, Fielder PJ, Khawli LA, Lin K (2011) Impact of drug conjugation on pharmacokinetics and tissue distribution of anti-STEAP1 antibody-drug conjugates in rats. Bioconjug Chem 22:1994–2004. https://doi.org/10.1021/bc200212a
18. Wilbur DS, Chyan M, Nakamae H, Chen Y, Hamlin DK, Santos EB, Kornblit BT, Sandmaier BM (2012) Reagents for astatination of biomolecules. 6. An intact antibody conjugated with a maleimido-closo-decaborate(2-) reagent via sulfhydryl groups had considerably higher kidney concentrations than the same antibody conjugated with an isothiocyanato-closo-de. Bioconjug Chem 23:409–420. https://doi.org/10.1021/bc200401b
19. Burns JA, Butler JC, Moran J, Whitesides GM (1991) Selective reduction of disulfides by tris(2-carboxyethyl)phosphine. J Org Chem 56:2648–2650
20. Nunes JPM, Morais M, Vassileva V, Robinson E, Rajkumar VS, Smith MEB, Pedley RB, Caddick S, Baker JR, Chudasama V (2015) Functional native disulfide bridging enables delivery of a potent, stable and targeted antibody-drug conjugate (ADC). Chem Commun (Camb) 51:10624–10627. https://doi.org/10.1039/c5cc03557k
21. Schumacher FF, Nunes JPM, Maruani A, Chudasama V, Smith MEB, Chester KA, Baker JR, Caddick S (2014) Next generation maleimides enable the controlled assembly of antibody-drug conjugates via native disulfide bond bridging. Org Biomol Chem 12:7261–7269. https://doi.org/10.1039/c4ob01550a
22. Maruani A, Smith MEB, Miranda E, Chester KA, Chudasama V, Caddick S (2015) A plug-and-play approach to antibody-based therapeutics via a chemoselective dual click strategy. Nat Commun 6:6645. https://doi.org/10.1038/ncomms7645
23. Lee MTW, Maruani A, Richards DA, Baker JR, Caddick S, Chudasama V (2017) Enabling the controlled assembly of antibody conjugates with a loading of two modules without antibody engineering. Chem Sci 8:2056–2060. https://doi.org/10.1039/c6sc03655d
24. Robinson E, Nunes JPM, Vassileva V, Maruani A, Nogueira JCF, Smith MEB, Pedley RB, Caddick S, Baker JR, Chudasama V (2017) Pyridazinediones deliver potent, stable, targeted and efficacious antibody-drug conjugates (ADCs) with a controlled loading of 4 drugs per antibody. RSC Adv 7:9073–9077. https://doi.org/10.1039/c7ra00788d
25. Smith MEB, Schumacher FF, Ryan CP, Tedaldi LM, Papaioannou D, Waksman G, Caddick S, Baker JR (2010) Protein modification, bioconjugation, and disulfide bridging using bromomaleimides. J Am Chem Soc 132:1960–1965. https://doi.org/10.1021/ja908610s

26. Morais M, Nunes JPM, Karu K, Forte N, Benni I, Smith MEB, Caddick S, Chudasama V, Baker JR (2017) Optimisation of the dibromomaleimide (DBM) platform for native antibody conjugation by accelerated post-conjugation hydrolysis. Org Biomol Chem 15:2947–2952. https://doi.org/10.1039/c7ob00220c
27. Miao Z, Chen G, Zhu T, Khasanov AB, Hong Y, Zang HD, Chucholowski A (2015) Drug-conjugates with a targeting molecule and two different drugs. US Patent 2015/0105540
28. Walsh SJ, Omarjee S, Galloway WRJD, Kwan TT-L, Sore HF, Parker JS, Hyvonen M, Carroll JS, Spring DR (2019) A general approach for the site-selective modification of native proteins, enabling the generation of stable and functional antibody–drug conjugates. Chem Sci 10:694–700. https://doi.org/10.1039/c8sc04645j
29. Badescu G, Bryant P, Bird M, Henseleit K, Swierkosz J, Parekh V, Tommasi R, Pawlisz E, Jurlewicz K, Farys M, Camper N, Sheng X, Fisher M, Grygorash R, Kyle A, Abhilash A, Frigerio M, Edwards J, Godwin A (2014) Bridging disulfides for stable and defined antibody drug conjugates. Bioconjug Chem 25:1124–1136. https://doi.org/10.1021/bc500148x
30. Bryant P, Pabst M, Badescu G, Bird M, McDowell W, Jamieson E, Swierkosz J, Jurlewicz K, Tommasi R, Henseleit K, Sheng X, Camper N, Manin A, Kozakowska K, Peciak K, Laurine E, Grygorash R, Kyle A, Morris D, Parekh V, Abhilash A, Choi JW, Edwards J, Frigerio M, Baker MP, Godwin A (2015) In vitro and in vivo evaluation of cysteine rebridged trastuzumab-MMAE antibody drug conjugates with defined drug-to-antibody ratios. Mol Pharm 12:1872–1879. https://doi.org/10.1021/acs.molpharmaceut.5b00116
31. Pabst M, McDowell W, Manin A, Kyle A, Camper N, De Juan E, Parekh V, Rudge F, Makwana H, Kantner T, Parekh H, Michelet A, Sheng X, Popa G, Tucker C, Khayrzad F, Pollard D, Kozakowska K, Resende R, Jenkins A, Simoes F, Morris D, Williams P, Badescu G, Baker MP, Bird M, Frigerio M, Godwin A (2017) Modulation of drug-linker design to enhance in vivo potency of homogeneous antibody-drug conjugates. J Control Release 253:160–164. https://doi.org/10.1016/j.jconrel.2017.02.027
32. Godwin A, Badescu G, Bird M, Bryant P, Morris D, Frigerio, M (2016) Process for the conjugation of a peptide or protein with a reagent comprising a leaving group including a portion of PEG - WO patent 2016/059377
33. Godwin A, Kyle A, Evans N (2017) Conjugates and conjugating reagents comprising a linker that includes at least two (-CH2-CH2-O-) units in a ring - WO Patent 2017/178828 A1
34. Godwin A (2017) Conjugates and conjugating reagents - WO Patent 2017/199046 A1

Chapter 9

Antibody Conjugations via Glycosyl Remodeling

Hanna Toftevall, Helén Nyhlén, Fredrik Olsson, and Jonathan Sjögren

Abstract

The antibody Fc-glycans are interesting targets for conjugation of cytotoxic compounds due to their localization and their chemical composition. In striving to obtain site-specific conjugates, the antibody Fc-glycans have been explored in numerous ways. Here we present a two-step enzymatic methodology coupled to click-chemistry for conjugation at the core GlcNAc of the Fc-glycan resulting in ADCs that are homogenous with a DAR 2.0, retain antigen binding, and display cytotoxic anti-tumor effects both in vitro and in vivo.

Key words ADC conjugation, Antibody glycosylation, Glycosyl remodeling, Site-specific conjugation, Click-chemistry

1 Introduction

Conjugation of cytotoxic payloads to antibodies to form antibody–drug conjugates (ADCs) has resulted in clinically improved therapeutic agents compared to native antibodies. The method and site of conjugation dramatically affects the characteristics and properties of the ADC. Classical methods of conjugating payloads to antibodies typically involve chemical conjugation to either disulfides using maleimide chemistry or lysines using amine coupling. The resulting ADC suffers from a heterogenous product profile and subpopulations that may result in shorter circulating half-life, lower efficacy, and off-target effects [1]. To address these issues a number of site-specific conjugation strategies have been developed, such as the introduction of unnatural amino acids, engineered cysteines, enzymatic ligation, and N-glycan remodeling [2, 3]. All human antibodies are glycoproteins and the most common therapeutic antibody, human IgG, carry a complex type N-glycan at position N297 of the Fc domain [4, 5]. The glycans of IgG result in a horseshoe-shaped form of the Fc and they are important for the interactions between IgG and its receptors [6]. The IgG Fc-glycans are of interest as a site for conjugation both because of their

L. Nathan Tumey (ed.), *Antibody-Drug Conjugates: Methods and Protocols*, Methods in Molecular Biology, vol. 2078,
https://doi.org/10.1007/978-1-4939-9929-3_9,

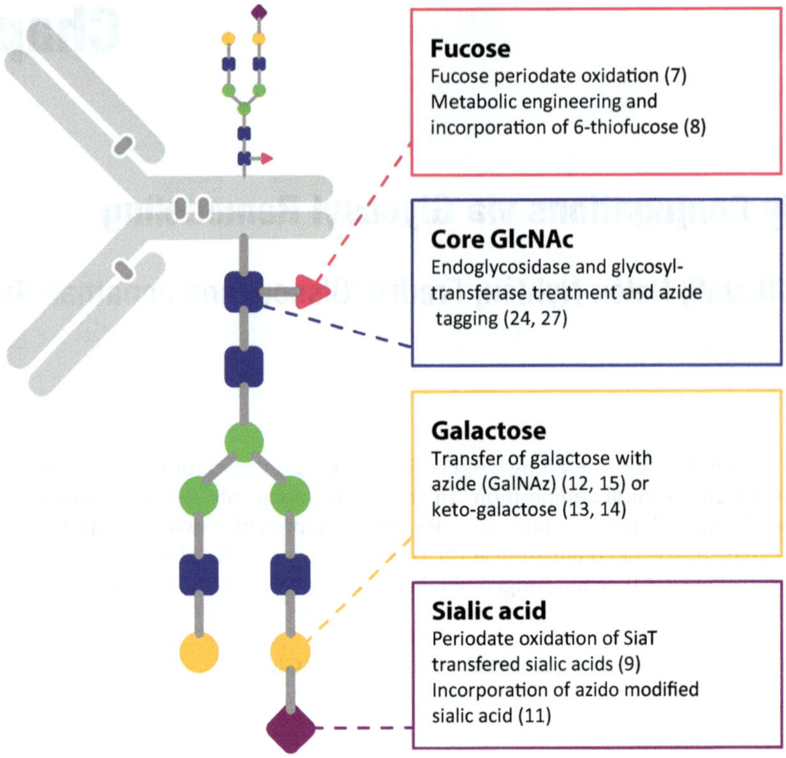

Fig. 1 Schematic representation of the available conjugation technologies targeting the conserved IgG Fc-glycan. The glycans are schematically depicted according to the SNFG symbol nomenclature

location, covered between the Fc domains and far from the antigen binding sites, and their different chemical composition compared to amino acids, making specific chemical modifications possible. The technologies for conjugation on the Fc-glycans available include glycan metabolic engineering, glycotransferase treatment combined with glycan oxidation, and endoglycosidase and transferase treatment coupled with keto- or azide tagging (Fig. 1).

The core fucose of the Fc-glycan can be modified using selective periodate oxidation followed by a reaction with hydrazide toxic compounds to form a hydrazone linked conjugate that displays intact immunoreactivity [7]. Metabolic glycan engineering has been achieved by supplementing 6-thiofucose peracetate in the cell culture medium and in this way incorporate a thiol-group at the core fucose of the N-glycan [8]. The resulting ADC proved cytotoxic and showed retained antigen binding and good stability profiles.

By using oxidation and oxime ligation, biologically active compounds can be conjugated to enzymatically added sialic acids at the native Fc-glycan. Sialic acids are rarely found on recombinant IgG and for this reason, transfer of galactose to obtain G2 glycans followed by transfer of sialic acid, are needed [9]. The sialic acids are exposed to periodate oxidation causing the formation of an aldehyde group that can be conjugated with aminooxy groups carrying a cytotoxic drug, a process that has been shown to induce methionine oxidation that may affect FcRn binding [3, 10]. An ADC constructed in this manner displayed a DAR of 1.6 and showed expected dose response curves as compared to thiol-conjugated ADCs both in vitro and in vivo [9]. A similar approach using enzymatic two-step transfer of galactose and azido-modified sialic acid allowed copper-free click-chemistry and an ADC with DAR 4.3 was obtained, somewhat surprising but explained by conjugation of Fab glycans [11].

The galactose residues can be used for modification that involves removal of the galactose sugars using beta-1,4 galactosidase followed by transfer of a derivative of galactose to the branched GlcNAc, using an engineered galactosyltransferase (GalT) [12]. Site-specific antibody conjugation using the engineered GalT has been described by use of a keto-tagged sugar followed by oximation [13, 14]. The engineered GalT was also used to transfer GalNAz to the branched GlcNAc [15] and this procedure is available as the SiteClick™ technology. A cyclooctyne-modified label can then be conjugated to the azide using strain-promoted copper-free click-chemistry [16, 17]. For imaging applications, this approach has proven successful when conjugating the antibody with chelators and radionucleotides such as copper-labeled tetrazine or a hybrid of zirconium and Alexa Fluor 680 [18, 19]. Recently, this technology has been applied to conjugate an antibody with a chelator and a cytotoxic drug to obtain combined positron emission tomography (PET) imaging with anti-tumor activity [20].

The discovery of IgG-specific endoglycosidases has made it possible to homogenize the glycan structures and expose the core GlcNAc of the native IgG glycan as a target for conjugation. EndoS and EndoS2 are both endoglycosidases from *Streptococcus pyogenes* and have been characterized to cleave the Fc-glycan in the chitobiose core leaving the GlcNAc attached to asparagine [21–23]. The combination of EndoS2, an engineered GalT and click-chemistry is commercially available as GlyCLICK® and the methodology for this conjugation technology is presented in this chapter. After endoglycosidase treatment the exposed GlcNAc is modified using the engineered galactosyl transferase GalT(Y289L) and UDP-GalNAz which results in an azide available for biocompatible copper-free strain-promoted azide–alkyne chemistry reaction (SPAAC) with a cyclooctyne functionalized label of choice (Fig. 2) [12, 17]. An undisclosed but likely similar approach has highlighted the conserved glycosylation site of IgG as the optimal conjugation site for this type of conjugation [24]. EndoS has also been mutated to drive transglycosylation and incorporation of synthetic N-glycans with unnatural sialic acids enabling

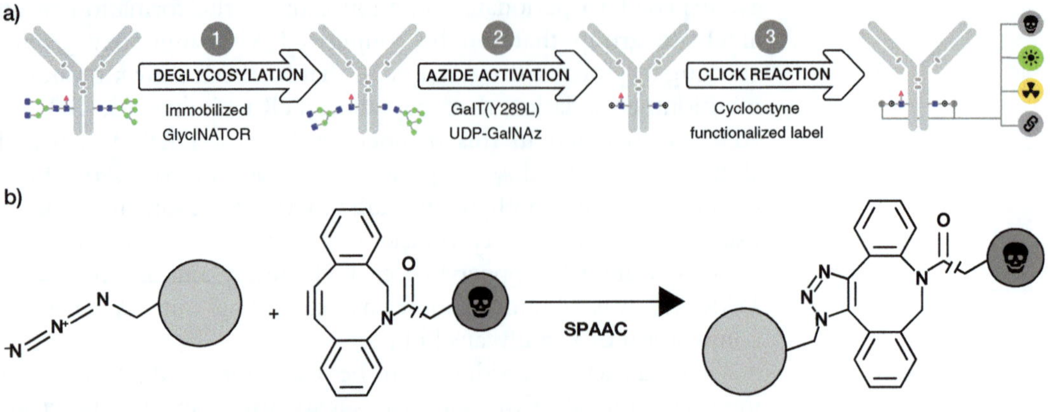

Fig. 2 GlyCLICK conjugation combines two enzymatic steps with a following copper-free azide–alkyne click-chemistry step. (**a**) Schematic presentation of the GlyCLICK conjugation process. (1) EndoS2 (as Immobilized GlycINATOR) hydrolyzes the Fc-glycans of IgG and exposes the core GlcNAc. (2) The engineered β-1,4-galactosyltransferase, GalT(Y289T), transfers GalNAz from UDP-GalNAz to the GlcNAc rendering an azide-activated IgG. (3) By a strain-promoted copper-free click-reaction using a cyclooctyne functionalized label, the label is conjugated to the two available azides of GalNAz at the Fc domains of the IgG. (**b**) The principle of strain-promoted azide–alkyne click-chemistry (SPAAC). An azide-activated protein (grey circle), as the Fc/2 part of an antibody, is reacting with a cyclooctyne-modified molecule resulting in a covalent conjugation linked via the triazole. In this example a dibenzocyclooctyne (DBCO) functionalized toxin molecule is shown

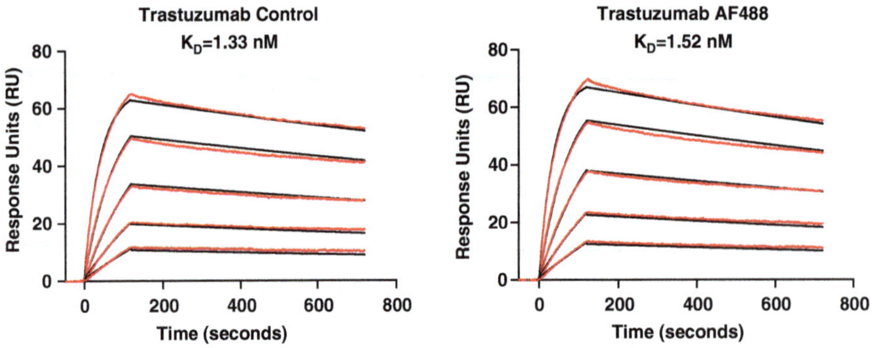

Fig. 3 Surface plasmon resonance (SPR) analysis of trastuzumab and a trastuzumab conjugate obtained by GlyCLICK. Trastuzumab control and trastuzumab-AlexaFluor488 conjugate displayed the same binding to antigen in the assay. Anti-Human IgG (Fc) was used as the capture molecule on the chips for sample analysis. HER2 was injected in a range 6.25–100 nM and data were fitted against a 1:1 mathematical model to determine the kinetic constants

conjugation at four terminal sialic acids [25]. Using the GlyCLICK technology shown in Fig. 2, the resulting conjugate displays intact immunoreactivity as demonstrated by SPR analysis (Fig. 3), a DAR of 2.0 located at the Fc-region (Fig. 4), and a homogenous HIC profile (Fig. 5). Importantly, the removal of the glycans disrupts the interactions with Fc-gamma receptors but retains binding to FcRn, an indication of potential for decreased off target effects while

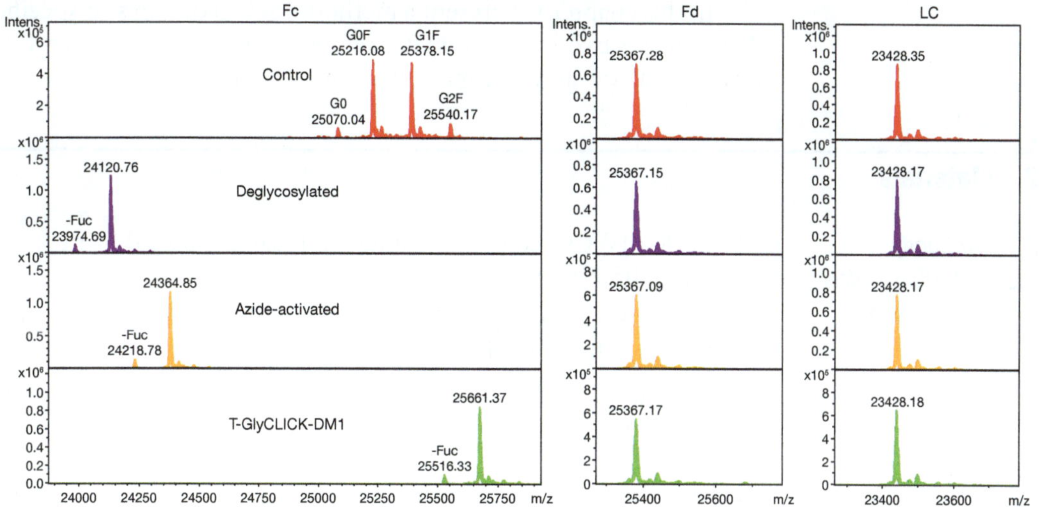

Fig. 4 MS analysis of a trastuzumab-DM1 toxin conjugate (T-GlyCLICK-DM1) showing the site-specific conjugation on Fc. Deconvoluted mass spectra from LC-MS analysis of subunits after different steps using the GlyCLICK conjugation method. The specific and complete shifts in mass were only seen on the Fc resulting in a DAR of 2.0 after the final conjugation step. The analyses were performed at nonreduced (for Fc) and reduced (for LC and Fd) conditions, respectively. Separation was performed by RP-HPLC and analyzed using an ESI- Q-TOF mass spectrometer (*see* **Note 7**)

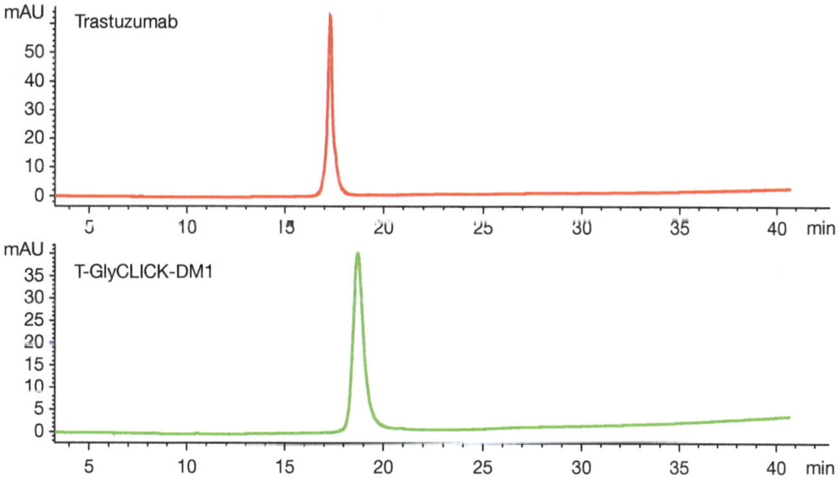

Fig. 5 Hydrophobic interaction analysis of trastuzumab control and a corresponding conjugate with DM1 toxin. The trastuzumab-DM1 (T-GlyCLICK-DM1) displayed a homogeneous peak and a minor shift in hydrophobicity as compared to the trastuzumab control (*see* **Note 16**)

retaining the expected pharmacokinetic profile [26]. An anti-uPARAP antibody conjugated to the highly potent pyrrolobenzo-diazepine (PBD) dimer payload using GlyCLICK has shown homogenous conjugates with potent tumor cell killing effect in vitro, efficacy on ex vivo sarcoma patient samples, and to cure mice with a single 2 mg/kg dose in vivo [27].

In this chapter we present a methodology to obtain site-specific ADCs using two step enzymatic remodeling of the Fc-glycan followed by azide–alkyne copper-free click-chemistry.

2 Materials

2.1 Antibody Concentration and/or Buffer Exchange

1. 50 K MWCO centrifugal filter unit, sample size 0.5 ml (cat# UFC505096, Merck Millipore).
2. Microspin desalting column 40 K, sample size 50–200 μl (cat# 87766, Thermo Scientific).
3. Centrifuge with fixed angle rotor that can accommodate 1.5–2 ml centrifuge tubes.

2.2 Modification of the Carbohydrate on Antibody Fc Domain

1. 100–250 μg of antibody in 25 mM TBS pH 7.4. It is important that the antibody is present in a non-phosphate buffer, preferably a Tris-based buffer, free of carrier proteins and/or azide (*see* **Note 1**).
2. GlyCLICK® Azide activation kit for activation of 250 μg antibody. (cat # L1-AZ1–025, Genovis AB) (*see* **Note 2**).
3. 25 mM Tris pH 7.4, 0.15 M NaCl (TBS) (*see* **Note 3**).
4. End-over-end mixer.

2.3 Azide Attachment

1. GlyCLICK Azide activation kit for activation of 250 μg antibody (cat # L1-AZ1–025, Genovis AB) (*see* **Note 2**).
2. 25 mM Tris pH 7.4, 0.15 M NaCl (TBS) (*see* **Note 3**).
3. Incubator or water bath for 30 °C.

2.4 Purification and Concentration of Azide-Modified Antibody

1. 50 K MWCO centrifugal filter unit, sample size 2 ml (cat# UFC 205024, Merck Millipore)
2. 25 mM Tris pH 7.4, 0.15 M NaCl (TBS) (*see* **Note 3**).
3. Centrifuge with swinging bucket rotor that can accommodate 17 mm × 100 mm centrifuge tubes.

2.5 Conjugation with Cyclooctyne-Modified Label

1. Cyclooctyne-modified label for copper-free click-chemistry (*see* **Note 4**).
2. Dimethyl sulfoxide (DMSO) (*see* **Note 5**).
3. Incubator or water bath for 25 °C.

2.6 Purification and Concentration of Antibody–Drug Conjugate

1. 50 K MWCO centrifugal filter unit, sample size 2 ml (cat# UFC 205024, Merck Millipore).
2. Appropriate buffer, for example PBS or TBS.
3. Centrifuge with swinging bucket rotor that can accommodate 17 mm × 100 mm centrifuge tubes.

3 Methods

The method described is based on using a GlyCLICK Azide activation kit (*see* **Note 2**) for 250 μg antibody.

3.1 Antibody Concentration and/or Buffer Exchange

A concentration step **is only required if** the volume of 250 μg antibody is more than 200 μl (*see* **Note 6**).

1. Rinse the 50 K MWCO centrifugal filter unit, sample size 0.5 ml, by adding 500 μl of ddH_2O and cap the device.
2. Centrifuge at 5000 × *g* for 6 min. Make sure that the cap strap and one membrane panel of the filter unit face the center of the rotor.
3. Discard the flow-through.
4. Add sufficient volume of antibody solution to contain 100–250 μg of antibody to the prerinsed 50 K MWCO centrifugal filter unit. For example, if the antibody concentration is 1 mg/ml, add 250 μl.
5. Centrifuge at 5000 × *g* for 2–6 min. Make sure that the cap strap and one membrane panel of the filter unit face the center of the rotor.
6. Discard the flow-through.
7. If the antibody volume in the filter unit is more than 200 μl, centrifuge for an additional 2 min at 5000 × *g*, or until the appropriate volume is achieved.
8. Invert the small filter unit into the collection tube.
9. Centrifuge at 1000 × *g* for 3 min to collect the concentrated antibody. After collection, the amount of concentrated Ab should be approximately 150–200 μl in the collection tube.

   A buffer exchange step **is required if** the sample contains phosphate and/or azide (*see* **Note 1**).
10. Break off the bottom closure of the microspin desalting column. Loosen the lid (**do not** remove the lid).
11. Place the column in a collection tube (1.5–2 ml) and centrifuge at 1500 × *g* for 1 min to remove the storage solution.
12. Discard the flow-through and place the column in the collection tube.
13. Add 300 μl TBS buffer on top of the resin. Centrifuge the column at 1500 × *g* for 1 min and discard the flow-through.
14. Repeat **step 13** two more times. Last spin for 2 min.
15. Blot the bottom of the column to remove excess liquid. Place the column in a new collection tube (1.5–2 ml).

16. Apply the antibody solution on top of the resin (100–200 μl).
17. Centrifuge at 1500 × *g* for 2 min to recover the flow-through with antibody in TBS buffer.

3.2 Modification of the Carbohydrate on the Antibody Fc Domain

GlycINATOR® (EndoS2) is an IgG-specific endoglycosidase that hydrolyzes all glycoforms present at the Fc-glycosylation site. The enzyme acts on the chitobiose core and leaves the core GlcNAc intact. GlycINATOR deglycosylates all human IgG subclasses and IgG from many other species, for example, mouse, rat, and monkey.

For this step a microspin column with Immobilized GlycINATOR from the GlyCLICK kit is used.

1. Break off the bottom plastic cap of the Immobilized GlycINATOR column and slightly open the lid. Save the cap. The lid and the cap of the spin column are used later during incubation.
2. Place the column in a 1.5–2 ml collection tube.
3. Centrifuge the column at 200 × *g* for 1 min to remove the storage solution.
4. Discard the flow-through.
5. Place the column in the collection tube.
6. Add 300 μl TBS buffer on top of the resin and reseal the column with the lid, loosen the lid slightly.
7. Centrifuge the column at 200 × *g* for 1 min and discard the flow-through.
8. Repeat the **steps 6** and 7 two more times.
9. Reinsert the bottom cap at the bottom of the spin column.
10. Immediately add the antibody solution (100–200 μl containing a maximum of 250 μg antibody) to the column and reseal the column with the lid.
11. Take care to fully suspend the media by manually turning the column end-over-end to make sure there is a flow in the column.
12. Incubate the column by end-over-end mixing at room temperature for 30 min.
13. Remove the bottom cap and place the column in a clean microcentrifuge tube (1.5–2 ml). Loosen the lid slightly.
14. Centrifuge the column at 1000 × *g* for 1 min to recover the antibody sample.
15. Attach the bottom cap. Add 50 μl TBS and seal the column with the lid.
16. Invert the column a couple of times.
17. Remove the bottom cap and place the column in a clean microcentrifuge tube (1.5–2 ml). Loosen the lid.

18. Centrifuge at 1000 × *g* for 1 min to recover the antibody sample.
19. Repeat **steps 15–18** once more.
20. Pool the collected antibody fractions.
21. Optional at this point is to verify the de-glycosylation by analyzing the sample by MS (Fig. 4) (*see* **Note 7**).

3.3 Azide Attachment

In this enzymatic step an engineered galactosyl transferase, GalT (Y289L) attaches a GalNAz to the inner core GlcNAc on the Fc N-glycan generated by GlycINATOR in Subheading 3.2 (*see* **Note 2**).

1. Prepare the azide modification solution by adding 30 μl of Buffer additive and the pooled solution containing the modified antibody from Subheading 3.2, **step 20** to the tube containing the lyophilized UDP-GalNAz (*see* **Note 8**).
2. Add TBS to a final volume of 375 μl.
3. Mix the solution by carefully pipetting up and down.
4. Add 25 μl of the GalT enzyme solution. The final reaction volume should be 400 μl (*see* **Note 2**). Unused enzyme can be stored at 2–8 °C.
5. Mix the solution by carefully pipetting up and down. Wrap the tube cap with Parafilm® or similar.
6. Incubate overnight, protected from light at 30 °C.

3.4 Purification and Concentration of the Azide-Modified Antibody

This step will remove excess UDP-GalNAz by diafiltration using spin filter devices. The conical collection tube is attached on the unit during centrifugation.

1. Remove the conical collection tube from the top of the 50 K MWCO centrifugal filter unit, sample size 2 ml.
2. Add 2 ml of TBS to the 50 K MWCO centrifugal filter unit.
3. Centrifuge at 1200 × *g* for 10 min. Make sure that one membrane panel of the filter unit faces the center of the rotor.
4. Discard the flow-through.
5. Add 1.6 ml TBS and 400 μl of the azide-modified antibody from Subheading 3.3, **step 6**, to the prerinsed 50 K MWCO centrifugal filter unit.
6. Centrifuge at 1200 × *g* for 6 min. Make sure that one membrane panel of the filter unit faces the center of the rotor.
7. Discard the flow-through.
8. Add sufficient volume of TBS to the retentate in the 50 K MWCO centrifugal filter unit to achieve a total volume of 2 ml.

9. Centrifuge at 1200 × *g* for 10 min. Make sure that one membrane panel of the filter unit faces the center of the rotor.
10. Discard the flow-through.
11. Repeat **steps 8–10** two more times.
12. If the antibody volume in the centrifugal filter unit is more than approximately 200 μl, the volume in the filter unit should be reduced by additional centrifugation, e.g., for an additional 5 min at 1200 × *g* or until the appropriate volume is achieved.
13. Remove the filtrate tube and invert the centrifugal filter unit with the antibody into the conical collection tube.
14. Centrifuge at 1000 × *g* for 3 min to collect the concentrated antibody.
15. Transfer the antibody from the conical collection tube to a 1.5 ml centrifuge tube (*see* **Note 9**).
16. Adjust the volume with TBS to 225 μl.
17. Optional at this point is to verify the azide activation (addition of GalNAz) at the Fc by analyzing the sample with MS (Fig. 4) (*see* **Note 7**).

3.5 Conjugation with Cyclooctyne-Modified Label

In this step the azide-activated antibody reacts with cyclooctyne-modified label in a strain-promoted, copper-free click-chemistry reaction to form an antibody conjugate.

1. Reconstitute the cyclooctyne-modified label in DMSO to a concentration of 2–5 mM (*see* **Notes 10** and **11**).
2. Add a maximum of 25 μl cyclooctyne-modified label to 225 μl azide-activated antibody in TBS from Subheading 3.4, **step 16**, in the 1.5 ml centrifuge tube. The amount of cyclooctyne-modified label to be added depends on the specific cyclooctyne-label used (*see* **Note 12**).
3. Mix by carefully pipetting up and down.
4. Close the tube and seal with Parafilm® or similar.
5. Incubate overnight, protected from light at 25 °C.

3.6 Purification of Antibody Conjugate

This step will remove excess cyclooctyne-modified label by diafiltration using spin filter devices. TBS or PBS may be used for the purification and collection of the modified antibody. The conical collection tube is attached on the unit during centrifugation.

1. Remove the conical collection tube from the top of the 50 K MWCO filter unit, sample size 2 ml.
2. Add 2 ml of the desired buffer, such as PBS or TBS, to the 50 K MWCO filter unit.
3. Centrifuge at 1200 × *g* for 10 min. Make sure that one membrane panel of the filter unit faces the center of the rotor.

4. Discard the flow-through.
5. Add 1.6 ml of the desired buffer, such as PBS or TBS, and the conjugated antibody from Subheading 3.5, **step 5**, to the pre-rinsed 50 K MWCO filter unit.
6. Centrifuge at 1200 × *g* for 10 min. Make sure that one membrane panel of the filter unit faces the center of the rotor.
7. Discard the flow-through.
8. Add the sufficient volume of the desired buffer, such as PBS or TBS, to the retentate in the 50 K MWCO centrifugal filter unit to achieve a total volume of 2 ml.
9. Centrifuge at 1200 × *g* for 10 min. Make sure that one membrane panel of the filter unit faces the center of the rotor.
10. Discard the flow-through.
11. Repeat **steps 8–10** two more times (*see* **Note 13**).
12. Remove the filtrate tube and invert the centrifugal filter unit with the antibody into the conical collection tube.
13. Centrifuge at 1000 × *g* for 3 min to collect the antibody conjugate.
14. Transfer the antibody conjugate from the conical collection tube to a 1.5 ml microcentrifuge tube. The antibody conjugate can now be stored protected from light at +4–8 °C (*see* **Note 14**).
15. If Nanodrop is available, determine the protein concentration (*see* **Note 15**).
16. It is possible at this stage to verify the complete conjugation and a DAR = 2 by analyzing the sample with MS (Fig. 4) (*see* **Note 7**).

4 Notes

1. It is important that the antibody is present in a non-phosphate buffer, free of carrier proteins and/or azide. Phosphate can cause precipitation during the azide attachment step. Free azide in the solution will compete for available reagent and cause an incomplete conjugation. For adjusting the antibody buffer *see* Subheading 3.1.
2. GlyCLICK Azide Activation kit (cat# L1-AZ1-025, Genovis AB) contains the reagents β-1,4-galactosyltransferase (Y289L) (GalT (Y289L)), UDP-GalNAz, Buffer additive, Immobilized GlycINATOR (EndoS2), and other components necessary for the conjugation protocol. GalT (Y289L) and UDP-GalNAz are components of SiteClick™, Life Technologies Corporation. GlyCLICK® technology is available from Genovis

AB. Azide activation kits for activation of larger amounts than 250 μg IgG is available.

3. The most convenient way of preparing 25 mM TBS pH 7.4 (25 mM Tris pH 7.4, 0.15 M NaCl) is to purchase stock solution 20× TBS (cat# 28358, Thermo Scientific) and prepare the buffer according to manufacturer's instructions.
4. The cyclooctyne-modified label can for example be a dibenzocyclooctyne (DIBO or DBCO). We have in this work used a DBCO-functionalized toxin molecule.
5. The DMSO is required for reconstitution of cyclooctyne-modified label.
6. The maximum volume of 200 μl of the antibody is critical to obtain the correct concentrations during the following steps to ensure complete reactions.
7. Sample preparation for MS analysis of de-glycosylation, azide activation and final ADC (Fig. 4).

   Antibody samples were mixed with FabRICATOR® (Genovis AB) in TBS and incubated for 30 min at 37 °C for generation of Fc and F(ab')2 fragments. For the reduced samples DTT and Guanidine hydrochloride were added, and the samples incubated for an additional 30 min at 37 °C. The FabRICATOR digested fragments were separated on an Acquity UPLC BEHC4 protein column, 300 Å, 1.7 μm 2.1 × 100 mm (Waters), using 0.1% FA in Milli Q water (solvent A) and 0.1% FA in 95% acetonitrile (solvent B). Injection was at 10% B, kept for 13 min to desalt the samples, followed by a 1 min increase to 25% B. Separation of the fragments was achieved between 25% B and 36% B for 12 min using a flow rate of 0.2 ml/min at 50 °C. The column was washed for 3 min at 90% B before reconditioning. The LC was connected to a Q-TOF Impact II (Bruker), equipped with an electrospray ionization source, and a resolving power of 50,000. The source was set to 4.5 kV capillary voltage, 220 °C dry temperature, 1.8 Bar nebulization gas pressure and 8 l/min nebulization gas flow rate. Mass range from 300 *m/z* to 3000 *m/z*. The obtained data was deconvoluted using the MaxEnt algorithm and the monoisotopic molecular weights of the subunits determined by the SNAP algorithm.
8. UDP-GalNAz provided in the GlyCLICK kit is lyophilized and the vial contains 0.22 mg. Unused reconstituted UDP-GalNAz can be stored at −20 °C.
9. At this stage, the antibody can be stored, protected from light, at 2–8 °C for conjugation of label at a later time.
10. It is important to take the appropriate safety precautions since the cyclooctyne-modified label is a toxic molecule. Make sure

to use adequate protective ware and follow the routines and regulations according to the safety data sheet of the reagent.

11. In our experiment we have used DBCO-PEG4-Ahx-DM1 (cat# SET030, Levena Biopharma).
12. The molar ratio between cyclooctyne-modified label and azide activated antibody depends on the label (cyclooctyne-linker-toxin) and the antibody to be conjugated. The molar ratio can vary between 10:1 up to 30:1. A label that is of more hydrophobic kind may cause precipitation if used with a to high ratio to the antibody. A small-scale test is recommended before performing a larger conjugation, for example, start with the ratio 10:1 (label:antibody) and analyze to evaluate the degree of conjugation by LC-MS (Fig. 4) (*see* **Note** 7).
13. If antibody concentration of more than 2 mg/ml is desired, the volume in the filter unit can be reduced by prolonged centrifugation, e.g., for an additional 5 min at 1200 × *g* or until the appropriate volume is achieved.
14. Do not freeze. Sodium azide or thimerosal may be added to a final conc. of 0.02% (w/v) for long-time storage, if preferred.
15. Protein concentration of the generated ADC can easily be measured by Abs 280 and the correct molar extinction coefficient. Measurement of the protein concentration by Abs 280 can be performed after the de-glycosylation step, Subheading 3.2, **step 20**, as well if needed. Measurement of the protein concentration by Abs 280 after the azide activation will be misleading since the azide will contribute to the absorbance at 280 nm.
16. The samples were analyzed on a TSKgel®ButylNPR HIC column (Tosoh Bioscience) in 25 mM sodium phosphate buffer pH 7.0, 1.5 M ammonium sulfate and eluted with decreasing salt gradient with 20% isopropanol.

References

1. Junutula JR, Raab H, Clark S, Bhakta S, Leipold DD et al (2008) Site-specific conjugation of a cytotoxic drug to an antibody improves the therapeutic index. Nat Biotechnol 26 (8):925–932. https://doi.org/10.1038/nbt.1480
2. Beck A, Goetsch L, Dumontet C, Corvaïa N (2017) Strategies and challenges for the next generation of antibody–drug conjugates. Nat Rev Drug Discov 16(5):315–337. https://doi.org/10.1038/nrd.2016.268
3. Chudasama V, Maruani A, Caddick S (2016) Recent advances in the construction of antibody–drug conjugates. Nat Chem 8 (2):114–119. https://doi.org/10.1038/nchem.2415
4. Arnold JN, Wormald MR, Sim RB, Rudd PM, Dwek RA (2007) The impact of glycosylation on the biological function and structure of human immunoglobulins. Annu Rev Immunol 25:21–50. https://doi.org/10.1146/annurev.immunol.25.022106.141702
5. Jefferis R (2009) Recombinant antibody therapeutics: the impact of glycosylation on mechanisms of action. Trends Pharmacol Sci 30(7):356–362. https://doi.org/10.1016/j.tips.2009.04.007

6. Nimmerjahn F, Ravetch JV (2007) Fc-receptors as regulators of immunity. Adv Immunol 96:179–204. https://doi.org/10.1016/S0065-2776(07)96005-8
7. Zuberbühler K, Casi G, Bernandes GJ, Neri D (2012) Fucose-specific conjugation of hydrazide derivatives to a vascular-targeting monoclonal antibody in IgG format. Chem Commun 48(56):7100–7102. https://doi.org/10.1039/c2cc32412a
8. Okeley NM, Toki BE, Zhang X, Jeffrey SC, Burke PJ, Alley SC, Senter PD (2013) Metabolic engineering of monoclonal antibody carbohydrates for antibody–drug conjugation. Bioconjug Chem 24(10):1650–1655. https://doi.org/10.1021/bc4002695
9. Zhou Q, Stefano JE, Manning C, Kyazike J et al (2014) Site-specific antibody–drug conjugation through glycoengineering. Bioconjug Chem 25(3):510–520. https://doi.org/10.1021/bc400505q
10. Wang W, Vlasak J, Li Y, Pristatsky P et al (2011) Impact of methionine oxidation in human IgG1 Fc on serum half-life of monoclonal antibodies. Mol Immunol 48 (6–7):860–866. https://doi.org/10.1016/j.molimm.2010.12.009
11. Li X, Fang T, Boons GJ (2014) Preparation of well-defined antibody-drug conjugates through glycan remodeling and strain-promoted azide-alkyne cycloadditions. Angew Chem Int Ed Engl 53(28):7179–7182. https://doi.org/10.1002/anie.201402606
12. Ramakrishnan B, Qasba PK (2002) Structure-based design of beta 1,4-galactosyltransferase I (beta 4Gal-T1) with equally efficient N-acetylgalactosaminyltransferase activity: point mutation broadens beta 4Gal-T1 donor specificity. J Biol Chem 277 (23):20833–20839. https://doi.org/10.1074/jbc.M111183200
13. Boeggeman E, Ramakrishnan B, Pasek M, Manzoni M, Puri A et al (2009) Site specific conjugation of fluoroprobes to the remodeled Fc N-glycans of monoclonal antibodies using mutant glycosyltransferases: application for cell surface antigen detection. Bioconjug Chem 20 (6):1228–1236. https://doi.org/10.1021/bc900103p
14. Zhu Z, Ramakrishnan B, Li J, Wang Y, Feng Y et al (2014) Site-specific antibody-drug conjugation through an engineered glycotransferase and a chemically reactive sugar. MAbs 6 (5):1190–1200. https://doi.org/10.4161/mabs.29889
15. Zeglis BM, Davis CB, Aggeler R, Kang HC et al (2013) An enzyme-mediated methodology for the site-specific radiolabeling of antibodies based on catalyst-free click chemistry. Bioconjug Chem 24(6):1057–1067. https://doi.org/10.1021/bc400122c
16. Agard NJ, Prescher JA, Bertozzi CR (2004) A strain promoted [3 +2] azide – alkyne cycloaddition for covalent modification of biomolecules in living systems. J Am Chem Soc 126:15046–15047. https://doi.org/10.1021/ja044996f
17. Jewett JC, Bertozzi CR (2010) Cu-free click cycloaddition reactions in chemical biology. Chem Soc Rev 39(4):1272–1279
18. Cook BE, Adumeau P, Membreno R, Carnazza KE, Brand C, Reiner T, Agnew BJ, Lewis JS, Zeglis BM (2016) Pretargeted PET imaging using a site-specifically labeled immunoconjugate. Bioconjug Chem 27(8):1789–1795. https://doi.org/10.1021/acs.bioconjchem.6b00235
19. Zeglis BM, Davis CB, Abdel-Atti D, Carlin SD et al (2014) Chemoenzymatic strategy for the synthesis of site-specifically labeled Immunoconjugates for multimodal PET and optical imaging. Bioconjug Chem 25 (12):2123–2128. https://doi.org/10.1021/bc500499h
20. Adumeau P, Vivier D, Sharma SK, Wang W, Zhang T, Chen A, Agnew BJ, Zeglis BM (2018) Site-specifically labeled antibody–drug conjugate for simultaneous therapy and immunoPET. Mol Pharm 15(3):892–898. https://doi.org/10.1021/acs.molpharmaceut.7b00802
21. Collin M, Olsén A (2001) EndoS, a novel secreted protein from *Streptococcus pyogenes* with endoglycosidase activity on human IgG. EMBO J 20(12):3046–3055. https://doi.org/10.1093/emboj/20.12.3046
22. Sjögren J, Struwe WB, Cosgrave EF, Rudd PM, Stervander M, Allhorn M, Hollands A, Nizet V, Collin M (2013) EndoS2 is a unique and conserved enzyme of serotype M49 group A *Streptococcus* that hydrolyses N-linked glycans on IgG and α_1-acid glycoprotein. Biochem J 455(1):107–118. https://doi.org/10.1042/BJ20130126
23. Sjögren J, Cosgrave EF, Allhorn M, Nordgren M, Björk S, Olsson F, Fredriksson S, Collin M (2015) EndoS and EndoS2 hydrolyze Fc-glycans on therapeutic antibodies with different glycoform selectivity and can be used for rapid quantification of high-mannose glycans. Glycobiology 25 (10):1053–1063. https://doi.org/10.1093/glycob/cwv047
24. van Geel R, Wijdeven MA, Heesbeen R, Verkade JM, Wasiel AA, van Berkel SS, van Delft FL (2015) Chemoenzymatic conjugation of

toxic payloads to the globally conserved N-glycan of native mAbs provides homogeneous and highly efficacious antibody–drug conjugates. Bioconjug Chem 26 (11):2233–2242. https://doi.org/10.1021/acs.bioconjchem.5b00224
25. Tang F, Yang Y, Tang Y, Tang S et al (2016) One-pot N-glycosylation remodeling of IgG with non-natural sialylglycopeptides enables glycosite-specific and dual-payload antibody–drug conjugates. Org Biomol Chem 14 (40):9501–9518. https://doi.org/10.1039/c6ob01751g
26. Gao P, Pinkston KL, Wilganowski N, Robinson H, Azhdarinia A, Zhu B, Sevick-Muraca EM, Harvey BR (2015) Deglycosylation of mAb by EndoS for improved molecular imaging. Mol Imaging Biol 17(2):195–203. https://doi.org/10.1007/s11307-014-0781-9
27. Hald A, Nielsen C, MacCann D, Doran N, Morgan H, Buick R, Behrendt N, Engelholm L (2018) Generation of an ADC against sarcoma and glioblastoma. Paper presented at 8th Annual World ADC Europe, Berlin, 26–28 Mar 2018

Chapter 10

ADC Analysis by Hydrophobic Interaction Chromatography

Ryan Fleming

Abstract

Hydrophobic interaction chromatography (HIC) is a traditional technique used for the separation, purification, and characterization of proteins. As the number of antibody–drug conjugates (ADCs) continues to increase in clinical trials, HIC and other orthogonal methods utilizing changes in hydrophobicity are being used for ADC characterization and analysis. Unlike other techniques, HIC uniquely allows for protein analysis under mild nondenaturing conditions that preserve the native structure and activity of the molecules. Analysis of the ADC in its native form is advantageous. Herein, we describe a generic HIC protocol for the screening, analysis, and characterization of ADCs using an ammonium sulfate buffer and a high-pressure liquid chromatography system. Parameters affecting data quality and interpretation are addressed. In addition, several recommendations are included for method optimization and troubleshooting.

Key words Hydrophobic interaction chromatography (HIC), Antibody–drug conjugates (ADCs), Hydrophobicity, Retention time, Drug-to-antibody ratio (DAR), Payload

1 Introduction

Hydrophobic interaction chromatography, as the name implies, is a liquid chromatography-based technique used to separate proteins based on their intrinsic hydrophobicity; it is widely used for the characterization and analysis of ADCs [1, 2]. The method was first described by Tiselius which he termed "protein salting out"; however, the actual HIC terminology was later coined by Hjerten describing the separation process of binding and eluting proteins from a solid matrix [3]. "Salting out" occurs when proteins are placed in a high molar salt solution causing them to lose their water hydration shell. The water molecules that form the hydration shell around the protein through association with charged amino acid side chains are lost as they preferably interact with the salt ions in solution [4]. This process leads to the net repulsion of the protein and the polar solvent ions, and the increased interaction of the hydrophobic amino acid residues between the protein molecules leads to "salting out" or precipitation due to protein–protein

L. Nathan Tumey (ed.), *Antibody-Drug Conjugates: Methods and Protocols*, Methods in Molecular Biology, vol. 2078,
https://doi.org/10.1007/978-1-4939-9929-3_10, © Springer Science+Business Media, LLC, part of Springer Nature 2020

association [4]. Salting out of proteins in this manner, within a solid phase matrix comprised of hydrophobic nonpolar alkyl functional groups, promotes the association of the protein's surface hydrophobic amino acids and the matrix's nonpolar chains [3]. Typically, the longer or more branched the functional groups on the column matrix, the stronger the interaction [4]. Consequently, the strength of the interaction is proportional to the net surface hydrophobicity of the protein. The interaction of the protein with the HIC matrix is usually reversible. Rehydration of the protein by reducing the ionic strength of the buffer to normal physiological conditions re-forms the hydration shell and as a result repels the protein from the matrix [5] Binding of a protein in mobile phase A (a high salt buffer) and elution using a linear gradient via mobile phase B (a low salt buffer) can be used to rank order proteins based on hydrophobicity. Less-hydrophobic molecules with weaker interactions elute sooner than tighter-binding more-hydrophobic species with longer retention times [1]. Either the retention time or amount of mobile phase B needed to elute a protein from the HIC column indirectly reveals the degree of hydrophobicity, and this property can be used to compare and characterize proteins and antibody–drug conjugates (ADCs) alike [5, 6].

ADCs are made by attaching a cytotoxic agent to a tumor antigen targeting antibody and are a rapidly growing class of drugs for cancer treatment in clinical evaluation [7]. To date, there are four ADCs approved in the United States: Brentuximab vedotin, Ado-trastuzumab entansine, Gemtuzumab ozogamicin, and Inotuzumab ozogamicin [8]. However, there are over 50 ADC drug candidates in clinical-phase trials and several have been fast-tracked by the Food and Drug Administration (FDA) [9]. The FDA requires a complete characterization of all new drug candidates when filing an Investigational-New-Drug application, before entering clinical trials [10]. HIC analysis is one of the primary methods used to characterize ADCs and is often cited in the candidate drug applications [2, 6].

ADC cytotoxic agents (payloads) must cross the lipid membrane to inhibit DNA replication, protein synthesis, enzymatic activity or cell division. To cross the membrane, the payload must be lipophilic and, therefore, hydrophobic in nature. The attachment of the payload to the antibody increases the hydrophobicity and this change can be detected via HIC as an increase in protein retention time [4]. This characteristic is used for ADC analysis [2]. The retention time of the ADC is affected by the payload in three ways. First, the number of payloads attached is proportional to the hydrophobicity and therefore retention time. Second, more hydrophobic payloads have longer retention times. Last, a payload conjugated to exposed amino acids on the antibody allows for more interaction of the payload with the column matrix resulting in a longer retention time. A combination of these three payload-related factors determine the overall hydrophobicity profile and relative HIC retention time of the ADC [6, 11]. The separation of each drug species through differences in hydrophobicity and the quantification of each population forms the bases of ADCs analysis by HIC [7].

HIC is mainly used in combination with other orthogonal methods like reverse phase and mass spectrometry for the monitoring of ADC conjugation reactions. HIC and all other liquid chromatography-based methods must be initially paired with mass spectrometry analysis to determine peak identity or drug-to-antibody ratio (DAR), because a shift in peak retention time will not convey the degree of drug loading [4]. However, HIC can quickly and accurately determine the ratio of each drug species and corresponding DAR once the peak identity is known. For this reason, HIC is the primary method used for quality assessment and reaction monitoring and can be used for analyzing ADCs with acid-labile linkers due to the mild nature of the separation process [7, 10].

HIC analysis is also used for candidate drug selection when attempting to minimize in vitro and in vivo toxicity due to nonspecific interactions. Hydrophobic molecules tend to associate more readily with the lipid bilayer of the cell membrane through nonspecific binding and may lead to unwanted toxicities [12, 13]. Because hydrophobicity is proportional to the retention time in HIC analysis, it is often used to rank antibodies and ADC candidates based on their retention times and consequently their hydrophobicity [14]. Efficacy and HIC ranking (hydrophobicity propensity) along with other criteria are considered in ADC candidate drug selection [15].

In this chapter, a generic HIC method is described utilizing the widely used Butyl-nonporous resin (4.6 μm ID × 3.5 cm, 2.5 μm) with an ammonium sulfate buffer system. ADCs are analyzed using an Agilent 1290 UHPLC instrument equipped with a diode array detector and fraction collector. Unconjugated antibodies and ADCs are prepared in standard formulation buffer and injected onto the HIC Butyl column pre-equilibrated with a high molar concentration of ammonium sulfate buffer. The protein is eluted from the column using a linear gradient of low salt Tris(hydroxymethyl)aminomethane hydrochloride (Tris–HCl)-based buffer that facilitates separation of the different hydrophobic species. DAR is determined by comparing the relative amount of each peak and the degree of payload conjugation. The HIC technique described provides a quick yet robust means to analyze and characterize ADCs. Generating optimized HIC data is often a highly empirical process due to the varying complexities of the ADC molecules, i.e., properties of the antibody, payload, attachment site, and conjugation chemistry. Many of the factors to be considered during this optimization process are discussed in the below sections.

Compared to other techniques used for the analysis and characterization of ADCs, HIC uniquely provides a quick method for analysis with several advantages. Other methods like mass spectrometry, reverse phase and hydrophilic-interaction chromatography (HILIC) rely on organic solvents as mobile phases; low or high pH; and elevated temperatures that may denature the ADCs or introduce artifacts. Modifications to these methods to solve these issues are time-consuming and often ADC-specific. For example, ADCs with acid labile linkers, like SN38, cannot be analyzed by traditional mass spectrometry and reverse phase techniques using acidic counter ions and therefore, method development to replace the counter ions is required. ADC fractions separated by HIC retain their activity and can be used for efficacy studies. Furthermore, HIC-HPLC instruments are often equipped with a fraction collector for peak identification by mass spectrometry (*see* Chapter 20). HIC cannot be used with some hydrophilic payloads. Also, very hydrophobic payloads can require extensive method development. HIC must be combined with mass spectrometry for positive peak species identification for accurate DAR calculation; otherwise, assumptions for the peak drug loading will have to be made. For hydrophobicity ranking of ADCs, HIC analysis is uniquely suited because column binding is driven by the proteins' hydrophobicity, which is proportional to retention time. There are no general rules for HIC method optimization and optimized methods are sample-specific. The method described herein utilizes a commonly available ammonium sulfate buffer system and butyl column for the characterization, ranking, and analysis of ADCs and is a good starting point when developing an optimized HIC method. Several references for method optimization and troubleshooting are listed below.

2 Materials

Appropriate lab personal protective equipment (PPE) should be used when preparing and handling reagents and especially ADCs. The use of double nitrile gloves and sleeve protectors is recommended to prevent exposure. Solutions are prepared with HPLC-grade reagents and were filtered (0.2 μm) prior to use. HPLC waste material should be disposed of appropriately in accordance with local regulations. All equipment and consumables are labeled appropriately to communicate potential hazard. Representative data were generated using the method described below unless otherwise specified.

2.1 Buffers

Mobile Phase A: 25 mM Tris–HCL, 1.5 M ammonium sulfate, pH 8.0. Fill a graduated cylinder with 700 mL of HPLC-grade water and add 198.2 g of ammonium sulfate. Next, add 25 mL of 1 M Tris–HCL pH 8.0; insert a stir bar and mix thoroughly. Check and adjust the pH to 8.0 as need with 0.1 M sodium hydroxide. Add HPLC-grade water to 1 L and mix. Remove buffer particulate by 0.2 μM filtration (*see* **Notes 1–8**).

Mobile Phase B: 25 mm Tris–HCl pH 8.0, 5% isopropanol: Add 25 mL of 1 M Tris–HCL, pH 8.0, 925 mL of HPLC-grade water and 50 mL of isopropanol to a to a 1-L graduated cylinder and mix well. Filter the solution through a 0.2 μm filter unit (*see* **Notes 1–8**).

2.2 HIC Column

Tosoh Bioscience 4.6 μm ID × 3.5 cm, 2.5 μm butyl-nonporous resin column (Cat: 14947) (*see* **Notes 2, 4, 5, 6, 8** and **9**).

2.3 Sample Preparation

Antibody and ADC samples are diluted into 1× PBS pH 7.2 to 1 mg/mL and are 0.2 μM spin filtered (*see* **Notes 10** and **11**).

2.4 HPLC Instrument

Agilent 1290 Infinity UHPLC equipped with quaternary pump, 1200 series high performance autosampler, diode array detector, and fraction collector using the Open Lab software (*see* **Notes 5, 12** and **13**).

3 Methods

3.1 Instrument Settings

3.1.1 Detector

Read absorbance at 280 nM and 214 nm and a peak width of >0.2 min (4 s response time) (1.25 Hz) (*see* **Notes 4** and **14**).

3.1.2 Flow Rate

0.8 mL/min at room temperature (*see* **Notes 6, 8** and **13**).

3.1.3 Gradient

Linear gradient from 95% mobile phase A to 100% mobile phase B over 13 min. *See* Table 1 for the instrument pump settings (*see* **Notes 7, 8** and **15**).

3.1.4 Peak Integration Perimeters

Set the instrument integration parameters as indicated in Table 2. *See* Fig. 4 for an example of peak integration (*see* **Notes 7, 9, 16** and **17**).

3.2 Samples Application

Add 200 μL of sample into a HPLC vial and inject 50 μL (50 μg) of sample onto the column (*see* **Notes 9, 11** and **19**).

3.3 Data Interpretation

See Fig. 1a for an example of a typical HIC trace of a site-specific ADC and Fig. 1a for the zoomed in image showing peak shape. Hydrophobicity rank is done by comparing the retention times of

Table 1
Instrument pump setting

Time (min)	Mobile phase A (%)	Mobile phase B (%)
0	99	1
2	99	1
3	95	5
16	0	100
18	0	100
18.1	99	1
25	99	1

Table 2
HIC method integration parameters

Integrations events	Values
Tangent skim mode	Standard
Tail peak skim height ratio	0
Front peak skim height ratio	0
Skim valley ratio	20
Baseline correction	Classical
Peak to valley ratio	500
25	99

Time	Integration events	Values
Initial	Slope sensitivity	1
Initial	Peak width	0.04
Initial	Area reject	1
Initial	Height reject	1.7
Initial	Shoulders	Off
2	Integration	On
20	Integration	Off

the main peak of each antibody or ADC (*see* **Notes 7, 15, 16, 17 20** and **21**).

See Figs. 2 and 3 for an example of a random and site-specific ADC compared with the unconjugated antibody, respectively. The ADC DAR is calculated from the sum of the weighted ratios of the

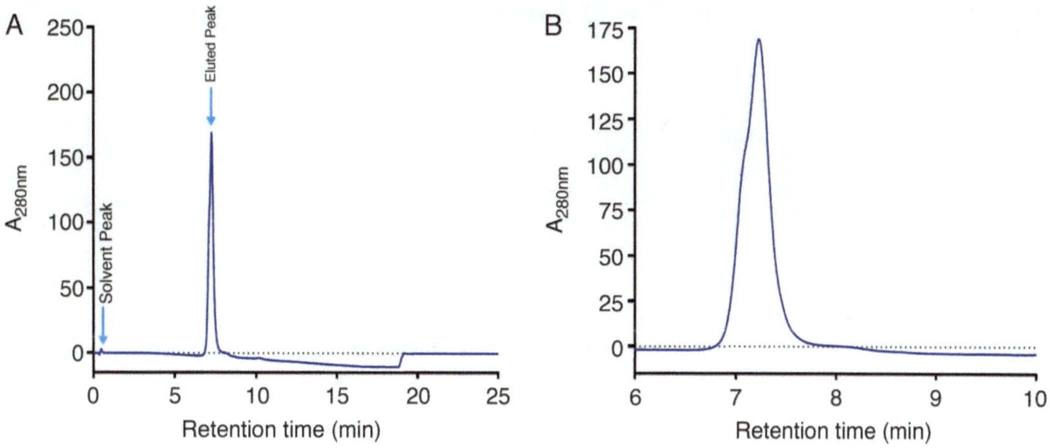

Fig. 1 Trace of ADC analyzed by hydrophobic-interaction chromatography. (**a**) Complete chromatogram highlighting the solvent peak, eluted peak, and the shift in baseline due to the ammonium sulfate buffer. (**b**) Zoomed in of the chromatogram showing peak shape

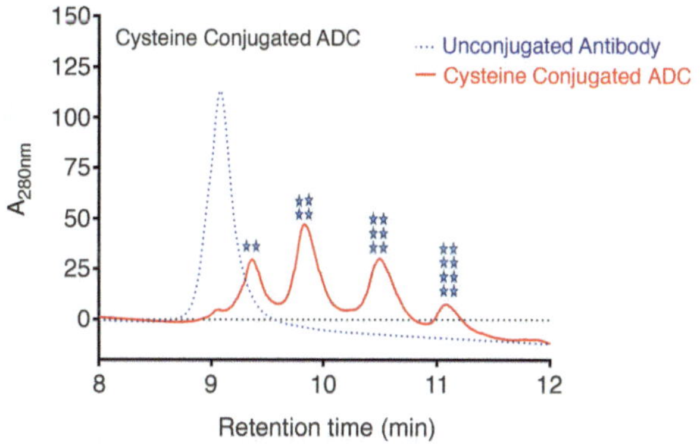

Fig. 2 HIC chromatogram of a Randomly Conjugated ADC at Hinge cysteines. Comparison of the ADC, in red, and unconjugated antibody, in blue. Drug loading per peak is indicated by the number of stars. The DAR is an average of four drug per antibody

area under the peak multiplied by the degree of payloads represented by that peak. An example of a DAR calculation is highlight in Fig. 4 (*see* **Notes 13**, **19**, and **20**).

4 Notes

1. Buffers can be stored at room temperature in tightly closed containers for up to 1 month. The 1.5 M ammonium sulfate solution, herein referred to as mobile phase A, if left exposed to air will crystalize and will have to be remade. Use only HPLC-grade reagents to prepare mobile phase solutions and 0.2 μm

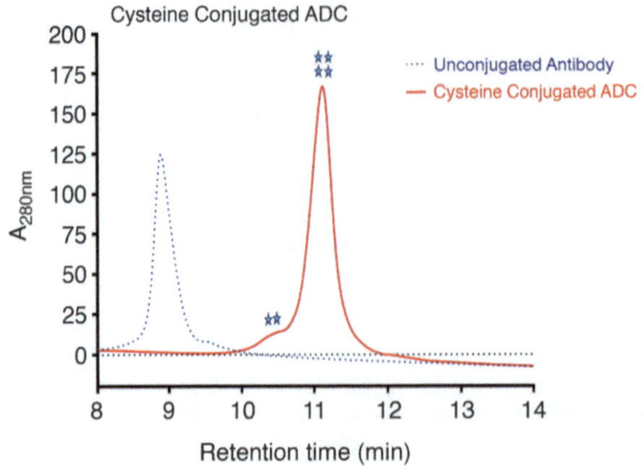

Fig. 3 HIC chromatogram of a site-specific conjugated ADC at engineered cysteines. Comparison of the ADC, in red, and unconjugated antibody, in blue. Drug loading per peak is indicated by the number of stars. Average DAR of 3.8 drugs per antibody. The four loaded species is shown with 4 stars and the two loaded species is shown with 2 stars. DAR = (Sum of the % AUC multiplied by peak drug loading)/100 for all peaks. DAR = [(3.39 × 0) + (19.19 × 2 + (35.15 × 4) + (28.89 × 6) + (13.38 × 8)]/100 = 4.59 drugs/antibody

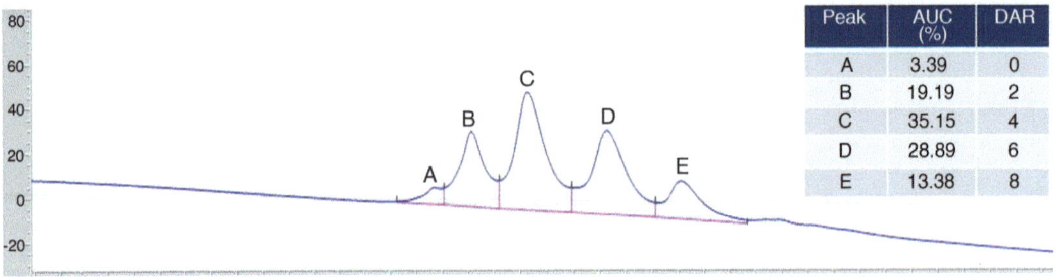

Fig. 4 HIC trace with integration area under the peaks for a random cysteine conjugated ADC. The AUC of each peak is calculated and used to determine the DAR for the ADC

filter all buffers to ensure data repeatability and reliability. Instrument clogs can result from particulates in the buffer which can also affect the back pressure, sample binding, and retention times. HIC buffer made with ammonium sulfate is the most commonly used mobile phase A and will give good results in as little as 25 min; however, any lyotropic salt that can "salt-out" proteins, such as ammonium acetate and sodium chloride, can be used. There are several advantages to using ammonium sulfate buffer. For example, mobile phase A made with less lyotropic salts will require a gradient that is twice as long, thus extending run times to around 1 h. Furthermore, higher molar salt concentrations are needed for ADC retention and this may affect column back pressure and increase the chance of salt precipitating in the instrument. Nonetheless, these mobile phases are considered when optimizing methods for peak shape and separation. In summary, ammonium acetate buffer is a good alternative, but will require molar concentration 2–3 times higher for the sample to bind to the same column.

2. Most payloads used today are hydrophobic in nature. The more hydrophobic, the stronger the potential column interaction and the longer the retention time. Very hydrophobic payloads may affect the ADC peak shape and elution propensity and may need organic modifiers to achieve complete column elution. Columns with nonbranched and shorter side chains should be considered when optimizing HIC methods for ADCs with very hydrophobic payloads.
3. Increasing the pH of the mobile phase buffers may help to improve binding of antibodies and ADCs; while decreasing the pH helps with protein elution and recovery. Most antibodies have an isoelectric point between 7 and 9. Therefore, a buffer pH closer to the pI will decrease the net surface charge and may promote a greater interaction with the column. Conversely, lowering the buffer pH, away from the pI, will increase the net surface charge and may help with protein elution. However, the effects of buffer pH change on ADC binding and elution is unpredictable and dependents on the resin type, buffer salts, and sample. Modifications in mobile phase buffer pH are often used for method optimization.
4. Sample that does not bind to the HIC column will flow through and elute with the solvent peak, resulting in an increase in solvent peak intensity. Increasing the ammonium sulfate concentration to 2 M and adjusting the pH closer to the pI of the ADC are strategies used to improve binding. However, testing columns with longer chains or more branched nonpolar groups may be necessary for some ADCs to be captured.
5. Poor sample recovery is not a common occurrence but can occasionally arise during HIC analysis of ADCs. ADCs not injected onto the HIC column can often be misinterpreted as not eluting from the column when in fact the ADC never bound to the column in the first place. Therefore, it is important to verify that the ADC did bind to the column and that the instrument is working properly. Also, ensure that the solvent peak intensity is not elevated. When ADCs do not elute, organic modifiers, such as isopropyl alcohol or acetonitrile, can be added to mobile phase B to facilitate release of the ADC from the column matrix. Organic modifiers can be added up to 15% v/v of mobile B; however, avoid buffer conditions that cause buffer salt precipitation or protein

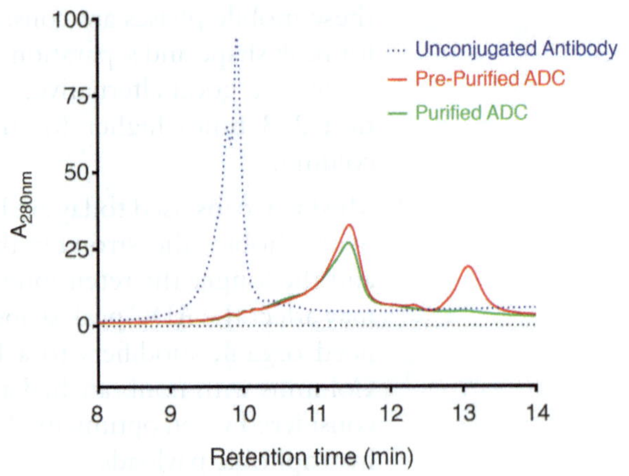

Fig. 5 HIC chromatogram of a site-specific conjugated ADC pre- and post payloads removal. Comparison of the unconjugated antibody, in blue, ADC pre-drug removal, in red, and ADC post drug removal in green

denaturation. Organic modifiers should never be used in mobile phase A. These modifiers help to elute protein by directly competing for binding to the column and by increasing the surface tension of the mobile phase, thus decreasing the hydrophobic interaction. Consequently, adding a modifier to mobile A increases the likelihood of the protein not binding to the column. Changing the mobile phase buffer pH and scouting HIC columns with shorter alkyl groups are also used to aid ADC elution. If other columns are used, first ensure that the unconjugated antibody binds and elutes in the first 25% of the gradient.

6. Peak baseline separation will generally not be achieved with generic methods for classically conjugated ADCs; however, good results are obtained for the more homogeneous site-specific conjugated ADCs, see Figs. 2 and 3, respectively. To achieve good peak separation, method optimization is needed. Optimization requires considering the flow rate, gradient, HIC column resin, and mobile phase composition. Optimized HIC methods are generally highly specific to a single ADC due to the complexity of the molecules.

7. Peak separation is another important parameter to inspect during data analysis. The number of expected peaks should be reflected on the trace. Missing or additional peaks are problematic for DAR calculation. For this reason, mass spectrometry analysis is needed to highlight the number of drug species and the degree of drug loading per peak to determine the adequacy of the method for peaks separation. Lengthening of the gradient is used to improve peak separation when considering

integration accuracy. Changing the mobile phase buffer salt, column type, and pH may also improve peak separation.

8. Gradient optimization can be done to improve peak shape and peak separation with the goal of improving data accuracy. Generally, peak separation and shape can be improved by increasing the length of the gradient. Gradient optimization parameters will have to be experimentally determined due to the complexity of ADCs. Gradient selection is mobile phase, flow rate, and HIC resin dependent. The gradient is shorter with ammonium sulfate buffer but must be extended when other buffer salts are used.
9. Butyl resins are the most widely used for HIC columns and are in mid-range for binding propensity due to resin chain length. Typical HIC columns have linear alkane chains or simple aromatic groups and may be further modified through branching. Butyl columns from individual manufactures may be customized differently, thus affecting the binding, peak separation, and elution profiles. Sample binding and retention is enhanced by using columns with longer or more branched chains and elution is conversely affected. Resin binding capacity is determined by chain length, with shorter chains having weaker binding capacities and vice versa. Some common resins, in order of chain length from lowest to highest and likewise binding capacity, are: methyl, ethyl, propyl, butyl, pentyl, hexyl, heptyl, and ocytyl.
10. Sample purity is critical for successful HIC analysis. All samples should be filtered, with free payload and aggregates removed to ensure high quality data is obtained. For small-scale conjugations ADCs can be purified using a buffer exchange column and for large-scale preparations ADCs can purified by Ceramic-Hydroxyapatite chromatography or tangential flow filtration to remove or minimize free payload contaminants and aggregates. Free payload, especially those that are very hydrophobic, will also bind to the HIC column, which may complicate data interpretation (Fig. 5). Protein aggregates tend to be more hydrophobic and will separate from the monomer, thus creating a separate peak. Because peak identification is critical for accurate data interpretation, all efforts should be made to eliminate peaks due to artifacts like aggregates and free drug.
11. Do not inject more than 100 μL of sample onto the column or the ADC may not bind. The method is designed to minimize sample preparation. If a large volume is injected, the salt concentration at the sample buffer interface will be too low and the ADC will not bind. Up to 50% v/v of mobile phase A can be added to the sample pre-injection to overcome this issue. Protein precipitation can occur when mobile phase A is

added directly to the sample and can affect the assay performance.

12. Make a note of the solvent peak retention time. A shift in the solvent peak retention time usually accompanies an increase in instrument back pressure. This suggest that there is restricted flow in the instrument, usually from salt precipitation. Flush the instrument as described above.
13. Record the initial instrument back pressure after column installation. An increase in back pressure will affect results. Remove residual salt from the instrument to prevent clogs or restricted flow by flushing the HPLC with 50 mL of water before and after running samples. The ammonium salt may precipitate within the instrument causing poor sample binding and recovery, shifts in retention times and incomplete sample elution, which will affect method optimization, data interpretation, and troubleshooting.
14. Changing the temperature of the column by adjusting the instrument column thermostat generally will not affect the binding, separation, or elution of the ADC from the column. In some cases, increasing the temperature results in better peak shape. Temperature modification should be the last parameter to consider during method optimization and troubleshooting. Temperatures above 30 °C can affect the stability of the ADC.
15. The ammonium sulfate buffer will cause a slight shift in the baseline through the gradient elution when monitoring the eluted peaks at A280nM. However, any absorbance wavelength that maximizes the signal to noise can be used. In some cases, the attached payload can absorb at a unique wavelength and monitoring with such a wavelength can discern conjugated from unconjugated peaks. For example, monitoring of Pyrrolobenzodiazepine conjugated ADCs at 330 nM will only detect peaks conjugated with the payload.
16. Integration of the area under the peak is necessary for DAR calculation and a good peak shape is important for the accuracy. Peak shape is primarily affected by the column and gradient selection. Accurate peak integration and the determination of the area under the peak can suffer if the peak is too broad or narrow. Lengthening the gradient can improve the shape of a narrow peak and shortening helps with broad peaks. Peak shape should only be altered to ensure integration accuracy. Changing the mobile phase composition, for example, by using ammonium acetate buffer or a different column type, may also improve peak shape.
17. ADCs with nonhydrophobic or hydrophilic payloads can have an uncharacteristic elution profile. These ADCs can elute with a shorter retention time or co-elute with the unconjugated

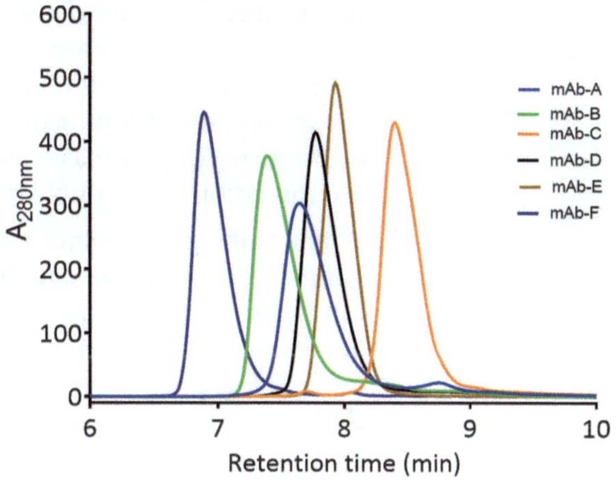

Fig. 6 HIC chromatogram of six antibodies. Hydrophobicity ranking of naked antibodies ADC candidates. Antibody F is the least hydrophobic and C is the most

antibody. If the ADCs and unconjugated antibody elute with the same retention time, HIC cannot be used for analysis and characterization.

18. Conjugation sites affect peak shape and the number of eluted peaks. To date, all approved ADCs use random conjugation methods on lysines or hinge cysteines. This conjugation method generates multiple peaks corresponding to the degree of drug loading and can be complicated to analyze (Fig. 2). Alternatively, several ADCs in clinical trials are site-specifically conjugated to one or more engineered sites. These site-specific ADCs are generally homogeneous and produce a single peak when analyzed by HIC and are less hydrophobic than their randomly conjugated counterparts. Some site-specific conjugation sites minimize the exposure of the payload and therefore reduce the hydrophobicity and retention time as compared to randomly conjugated ADCs.
19. Record the initial solvent peak intensity. An increase in the solvent peak intensity is indicative of incomplete sample binding. The solvent peak intensity is very useful for troubleshooting ADC binding issues and will indicate whether sample binding is improving. Keeping track of the solvent peak intensity is invaluable when testing columns or mobile phases during method optimization.
20. HIC analysis of some ADCs generates double peaks. For example, double peaks have been noticed with site-specific conjugated ADCs generated utilizing the Thr289Cys (Kabat numbering) substitution in human IgG1 or with payloads that contain enantiomers (Fig. 6 respectively). Double peaks

may be due the result of interactions with the column matrix as a function of conjugation site or payload structural differences. Payloads that create double peaks, will do so regardless of the site or method of conjugation. Verifying the mass and number of drug species, via mass spectrometry, is very useful for data interpretation with double peaks.

21. When ranking antibodies and ADCs for hydrophobicity, the sample concentration and buffer should be matched. Drug candidate ranking based on hydrophobicity is important because of the link between hydrophobicity and off-target toxicity. Figure 6 shows a HIC analysis of six antibodies against the same tumor-specific antigen being considered for ADC drug candidate. In this case, mAb-A is the least hydrophobic. When analyzing ADC for hydrophobicity ranking, the antibody, conjugation site, conjugation method, and payload all affect the retention time.

Acknowledgments

I thank Dr. Nazzareno Dimasi, Dr. Amit Kumar, and Benjamin Ruddle for useful discussion, critical review, and comments.

References

1. Cusumano A, Guillarme D, Beck A et al (2016) Practical method development for the separation of monoclonal antibodies and antibody-drug-conjugate species in hydrophobic interaction chromatography, part 2: optimization of the phase system. J Pharm Biomed Anal 121:161–173
2. Rodriguez-Aller M, Guillarme D, Beck A (2016) Practical method development for the separation of monoclonal antibodies and antibody-drug-conjugate species in hydrophobic interaction chromatography, part 1: optimization of the mobile phase. J Pharm Biomed Anal 118:393–403
3. Queiroz JA, Tomaz CT, Cabral JMS (2001) Hydrophobic interaction chromatography of proteins. J Biotechnol 87(2):143–159
4. Fekete S, Veuthey JL, Beck A et al (2016) Hydrophobic interaction chromatography for the characterization of monoclonal antibodies and related products. J Pharm Biomed Anal 130:3–18
5. Alley SC, Anderson KE (2013) Analytical and bioanalytical technologies for characterizing antibody–drug conjugates. Curr Opin Chem Biol 17(3):406–411
6. Wakankar A et al (2011) Analytical methods for physicochemical characterization of antibody drug conjugates. MAbs 3(2):161–172
7. Chen T, Chen Y, Stella C et al (2016) Antibody-drug conjugate characterization by chromatographic and electrophoretic techniques. J Chromatogr B 1032:39–50
8. Egloff H, Kidwell KM, Schott A (2018) Ado-trastuzumab emtansine-induced pulmonary toxicity: a single-institution retrospective review. Case Rep Oncol 11(2):527–533
9. Dan N, Setua S, Kashyap VK et al (2018) Antibody-drug conjugates for cancer therapy: chemistry to clinical implications. Pharmaceuticals (Basel) 11(2):32
10. McCombs JR, Owen SC (2015) Antibody drug conjugates: design and selection of linker, payload and conjugation chemistry. AAPS J 17 (2):339–351
11. Tomaz CT, Queiroz JA (2013) Chapter 6 - Hydrophobic interaction chromatography. In: Liquid chromatography. Elsevier, Amsterdam, pp 121–141
12. Donaghy H (2016) Effects of antibody, drug and linker on the preclinical and clinical

toxicities of antibody-drug conjugates. MAbs 8 (4):659–671
13. Hoffmann RM, Coumbe BGT, Josephs DH et al (2017) Antibody structure and engineering considerations for the design and function of antibody drug conjugates (ADCs). Oncoimmunology 7(3):e1395127
14. Estep P, Caffry I, Yu Y et al (2015) An alternative assay to hydrophobic interaction chromatography for high-throughput characterization of monoclonal antibodies. MAbs 7 (3):553–561
15. Haverick M, Mengisen S, Shemeem M et al (2014) Separation of mAbs molecular variants by analytical hydrophobic interaction chromatography HPLC: overview and applications. MAbs 6(4):852–858

Chapter 11

Two-Dimensional Liquid Chromatography Coupled to High-Resolution Mass Spectrometry for the Analysis of ADCs

Soraya Chapel, Florent Rouvière, Morgan Sarrut, and Sabine Heinisch

Abstract

From a structural point of view, the complete characterization of ADCs is a challenging task due to their high complexity. ADCs combine the heterogeneity of the initial antibody to the variability associated with the conjugation strategy, the manufacturing process, and the storage. Given the inherent complexity of these biomolecules, online comprehensive two-dimensional liquid chromatography (LC × LC) is an attractive technique to address the challenges associated with ADC characterization. Compared to conventional one-dimensional liquid chromatography techniques (1D-LC), LC × LC combines two different and complementary separation systems. In the context of ADC analysis, LC × LC has been proven to be a rapid and efficient analytical tool: (1) to provide a higher resolving power by increasing the overall peak capacity and thus allowing to gain more information within a single run and (2) to allow mass spectrometry (MS) coupling with some chromatographic techniques that are not MS-compatible and hence to facilitate the structural elucidation of ADCs. In this chapter, we present the coupling of different chromatographic techniques including hydrophobic interaction chromatography (HIC), reversed phase liquid chromatography (RPLC), size exclusion chromatography (SEC), ion exchange chromatography (IEX), and hydrophilic liquid chromatography (HILIC). The interest of HIC × SEC, SEC × SEC, HIC × RPLC, IEX × RPLC, RPLC × RPLC, and HILIC × RPLC, all hyphenated to high-resolution mass spectrometry (HRMS), is discussed in the context of the characterization of ADCs.

Key words Antibody–drug conjugate, ADC, Online two-dimensional liquid chromatography, LC × LC, Cysteine-linked ADC, Lysine-linked ADC, Peptide mapping, High-resolution mass spectrometry, Intact protein analysis, Ion mobility

1 Introduction

Antibody–drug conjugates (ADCs) are one of the most promising classes of human therapeutics [1, 2]. Their technology combines the specificity of a monoclonal antibody (mAb) with a potent cytotoxic drug covalently bonded to the mAb via a stable linker. The resulting therapeutic biomolecule is designed to improve treatment efficacy compared to the first generation of mAbs while lowering the side effects encountered with classical chemotherapy.

L. Nathan Tumey (ed.), *Antibody-Drug Conjugates: Methods and Protocols*, Methods in Molecular Biology, vol. 2078, https://doi.org/10.1007/978-1-4939-9929-3_11,

4 ADCs are currently marketed and more than 60 clinical trials are ongoing [3].

The characterization of such formats is of prime importance to study their structure–function relationship by identifying microvariants, 3D-structures, drug loading, and conjugation sites in order to investigate their influence on antigen binding, pharmacokinetics, pharmacodynamics, stability [4], and also to prove that ADC manufacturing and stability can be managed in the frame of clinical studies with respect to the critical quality attributes (CQAs), to ensure both treatment efficacy and patient safety.

From a structural point of view, the complete characterization of ADCs is a challenging task due to their high complexity. In addition to the heterogeneity of the initial mAb, the conjugation strategy brings an additional degree of variability [5]. Although several conjugation chemistries exist to bind a cytotoxic drug to an mAb [3, 5], in this chapter we will focus on two marketed ADCs, brentuximab vedotin and ado-trastuzumab emtansine, which are respectively cysteine and lysine-based ADCs. Brentuximab vedotin is made by the chemical conjugation of cytotoxins to mAbs, by reducing the cysteine residues that form interchain disulfide bonds, followed by the conjugation of the resulting free thiols with drugs. This process leads to heterogeneous population of conjugated products that contains species with various numbers of drugs per antibody, usually an even number (0, 2, 4, 6, 8) [6]. In the case of ado-trastuzumab emtansine, the conjugation takes place on the amino groups of lysine. Since 80–100 lysines are available (vs. only 8 interchain cysteines), the lysine conjugation leads to a more heterogeneous mixture of species compared to cysteine conjugation, in spite of a similar overall level of drugs incorporated per antibody (between 0 and 8 with an average of 3–4) [5, 7].

To face the complexity of such highly heterogeneous species, numerous analytical techniques are needed [4]. In this context, liquid chromatography (LC) and high-resolution mass spectrometry (HRMS) are the most used tools since they allow to get orthogonal information in both native and denaturing conditions while using intact, top-down, middle-up (protein level), and bottom-up approaches (peptide level) [8].

As an example, ion exchange chromatography (IEX), size-exclusion chromatography (SEC), hydrophobic interaction chromatography (HIC), and hydrophilic interaction liquid chromatography (HILIC) can be used to study charge variants, protein aggregation, drug load distribution, and glycoforms respectively. Reversed phase liquid chromatography (RPLC) coupled to HRMS is currently the technique of choice to get access to the primary structure of the protein via peptide mapping (bottom-up approach) or to separate and identify large protein fragments obtained after digestion (middle-up approach) [8]. Lastly, ion mobility coupled to

MS (IM × MS) has been reported as an interesting tool to characterize conformational changes in the proteins [9].

In spite of this large panel of analytical techniques, some challenges still need to be addressed such as (a) improving the separation power to facilitate both structural elucidation by MS and in-depth comparison between samples, (b) crossing data from different techniques, and/or (c) making the chromatographic techniques using large amounts of salts (HIC, IEX, and SEC), MS-compatible.

In this context, online comprehensive two-dimensional liquid chromatography (LC × LC) is an attractive technique to tackle these challenges [10]. It allows, in one single run, (a) to couple two orthogonal techniques, therefore drastically increasing the peak capacity [11], (b) to allow the direct coupling of the first dimension with MS, by means of a second MS compatible dimension, (c) to avoid off-line sample treatments thereby preventing any sample loss or degradation, and (d) to cross, within one single run, the information provided by two different techniques while reducing sample consumption.

This chapter reports different applications using online LC × LC-HRMS for the characterization of ADCs: (a) at intact level by HIC × SEC-IM × MS and SEC × SEC-IM × MS, allowing structural elucidation of ADCs in native conditions, (b) in denaturing conditions by HIC × RPLC-UV-MS, IEX × RPLC-UV-MS and HILIC × RPLC-UV-MS to simultaneously obtain information on mAb heterogeneity, drug-to-antibody ratio (DAR) and drug load position, (c) at peptide level with a bottom-up approach by RPLC × RPLC-MS, IEX × RPLC-MS, and HILIC × RPLC-MS.

2 Principles of Two-Dimensional Liquid Chromatography

The main concept in 2D-LC is that one separation obtained in a first dimension is transferred to a second column to undergo a second separation, in which ideally all the unresolved analytes are further separated. In order to successfully achieve this goal, the two coupled separation dimensions must be complementary by offering different selectivities towards the compounds. Using the nomenclature defined by Marriott et al. [12], the first separation system is referred to as the first dimension and is denoted as ^{1}D and the second separation system is referred to as the second dimension denoted as ^{2}D. In a 2D-LC system the two dimensions can be coupled either off-line or online. In the off-line mode, fractions of the first dimension separation are collected and stored into vials until reinjection at a later time into the second dimension. The same instrument (pump system, sample manager, and detector) can be used for both dimensions by only changing the stationary phase and/or the mobile phase. In the online mode, collection, transfer

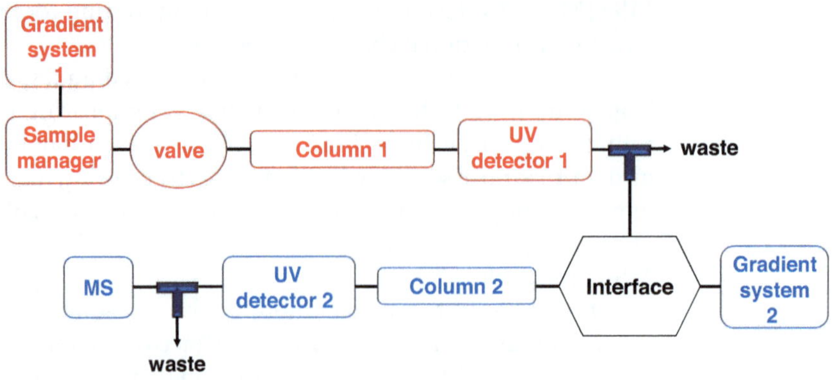

Fig. 1 Generic scheme of online 2D-LC-UV/HRMS instrumentation (*see* text for explanation)

and reinjection are conducted continuously in real time. The implementation is therefore more complex and requires two different chromatographic instruments connected via a suitable interface (Fig. 1). The interface generally consists in one or several automated two-positions switching valves with identical sample loops to ensure continuous fractioning of the first dimension eluent before transferring into the second dimension column. While one loop stores the first dimension fraction, the second loop sends the preceding stored fraction in the second dimension and vice versa. Since both dimensions are interconnected, flow splitting is sometimes required to decrease the flow rate entering the interface and hence to decrease the injection volume in the second dimension. Similarly, a second flow splitter may be necessary to send MS-compatible flow rates into the mass spectrometer. Both online and off-line transfer approaches display their own sets of strengths and weaknesses which were extensively highlighted in detailed reviews [13, 14]. Compared to off-line methods, online ones are more advantageous, because they avoid the risk of sample loss, sample contamination, and sample degradation. In addition, they are less time-consuming. However, online sample-handling can lead to serious issues due to the interdependence of the two dimensions, resulting in much more complex implementation. As a consequence, specific method development and optimization are mandatory.

2D-LC methods can be divided into two main modes as illustrated in Fig. 2. The simplest and easiest to be implemented is the heart-cutting mode denoted as LC-LC, in which large volumes of selected portions of ^{1}D are considered. This approach can involve either a single fraction or several fractions along the ^{1}D chromatogram. In this latter case it is referred to as multiple heart-cutting denoted as mLC-LC. The heart-cutting approach can be used to increase the resolution of a given unresolved pair of peaks in the first dimension, but it is not designed to increase the overall peak

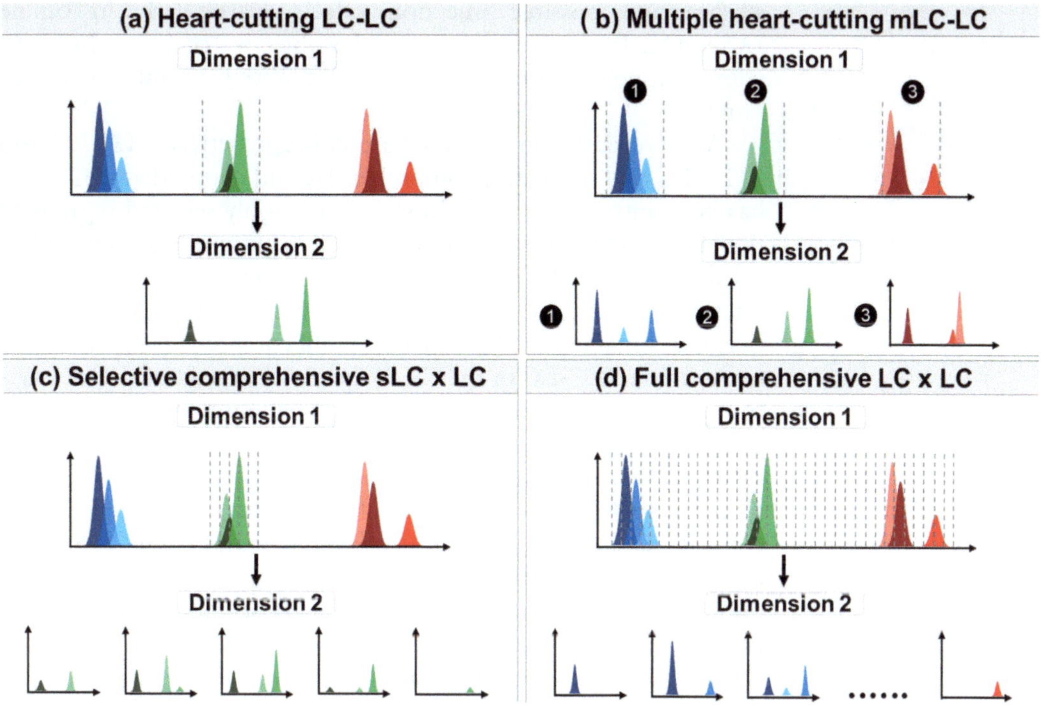

Fig. 2 Illustrative representation of four possible 2D-LC separations: (**a**) heart-cutting, (**b**) multiple heart-cutting, (**c**) selective comprehensive, and (**d**) full comprehensive (*see* text for explanation)

capacity of the 2D-LC method. For this reason, LC-LC or mLC-LC are more commonly used for targeted analysis of a small number of compounds. As an example in the field of ADCs, Li et al. [15] have developed a two-dimensional heart-cutting method involving SEC in ^{1}D coupled to RPLC in ^{2}D, to separate unconjugated small molecules drugs and their related impurities in ADC samples. In this approach, SEC was used to separate the small molecules of interest (free drug, linker, and process-related impurities) from ADC and other high molecular weight species (HMWS), whereas in RPLC, all the co-eluting small species were separated from a single collected fraction. A similar approach was reported by Goyon and coworkers [16] in multiple heart-cutting mSEC-RPLC, for the separation of free drugs, linker, and linker-drug from the monomeric ADC in different ADC samples.

In fully comprehensive 2D-LC denoted as LC × LC, the entire sample is subject to a separation in both dimensions with relatively small fractions transferred. Small fractions of ^{1}D are collected in order to overall maintain the resolution obtained in the first separation. Since the entire sample is subjected to two different separations, impressive peak capacities are expected. The theoretical peak capacity is the product of the peak capacities in each dimension but the effective peak capacity is usually much lower due to undersampling of first dimension peaks, partial coverage of the retention surface and possible injection effects, particularly in online LC × LC. In most applications, the objective of LC × LC is to gain as much information as possible about a highly complex sample.

Very recently, an intermediate concept between LC-LC and LC × LC called selective comprehensive and denoted as sLC × LC has been introduced [17]. In sLC × LC, only selected regions of the ^{1}D chromatogram are sent to the ^{2}D column. However, unlike mLC-LC where the fractions are quite large, in sLC × LC small fractions are sampled so that the resolution obtained in ^{1}D can be overall maintained in ^{2}D, similarly to full comprehensive LC × LC. Compared to LC-LC or mLC-LC the major benefit of sLC × LC is to minimize undersampling, thereby providing a higher resolution power in the first dimension and hence in the overall 2D-LC separation. This is a good alternative for LC × LC when the targeted analysis of one or several compounds is needed. In the context of ADC synthesis control, Venkatramani et al. [18] have demonstrated the applicability of sLC × LC with RPLC in both dimensions for qualitative and quantitative studies of the impurity profile of key linker-drug intermediates.

The appropriate selection among these 2D-LC approaches depends on both application scope and sample complexity.

3 Analysis at the Intact Level (Top-Down Approach)

The characterization of ADCs at the intact level requires the use of nondenaturing analytical techniques to maintain the structural and conformational form of the protein during the analysis. Denaturing conditions include physical parameters (heat, pH, radiations, etc.) and/or chemical parameters (reducing agents such as dithiothreitol (DTT), strong acid or base, high organic solvent content) which may lead to the dissociation of weak noncovalent binding between ADC subunits and to the loss of the three-dimensional structure of the protein. Various chromatographic techniques are essentially carried out in aqueous solvents and hence, suitable for mAb or ADC analysis at the intact level. Those include HIC, IEX, most often cation exchange (CEX), and SEC. Native MS performed under nondenaturing ionization conditions was also proved to be a valuable tool for the structural characterization of intact mAbs and ADCs, as it allows the direct observation of the protein structure by preserving its intact form [9, 19–24].

3.1 HIC × SEC

The top-down approach, which consists in analyzing the protein by starting from its intact form, is a powerful tool to obtain information about ADC sample purity. HIC coupled to ultraviolet (UV) detection (HIC-UV) is the gold-standard analytical technique for separating the different DARs (drug-to-antibody-ratio)

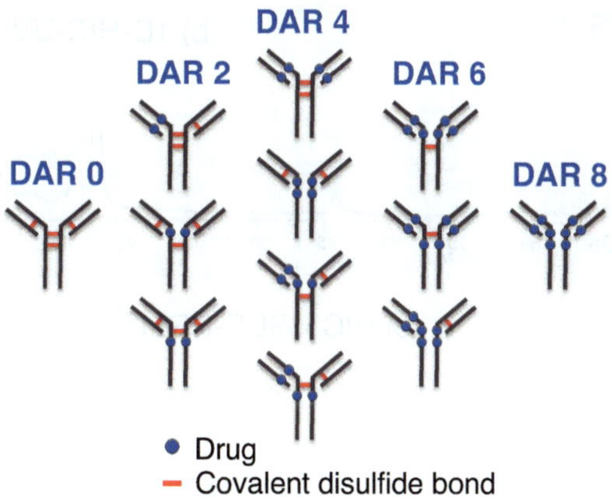

Fig. 3 Schematic representation of the possible positional isomers resulting from the drug conjugation of a cysteine conjugated ADC

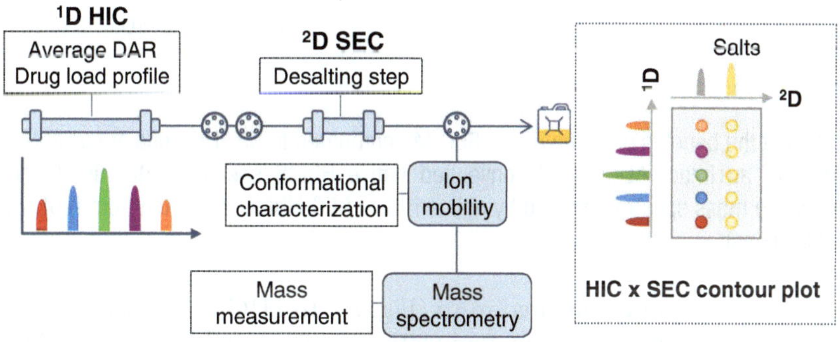

Fig. 4 Schematic representation of the setup for the online HIC × SEC-IM × MS analysis of cysteine-linked ADCs. (Adapted from [26, 27] with permission from ACS Publications)

of ADCs based on the interchain cysteines. DAR can be defined as the number of cytotoxic drug conjugated to a specific mAb. For cysteine-linked ADCs, the conjugation process usually results in the formation of DAR species with an even distribution of 0, 2, 4, 6 or 8 drugs incorporated per antibody, due to the presence of four disulfide bridges on the protein (Fig. 3). In the context of ADC synthesis, it should be noted that DAR 0 is considered as an impurity, since no drugs are linked, whilst DARs with odd number (DAR 1, DAR 3...) are degradation products. The precise characterization of the different DAR species present in an ADC sample is of prime importance in quality control because different isoforms may have different toxicological and/or pharmacokinetic properties and hence may affect the overall ADC efficacy and safety. In HIC, the proteins are separated by their hydrophobic interactions with the ligands present on the stationary phase surface. As a result, the retention increases with the protein hydrophobicity. The conjugation of hydrophobic payloads (or drugs) on mAb leads to the creation of species of increasing hydrophobicity compared to the

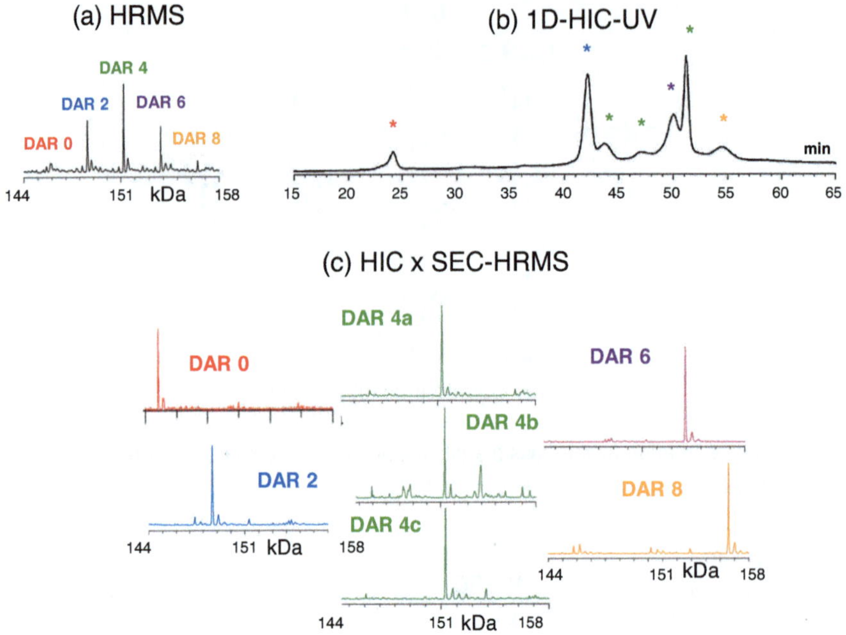

Fig. 5 Illustration of the benefits of online HIC × SEC-MS compared to HIC-UV alone or native MS alone for the characterization of an intact ADC: (**a**) deconvoluted native HRMS spectrum, (**b**) HIC-UV profile, and (**c**) deconvoluted native mass spectra obtained by online HIC × SEC-HRMS. (Adapted from [26] with permission from ACS Publications)

unconjugated mAb (Fig. 3). In HIC, ADCs can thus be separated by increasing conjugation payloads, which leads to the differentiation of the different DARs based on the number of attached drugs and their apparent hydrophobicity. In addition, changes in the protein structure, including posttranslational modifications (PTMs) such as deamidation and oxidation, or even glycosylation can be differentiated using HIC, since these changes directly affect the overall hydrophobicity of the molecule [25]. In the context of ADC characterization at the intact level, the coupling of the HIC separation with the structural identification power of MS detection, and especially HRMS may be a powerful tool. Peak overlapping or poor resolution can lead to misleading information when using HIC-UV alone, while the sole use of HRMS does not allow the distinction between different positional isomers (or isoforms) of the same DAR. The online coupling of HIC for the separation of DAR species, to nondenaturing native MS is therefore of great interest for ADC characterization at the intact level. However, the separation mechanism in HIC requires the use of high concentration of nonvolatile salts buffers in the mobile phase, which are not compatible with MS detection. The collection of HIC fractions followed by subsequent sample treatment in order to eliminate the nonvolatile salts from the sample, followed by redissolution in a more friendly solvent prior to reinjection in HRMS was performed [9]. However, such off-line analysis is labor-intensive, time-consuming (sample preparation and multiple injections), and can hardly be automated, which is a major drawback for high-throughput analysis in the context of research and development of ADCs. From this perspective, two-dimensional liquid chromatography is a clever solution to achieve the direct interfacing of HIC with MS, by incorporating an online fast desalting step in the second dimension. To have an efficient analytical technique, the second dimension must be compatible with MS detection and must use nondenaturing conditions in order to keep the protein intact. Such strategy was reported by Ehkirch et al. [26] for the analytical characterization of a marketed cysteine-linked ADC (brentuximab vedotin). HIC and IM × MS were hyphenated by using an online LC × LC setup involving HIC in 1D and SEC in 2D (online HIC × SEC-IM × MS) resulting in an analytical technique performed under entirely nondenaturing conditions. The schematic representation of the setup is presented in Fig. 4. The online LC × LC instrument consisted of two independent LC systems from Waters Corporation (Milford, MA, USA), including an Acquity H-Class in ^{1}D and an Acquity I-Class in ^{2}D, both connected by two 6-port high pressure two-position valves acting as interface between the two dimensions. In the first HIC dimension, a gradient of mobile phase containing 2.5 M of ammonium acetate and 0.1 M of phosphate buffer was used for the separation of the DAR species. Such a high volatile salt concentration, along with the use of a nonvolatile phosphate buffer, makes the direct hyphenation of HIC with MS impossible. In the second dimension, SEC was used as a simple desalting step with a more compatible isocratic mobile phase containing 100 mM of ammonium acetate. In this configuration, SEC, as size-based separation, was used as a fast online desalting step before MS, thereby allowing the differentiation between HIC salts of low molecular weight (MW < 100 Da) and ADC isoforms of high molecular weight (MW > 150 kDa). The first part of the SEC chromatogram, corresponding to the DAR species, was sent to HRMS while the later eluted salts could be directed towards the waste via a 6-port two-position switching valve.

In this analysis, fractions of 150 μL (representing 2–3 fractions per ^{1}D peak) allowed to maintain the integrity of the ^{1}D-HIC separation by keeping the resolution acquired in the first dimension. All detected peaks in HIC were unambiguously identified as even drug load species from DAR 0 to DAR 8, which led to an average DAR (avDAR) calculation of 4 in agreement with expected values. In addition to the structural peak identification by HRMS, ion mobility spectrometry (IMS) was used to confirm the conformational homogeneity of each individual HIC fraction. In native HRMS the detection of different positional isomers of identical masses was not possible (Fig. 5a). In 1D-HIC-UV, the unambiguous identification of all peaks, based on their retention only, was not possible (Fig. 5b). Compared to these analytical methods, the online HIC × SEC-IM × MS analysis allowed to demonstrate the presence of positional isomers of DAR 4 (Fig. 5c). In addition, the simplification of the ADC matrix entering the ionization source resulted in a significant increase in MS sensitivity, thereby supporting detection and unambiguous identification of minor species such as DAR 0 and DAR 8, much less sensitive in native HRMS (Fig. 5a, c). This online LC × LC approach highlights the possibility to have, within a single run, an analytical characterization of ADCs with different information levels. Those include drug profile and average DAR (both in HIC) and accurate identification of the drug load distribution through the mass measurement in HRMS. In addition to the ability to directly hyphenate two analytical techniques (HIC and HRMS), the indisputable advantage of online HIC × SEC-HRMS for ADC characterization at the intact level is the substantial improvement of sensitivity in MS, which is essential for the unambiguous identification of all detected species.

3.2 SEC × SEC

Besides the determination of drug conjugation in ADC samples (average DAR and their drug load distribution), online LC × LC may be used in the top-down approach to investigate other critical quality attributes (CQAs) such as size variants. The characterization of the size heterogeneity in mAb or ADC samples mostly relies on SEC and native MS. As opposed to HIC, SEC can be performed with either volatile or nonvolatile salts, but lower performance was reported for mAb analysis in SEC with nondenaturing MS compatible conditions (e.g. with ammonium acetate buffers) compared to more classical nondenaturing conditions using nonvolatile phosphate buffers [27]. The limited performance observed in SEC with ammonium acetate buffers can be attributed to the multimodal nature of the elution mechanism (separation not only based on size but also on ionic interactions, adsorption, and hydrophobicity) when using a low ionic strength buffer, which results in longer retention times, broader peaks, and lower sensitivity for basic and/or hydrophobic compounds. In order to keep optimal performances for mAb or ADC analysis, SEC has therefore to be performed with non-MS-compatible salts, making its direct hyphenation to MS impossible. Similarly to above HIC × SEC-IM × MS, a second dimension was used as desalting step to allow the hyphenation of SEC to MS detection. An online four-dimensional approach combining two SEC dimensions, ion mobility and HRMS (4D-SEC × SEC-IM × MS) was reported for the structural characterization of a wide range of mAbs [27] (adalizumab, pembrolizumab, and bevacizumab) under nondenaturing conditions. Nonvolatile salts (50 mM phosphate buffer and 250 mM potassium chloride) were used in the first SEC dimension for optimum separation of size variants, whereas in the second SEC dimension a nonvolatile buffer composed of 100 mM of

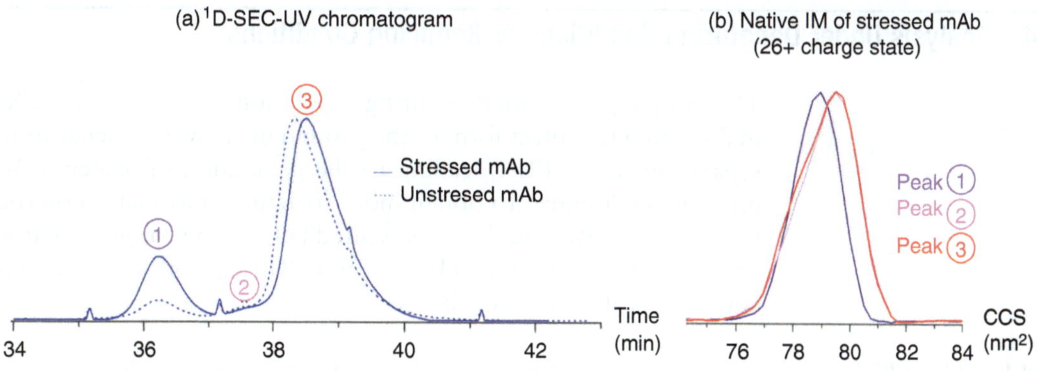

Fig. 6 Online SEC × SEC-IM × MS analysis of pembrolizumab. (**a**) Overlaid 1D-SEC-UV chromatograms of unstressed (dotted lines) and stressed (solid line) pembrolizumab. (**b**) Ion mobility collision cross sections (CCSs) of 26+ charge state of the monomeric species detected in 1D-SEC-UV. (Adapted from [27] with permission from ACS Publications)

ammonium acetate was used to allow the compatibility with MS. The online LC × LC instrument was the same as reported above for HIC × SEC and the setup was similar to that presented in Fig. 4, with an SEC column in the first dimension for size separation instead of a HIC column. The benefit of online SEC × SEC-IM × MS was proven by the comparison of stressed and unstressed mAb samples. Unexpected species, which could not be correctly identified in SEC-UV alone, were identified. A representative example of this approach is given in Fig. 6. With the sole use of ^{1}D-SEC-UV (Fig. 6a), peaks #1 and #2, eluted before the most intense peak of monomer (peak #3), would have been attributed to high molecular weight species (HMWS). Surprisingly, similar MS spectra were observed for the three peaks, suggesting that peaks #1 and #2 correspond to a monomer specie instead of dimer or trimer species. Considering this unambiguous identification, it could be stated that the amount of monomer was significantly increased under thermal stress (from 7% to 19.8%). Furthermore, the measurement of the collision cross sections (CCS) (26+ charge state) in IMS (Fig. 6b) not only confirmed the existence of unexpected monomer species but also suggested that the less retained monomer specie had a different conformation compared to the other two, considering the slight difference in CCS values (78.9 vs. 79.5 nm^2). By combining the information provided by the SEC separation with the intact mass measurement in native MS and with the CCS values provided by IMS, the online SEC × SEC-IM × MS analysis allowed the simultaneous HMWS and low molecular weight species (LMWS) profiling, their accurate relative quantitation and the unambiguous identification of each size variants. Although this 4D-approach was applied to mAbs in this reported study, it should also be very attractive in the case of ADCs.

4 Analysis Under Denaturing Conditions or Reducing Conditions

The coupling of a nondenaturing separation (e.g. HIC or CEX) maintaining the intact form of the protein in ^{1}D, with a denaturing separation (e.g. RPLC) leading to the generation of protein subunits in ^{2}D designed to obtain more structural information on the formerly separated species, is presented below. The coupling of two orthogonal techniques, HILIC and RPLC, for a middle-up approach is also discussed below.

4.1 HIC × RPLC

Compared to online HIC × SEC or online SEC × SEC, where ^{2}D-SEC is only a desalting step, the use of RPLC in ^{2}D extends the level of peak information in top-down approach. In RPLC, denaturing conditions (acidic pH, high organic content, elevated temperature...) lead to the dissociation of the weak noncovalent bonds in case of cysteine-linked ADC and hence to the formation of smaller subunits. RPLC in ^{2}D, prior to HRMS and after HIC, SEC or CEX results in more precise structural elucidation of the separated species.

A single heart-cutting HIC-RPLC-UV-HRMS was proposed by Birdsall et al. [28] to identify even DARs in a nontoxic drug mimic. In addition to the fact that the heart-cutting mode requires as many injections as ^{1}D-peaks to analyze and can therefore be time-consuming, it cannot provide information on the entire HIC separation, hence missing some potential important zones of the chromatogram.

In two recent studies, Sarrut et al. [29, 30] proposed an online HIC × RPLC-UV-HRMS method for the analysis of brentuximab vedotin. The online LC × LC instrument consisted of a Waters Acquity 2D-I-Class system (Milford, MA, USA) which includes two high-pressure binary pumps, an auto-sampler, a column manager with two independent column ovens and two 6-port two-position high-pressure valves. The first HIC dimension allowed to separate the different DAR species while maintaining the native form of the proteins. The second RPLC dimension, carried out under MS-compatible conditions (0.05% trifluoroacetic acid +0.1% formic acid in water-acetonitrile mobile phase), allowed the removal of the nonvolatile salts used in the first HIC dimension (2.5 M ammonium acetate and 0.1 M phosphate buffer), by redirecting the salt plug to the waste after each ^{2}D-injection, according to the setup presented in Fig. 4. In order to maximize the separation power, several parameters were optimized in both ^{1}D and ^{2}D, including nature of injection solvent, stationary phases, type of salts, salt concentration, and gradient conditions. In particular, significant peak shape improvement was obtained in ^{1}D by adding salt in the aqueous sample solvent to reduce its eluent strength in HIC. It is worth noting that the reduction of possible deleterious

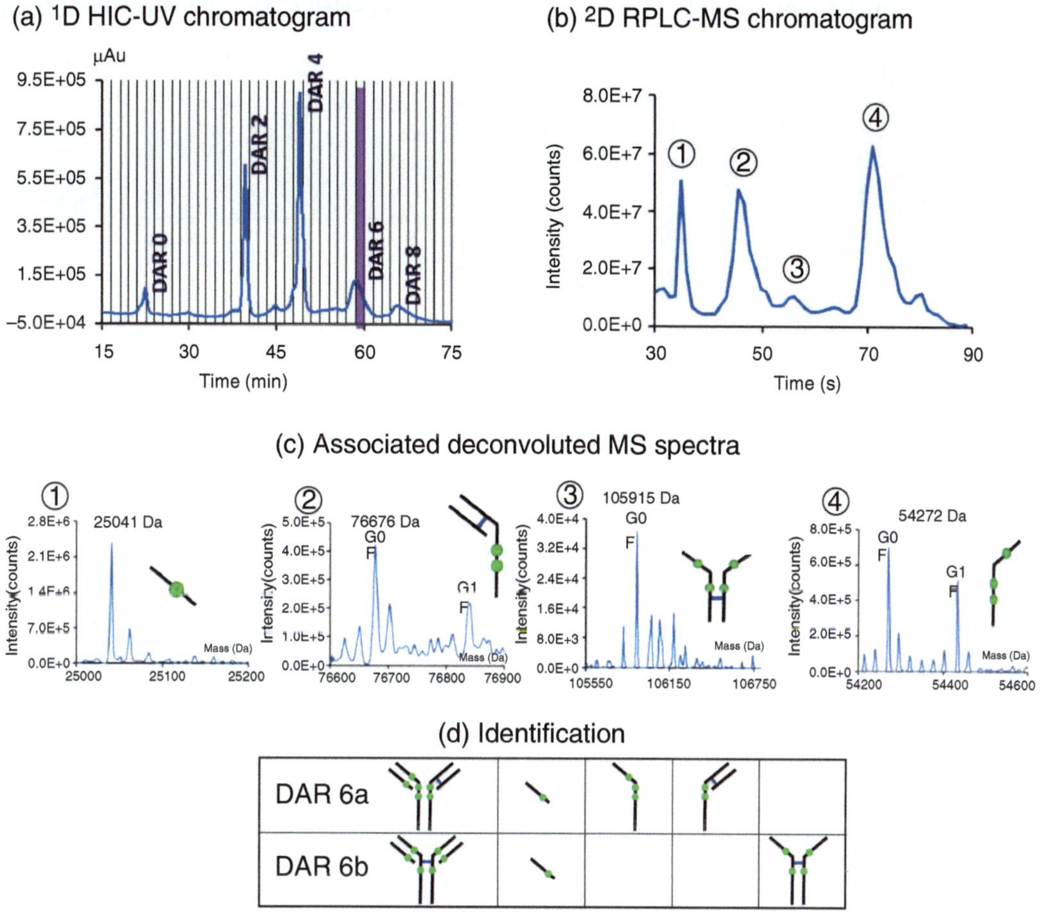

Fig. 7 Illustration of the successive steps for identifying the different DAR species in online HIC × RPLC-UV-HRMS. Example of the identification of DAR 6 and its subunits. (**a**) First dimension HIC-UV separation (the purple dashed area corresponds to one fraction sent in the second dimension). (**b**) 2nd dimension RPLC-MS-TIC chromatogram of the preceding fraction. (**c**) Deconvoluted mass spectra of the 4 labeled peaks allowing the identification of 4 subunits. (**d**) Assignation of the subunits to two different isoforms of DAR 6. (Adapted from [30] with permission from Elsevier)

injection effects in ²D is a key step in online LC × LC method development since noncompatible mobile phases may lead to peak broadening or even peak distortion which in turn leads to a decrease in both overall peak capacity and peak intensity. In this study, the precipitation, in ²D, of the injection plug rich in salts was avoided by bracketing the gradient elution with two water steps (sandwich injection), designed to minimize the contact of ¹D-HIC salt plug with ²D-hydro-organic solvent. Unlike other analytical methods used for ADC characterization, this optimized online HIC × RPLC-UV-HRMS method was able to unambiguously identify the positional isomers of the different DARs observed in HIC. The methodology is presented in Fig. 7, through the

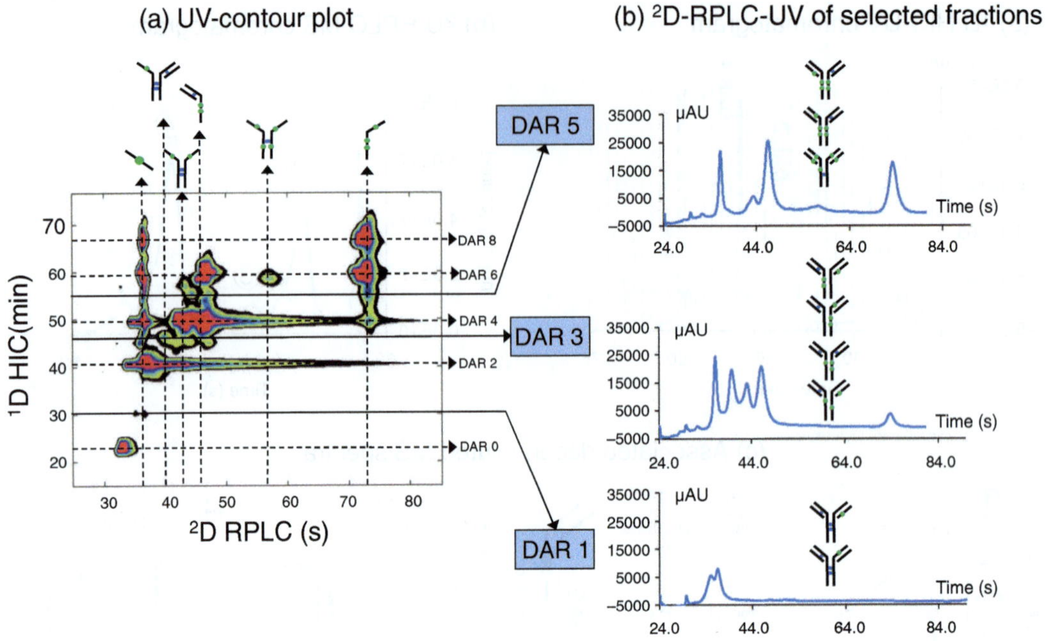

Fig. 8 Structural elucidation of odd DARs of brentuximab vedotin in online HIC × RPLC-HRMS. (**a**) UV contour plot of the online HIC × RPLC separation. The subunits, separated in RPLC, are indicated on the top of the contour plot; the DAR species, separated in HIC, are indicated on the right side of the contour plot. (**b**) 2D RPLC-separations of subunits corresponding to the most concentrated fractions in 1D for subsequent identification of DAR 1, 3 and 5. Identified isoforms are represented for each odd DAR. (Adapted from [30] with permission from Elsevier)

illustration of DAR 6 characterization. After the separation of DAR species in the first HIC dimension (Fig. 7a), each fraction was sent in the second RPLC dimension. The denaturing conditions led to the formation of subunits, further separated in RPLC according to their hydrophobicity (Fig. 7b). The separated subunits were then identified after deconvolution of their MS spectra (Fig. 7c). The presence of the four expected subunits of DAR 6 led to the unambiguous identification of the two positional isomers of DAR 6 as shown in Fig. 7. In addition to achieving online desalting of the first HIC separation, mandatory for the hyphenation to HRMS, RPLC was also very useful to gain information about the structure of the DAR species separated in HIC. With such approach, not only even DARs could be identified, but also odd DARs. The contour plot presented in Fig. 8 summarizes the structural elucidation of both even and odd DARs, with horizontal dotted lines showing the DAR species separated in HIC and dotted vertical lines showing the different subunits separated in RPLC. Using the methodology illustrated in Fig. 7, odd DARs (1, 3 and 5) and most of their related positional isomers could be unambiguously identified. Very large subunits (MW > 100 kDa) were more difficult to ionize and hence to detect in MS. However, subunit identification could

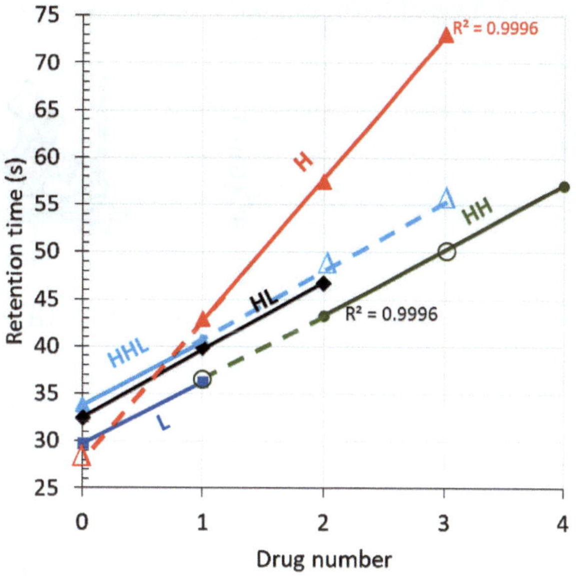

Fig. 9 Illustration of the potential of retention data in RPLC to predict the retention times of nonidentified subunits (empty symbols) considering the plot of retention times of identified subunits (full symbols) as a function of drug load number. H and L stand for heavy and light chains respectively. The coefficient of determination is given for HL and H for (with 3 identified subunits). (Adapted from [30] with permission from Elsevier)

be completed by crossing information from both retention and MS data, thereby making the prediction of the retention times of the different subunits possible as shown by the plots of the retention times of identified subunits against the drug load number (Fig. 9). As pointed out, experimental data were well fitted by straight lines ($R^2 > 0.99$). The good correlation between subunit retention time and conjugated drug number suggests that this latter is the driving force for retention in RPLC. From these different straight lines, it is possible to predict the retention time of any nonidentified subunit (empty symbols in Fig. 9) by interpolation or even extrapolation of the fitted straight line. Finally, the excellent repeatability obtained in HIC × RPLC-UV makes the related 2D-contour plots very convenient for assessing the conformity of ADCs in their later stage of development as well as in quality control. A visual comparison between nonconform and conform batches can be rapidly performed from 2D-UV contour plots shown in Fig. 10.

Online HIC × RPLC-UV-HRMS appears to be a powerful technique for fast and extensive characterization of cysteine-linked ADC.

4.2 CEX × RPLC

CEX was also coupled to RPLC in full comprehensive and selective comprehensive for mAbs [31, 32], and in multiple heart-cutting for lysine-conjugated ADCs [7]. CEX, performed with pH gradients,

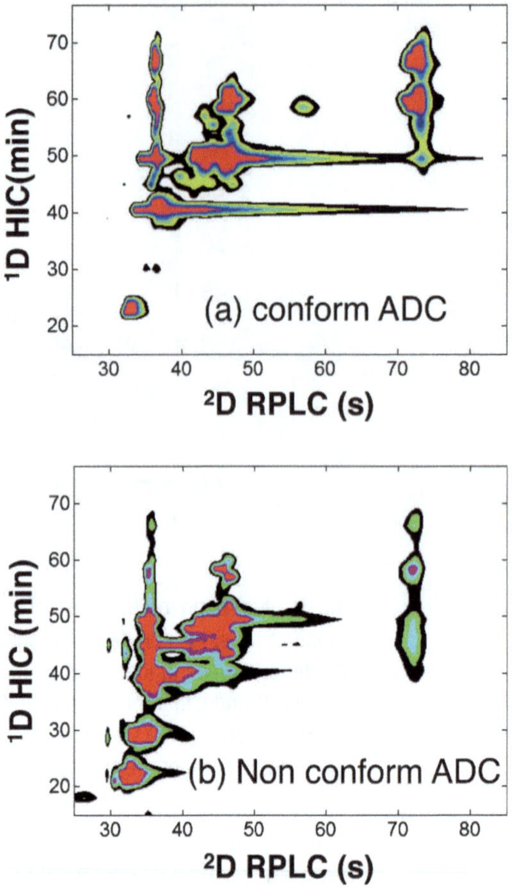

Fig. 10 Contour plots of HIC × RPLC-UV separations of nonstressed (top) and 2-months stressed (bottom) brentuximab vedotin illustrating the possibility of visual assessment of its conformity. (Adapted from [30] with permission from Elsevier)

can separate charge variants. The positive charges of the protein interact with the negative charges of the stationary phase, resulting in increased retention with increased protein charge. A positive charge is removed per lysine residue conjugated, which leads to a decrease in retention when the drug conjugation of lysine-linked ADCs increases. Drug conjugation, glycan variants, as well as PTMs (such as deamidation or oxidation) can alter the overall charge, thus changing the retention. In RPLC, the conjugation of hydrophobic drugs shifts the retention towards higher retention times, making the combination of CEX and RPLC, a good option to characterize these ADCs. CEX requires mobile phase salt buffers, usually not compatible with MS. The first role of RPLC is thus to remove salts prior to MS.

Sandra et al. [7] used multiple heart-cutting mCEX-RPLC-UV-HRMS for the characterization of the lysine-conjugated ADC ado-trastuzumab emtansine, commercialized as Kadcyla. The analyses were carried out with a commercially available Agilent 1290 Infinity 2D-LC system (Agilent Technologies, Waldbronn, Germany), with a set of 3 external valves for the mLC-LC configuration, including a 2-position/4-port duo valve and two "sampling deck" valves ensuring the multiple storage of fractions in mLC-LC. Top-down (protein level) and middle up (partially IdeZ digested protein) approaches were considered in this study. Partial digestion with IdeZ cleaves the protein below the hinge region, leading to two identical Fc/2 fragments and one $F(ab')_2$ fragment. CEX and RPLC were found to be complementary. More conjugated DARs are less retained in CEX while more retained in RPLC. Drug loading distribution from DAR 0 to DAR 8 could be assessed considering both the retention data and the structural information gained from the deconvolution of the MS spectra. Compared to the top-down approach, the analysis of IdeZ treated samples provided more information such as the presence of linker molecules alone and the distribution of drugs on the protein backbone via lysine linkages. Although this 2D-separation was carried out in multiple heart-cutting, one could easily imagine the additional information that online comprehensive CEX × RPLC could provide.

It should be noted that top-down and middle-up approaches were also considered for the characterization of different mAbs (rituximab, atezolizumab, obinutuzumab, trastuzumab, infliximab and cetuximab) by selective comprehensive (sCEX × RPLC-UV-HRMS) and full comprehensive (CEX × RPLC-UV-HRMS) approaches [31, 32]. In those cases, analyses were performed with 2D-LC Agilent 1290 Infinity line (Waldbronn, Germany) including a 2-position/4-port duo valve. Two "sampling deck" valves were used for sLC × LC. Using middle-up approach, mAbs were analyzed after partial digestion with IdeS, followed by reduction of disulfide bonds with DTT, leading to small fragments of about 25 kDa. The observed CEX peaks of intact mAb as well as of digested and digested/reduced mAb could be identified by HRMS. Furthermore, the authors drew attention to the increase in peak capacity brought by the second RPLC dimension, particularly relevant when analyzing mAb fragments.

4.3 HILIC × RPLC

HILIC involves the use of highly denaturing mobile phases (i.e. high organic content and most often acidic or basic pH). Yet, this technique may be attractive for mAbs or ADCs. In HILIC, the compounds are separated by their increased hydrophilicity, polarity and/or charge. HILIC can therefore be considered as quite complementary to RPLC. Stoll et al. [33] highlighted the potential of online comprehensive HILIC × RPLC for the separation of IdeS-digested and IdeS-digested/DTT-reduced mAbs. The benefit of the method was illustrated by analyzing three mAbs which differed by their extent of N-glycosylation which could be revealed on the

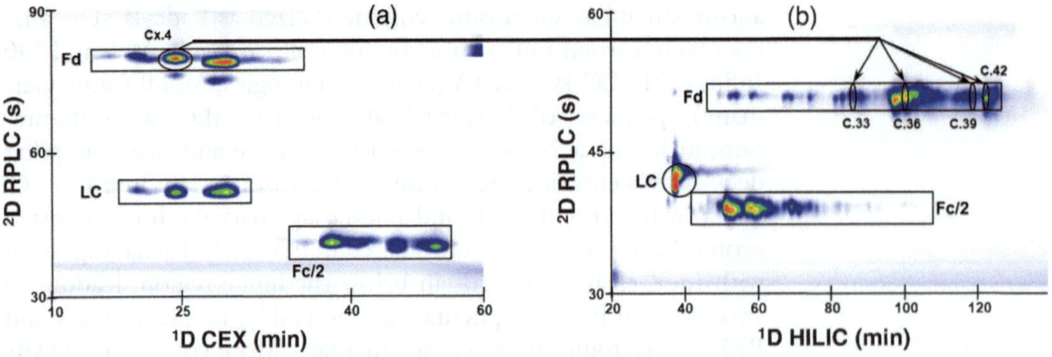

Fig. 11 Comparison of (**a**) online CEX × RPLC and (**b**) online HILIC × RPLC for the analysis of rituximab. (Adapted from [33] with permission from ACS Publications)

Fc/2 and Fd subunits of each mAb. The glycosylation profile of mAbs and ADCs is part of the CQAs that must be monitored during process development because it may affect the stability, the efficacy and the safety of the protein. The interest of 1D-HILIC had already been shown for the separation of protein glycoforms by differentiating according to glycan size [34–38]. In protein analysis, HILIC usually requires the use of trifluoroacetic acid (TFA) in the mobile phase, acting as an ion-pairing agent in order to maintain good peak shapes [34]. However, compared to weaker acids such as formic acid, TFA leads to lower protein MS signal. A second RPLC dimension is a clever way to combine the chromatographic resolution of HILIC, with an improved MS signal thanks to formic acid in the mobile phase. Moreover, given the inherent complementarity of these two chromatographic modes, the value of adding RPLC after a first HILIC separation is to gain more information on the separated species by increasing the separation space coverage. Experimentally, the online coupling of HILIC and RPLC is challenging because of injection effects resulting from solvent strength mismatch between both mobile phases. In their study, the authors circumvented the deleterious effects on the separation by online diluting the first dimension solvent with a weak solvent prior to injection in RPLC. The comparison of online CEX × RPLC [31] as discussed earlier, and HILIC × RPLC [33], both performed on an Agilent 2D-LC Infinity line, is given in Fig. 11. HILIC × RPLC was found to be more selective for the separation of the glycoforms of heavily glycosylated species as highlighted by the arrows in Fig. 11.

5 Bottom-Up Approach (RPLC × RPLC)

With bottom-up approach, also known as peptide mapping, the protein undergoes total digestion, typically with trypsin, resulting in small peptide fragments. Unlike middle-up, bottom-up

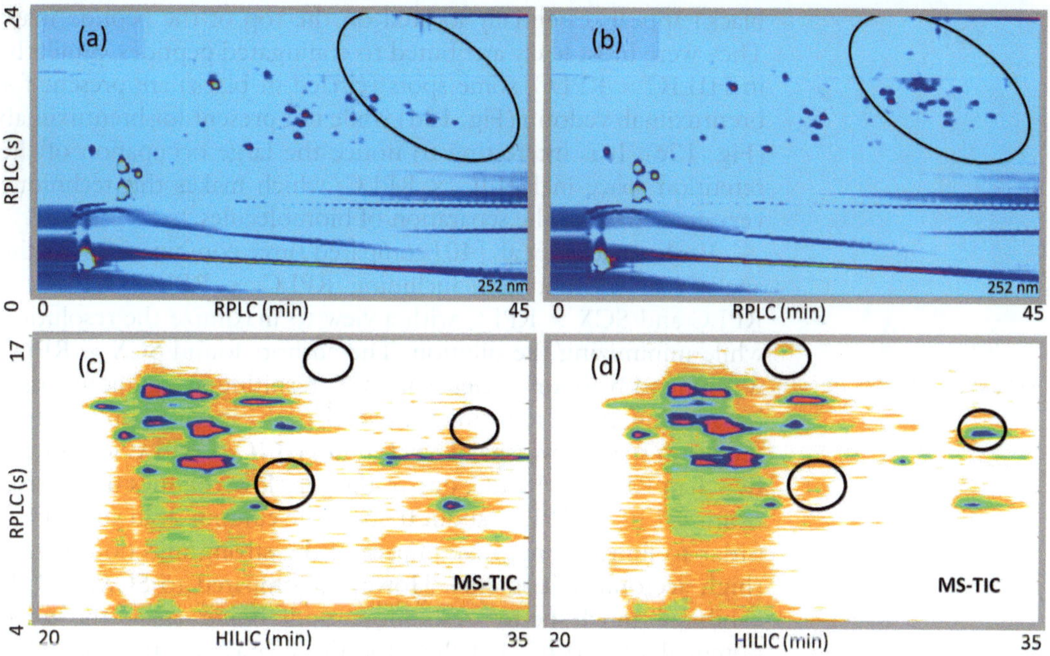

Fig. 12 Peptide maps in RPLC × RPLC-UV of (**a**) trastuzumab and (**b**) ado-trastuzumab emtansine, and in HILIC × RPLC-MS-TIC of (**c**) brentuximab and (**d**) brentuximab vedotin. Differences between mAb and ADC are circled in black. ((**a**, **b**) Adapted from [7] with permission from Elsevier. (**c**, **d**) Adapted from [39])

approach is used to obtain more precise information on the amino acid sequence and on the specific locations of any posttranslational or other modifications in the amino-acid chain of the protein [8]. For very large proteins such as mAbs or ADCs, tryptic digest leads to a large number of peptides, underlining the interest of online LC × LC for peak capacity enhancement. Figure 12 shows two different online LC × LC-UV-HRMS analyses of tryptic digests performed on similar 2D-LC Agilent 1290 Infinity lines as mentioned earlier. They were carried out to obtain structural information about the location of the conjugation sites on the proteins. A digest of traztuzumab (Fig. 12a) and a digest of its related lysine-linked ADC (ado-traztuzumab emtansine) (Fig. 12b) were separated in online RPLC × RPLC with different mobile phase pH between ^{1}D and ^{2}D (10 mM NH4-bicarbonate pH 8.2 in ^{1}D and 0.1% formic acid in ^{2}D) [7]. A digest of brentuximab (Fig. 12c) and a digest of its related cysteine-linked ADC (brentuximab vedotin) (Fig. 12d) were separated in HILIC × RPLC with 10 mM ammonium acetate in ^{1}D-HILIC and 0.1% formic acid in ^{2}D-RPLC [39]. In both cases, the direct comparison of the 2D-contour plots (Fig. 12) provides valuable insights on sample drug conjugation. In RPLC × RPLC, a large part of the peptide map is similar for mAb (Fig. 12a) and ADC (Fig. 12b) due to the fact that most peptides are identical. However, some additional spots (circled in black) appear, essentially located on the top of the peptide map. They were most likely attributed to conjugated peptides. Similarly, in HILIC × RPLC, some spots (circled in black) are present for brentuximab vedotin (Fig. 12d) while not present for brentuximab (Fig. 12c). It is interesting to notice the large occupation of the retention space in HILIC × RPLC, which makes this technique very attractive for the separation of biomolecules.

Vanhoenacker et al. [40] compared three combinations for the analysis of trastuzumab, including RPLC × RPLC, HILIC × RPLC and SCX × RPLC with a view to maximize the resolution while minimizing the dilution. The authors found SCX × RPLC was limited by poor efficiency in SCX, resulting in significant band broadening, hence reducing the overall peak capacity despite a large retention space coverage. They found HILIC × RPLC less attractive than RPLC × RPLC, due to the very low volumes transferred from HILIC to RPLC (about 0.5% of the column dead volume) in order to limit the negative impact of the strong injection solvent (high acetonitrile content). However, compared to SCX, HILIC exhibited much better resolution, underlining again the great potential of HILIC × RPLC for the characterization of mAbs or ADCs.

6 Conclusion

Antibody–drug conjugates are large and heterogeneous biomolecules. Their inherent complexity needs multiple complementary analytical approaches to achieve their comprehensive characterization, among which are liquid chromatography and mass spectrometry. Compared to 1D-LC, 2D-LC is a very attractive technique, since it enables to combine two chromatographic separations, hence maximizing the information gained during a single analysis. In the context of ADC analysis, the comprehensive approach is the most efficient way to benefit from extensive information on the complete sample. This chapter gives an overview of the different online LC × LC techniques that have been used for ADC analysis. Different orthogonal combinations were proven to be highly valuable for ADC characterization at different levels (intact ADC analysis, top/middle-down, middle-up and bottom-up approaches). Those include online HIC × SEC, SEC × SEC, HIC × RPLC, CEX × RPLC, HILIC × RPLC and RPLC × RPLC. In most reported studies, commercially available 2D-LC instruments were used. However, online LC × LC can also be carried out by combining two independent LC instruments, as online HIC × SEC or online SEC × SEC presented in Subheading 2. At first instance, 2D-LC may be used as a rapid way to enable the online coupling of noncompatible chromatographic separations with MS detection by providing a desalting step in the second dimension. This strategy was used with HIC, SEC and CEX in the first dimension. In addition, a second dimension offers more information on the formerly separated species by increasing the chromatographic separation space. Finally, the versatility of online LC × LC hyphenated to HRMS and also IMS makes it a powerful analytical tool for an extensive characterization of ADCs.

References

1. Beck A, Wurch T, Bailly C, Corvaia N (2010) Strategies and challenges for the next generation of therapeutic antibodies. Nat Rev Immunol 10:345–352. https://doi.org/10.1038/nri2747
2. Beck A, Reichert JM (2014) Antibody-drug conjugates: present and future. MAbs 6:15–17. https://doi.org/10.4161/mabs.27436
3. Beck A, Goetsch L, Dumontet C, Corvaïa N (2017) Strategies and challenges for the next generation of antibody-drug conjugates. Nat Rev Drug Discov 16:315–337. https://doi.org/10.1038/nrd.2016.268
4. Beck A, Wagner-Rousset E, Ayoub D, Van Dorsselaer A, Sanglier-Cianférani S (2013) Characterization of therapeutic antibodies and related products. Anal Chem 85:715–736. https://doi.org/10.1021/ac3032355
5. Panowski S, Bhakta S, Raab H, Polakis P, Junutula JR (2013) Site-specific antibody drug conjugates for cancer therapy. MAbs 6:34–45. https://doi.org/10.4161/mabs.27022
6. Le LN, Moore JMR, Ouyang J, Chen X, Nguyen MDH, Galush WJ (2012) Profiling antibody drug conjugate positional isomers: a system-of-equations approach. Anal Chem 84:7479–7486. https://doi.org/10.1021/ac301568f
7. Sandra K, Vanhoenacker G, Vandenheede I, Steenbeke M, Joseph M, Sandra P (2016) Multiple heart-cutting and comprehensive two-dimensional liquid chromatography hyphenated to mass spectrometry for the characterization of the antibody-drug conjugate ado-trastuzumab emtansine. J Chromatogr B 1032:119–130. https://doi.org/10.1016/j.jchromb.2016.04.040
8. Fekete S, Guillarme D, Sandra P, Sandra K (2016) Chromatographic, electrophoretic, and mass spectrometric methods for the analytical characterization of protein biopharmaceuticals. Anal Chem 88:480–507. https://doi.org/10.1021/acs.analchem.5b04561
9. Debaene F, Bœuf A, Wagner-Rousset E, Colas O, Ayoub D, Corvaïa N, Dorsselaer AV, Beck A, Cianférani S (2014) Innovative native MS methodologies for antibody drug conjugate characterization: high resolution native MS and IM-MS for average DAR and DAR distribution assessment. Anal Chem 86:10674–10683. https://doi.org/10.1021/acs.analchem.502593n
10. Stoll D, Danforth J, Zhang K, Beck A (2016) Characterization of therapeutic antibodies and related products by two-dimensional liquid chromatography coupled with UV absorbance and mass spectrometric detection. J Chromatogr B 1032:51–60. https://doi.org/10.1016/j.jchromb.2016.05.029
11. Sarrut M, Rouvière F, Heinisch S (2017) Theoretical and experimental comparison of one dimensional versus on-line comprehensive two dimensional liquid chromatography for optimized sub-hour separations of complex peptide samples. J Chromatogr A 1498:183–195. https://doi.org/10.1016/j.chroma.2017.01.054
12. Schoenmakers PJ, Mariott P (2003) Nomenclature and conventions in comprehensive multidimensional chromatography. LCGC Europe 16:335–339
13. Guiochon G, Marchetti N, Mriziq K, Shalliker RA (2008) Implementations of two-dimensional liquid chromatography. J Chromatogr A 1189:109–168. https://doi.org/10.1016/j.chroma.2008.01.086
14. Bedani F, Schoenmakers PJ, Janssen H-G (2012) Theories to support method development in comprehensive two-dimensional liquid chromatography – a review. J Sep Sci 35:1697–1711. https://doi.org/10.1002/jssc.201200070
15. Li Y, Gu C, Gruenhagen J, Zhang K, Yehl P, Chetwyn NP, Medley CD (2015) A size exclusion-reversed phase two dimensional-liquid chromatography methodology for stability and small molecule related species in antibody drug conjugates. J Chromatogr A 1393:81–88. https://doi.org/10.1016/j.chroma.2015.03.027
16. Goyon A, Sciascera L, Clarke A, Guillarme D, Pell R (2018) Extending the limits of size

exclusion chromatography: simultaneous separation of free payloads and related species from antibody drug conjugates and their aggregates. J Chromatogr A 1539:19–29. https://doi.org/10.1016/j.chroma.2018.01.039

17. Groskreutz SR, Swenson MM, Secor LB, Stoll DR (2012) Selective comprehensive multidimensional separation for resolution enhancement in high performance liquid chromatography. Part I: principles and instrumentation. J Chromatogr A 1228:31–40. https://doi.org/10.1016/j.chroma.2011.06.035
18. Venkatramani CJ, Huang SR, Al-Sayah M, Patel I, Wigman L (2017) High-resolution two-dimensional liquid chromatography analysis of key linker drug intermediate used in antibody drug conjugates. J Chromatogr A 1521:63–72. https://doi.org/10.1016/j.chroma.2017.09.022
19. Marcoux J, Champion T, Colas O, Wagner-Rousset E, Corvaïa N, Dorsselaer AV, Beck A, Cianférani S (2015) Native mass spectrometry and ion mobility characterization of trastuzumab emtansine, a lysine-linked antibody drug conjugate. Protein Sci 24:1210–1223. https://doi.org/10.1002/pro.2666
20. Chen J, Yin S, Wu Y, Ouyang J (2013) Development of a native nanoelectrospray mass spectrometry method for determination of the drug-to-antibody ratio of antibody–drug conjugates. Anal Chem 85:1699–1704. https://doi.org/10.1021/ac302959p
21. Rosati S, Yang Y, Barendregt A, Heck AJR (2014) Detailed mass analysis of structural heterogeneity in monoclonal antibodies using native mass spectrometry. Nat Protoc 9:967–976. https://doi.org/10.1038/nprot.2014.057
22. Rosati S, Rose RJ, Thompson NJ, van Duijn E, Damoc E, Denisov E, Makarov A, Heck AJR (2012) Exploring an orbitrap analyzer for the characterization of intact antibodies by native mass spectrometry. Angew Chem Int Ed 51:12992–12996. https://doi.org/10.1002/anie.201206745
23. Thompson NJ, Rosati S, Heck AJR (2014) Performing native mass spectrometry analysis on therapeutic antibodies. Methods 65:11–17. https://doi.org/10.1016/j.ymeth.2013.05.003
24. Campuzano IDG, Netirojjanakul C, Nshanian M, Lippens JL, Kilgour DPA, Van Orden S, Loo JA (2018) Native-MS analysis of monoclonal antibody conjugates by Fourier transform ion cyclotron resonance mass spectrometry. Anal Chem 90:745–751. https://doi.org/10.1021/acs.analchem.7b03021
25. Li W, Kerwin JL, Schiel J, Formolo T, Davis D, Mahan A, Benchaar SA (2015) Structural elucidation of post-translational modifications in monoclonal antibodies. In: State-of-the-art and emerging technologies for therapeutic monoclonal antibody characterization volume 2. Biopharmaceutical characterization: the NISTmAb Case Study. American Chemical Society, Washington, DC 20036, USA pp 119–183. https://doi.org/10.1021/bk-2015-1201.ch003
26. Ehkirch A, D'Atri V, Rouviere F, Hernandez-Alba O, Goyon A, Colas O, Sarrut M, Beck A, Guillarme D, Heinisch S, Cianferani S (2018) An online four-dimensional HIC×SEC-IM×MS methodology for proof-of-concept characterization of antibody drug conjugates. Anal Chem 90:1578–1586. https://doi.org/10.1021/acs.analchem.7b02110
27. Ehkirch A, Goyon A, Hernandez-Alba O, Rouviere F, D'Atri V, Dreyfus C, Haeuw J-F, Diemer H, Beck A, Heinisch S, Guillarme D, Cianferani S (2018) A novel online four-dimensional SEC×SEC-IM×MS methodology for characterization of monoclonal antibody size variants. Anal Chem 90:13929–13937. https://doi.org/10.1021/acs.analchem.8b03333
28. Birdsall RE, Shion H, Kotch FW, Xu A, Porter TJ, Chen W (2015) A rapid on-line method for mass spectrometric confirmation of a cysteine-conjugated antibody-drug-conjugate structure using multidimensional chromatography. MAbs 7:1036–1044. https://doi.org/10.1080/19420862.2015.1083665
29. Sarrut M, Fekete S, Janin-Bussat M-C, Colas O, Guillarme D, Beck A, Heinisch S (2016) Analysis of antibody-drug conjugates by comprehensive on-line two-dimensional hydrophobic interaction chromatography x reversed phase liquid chromatography hyphenated to high resolution mass spectrometry. II- Identification of sub-units for the characterization of even and odd load drug species. J Chromatogr B 1032:91–102. https://doi.org/10.1016/j.jchromb.2016.06.049
30. Sarrut M, Corgier A, Fekete S, Guillarme D, Lascoux D, Janin-Bussat M-C, Beck A, Heinisch S (2016) Analysis of antibody-drug conjugates by comprehensive on-line two-dimensional hydrophobic interaction chromatography x reversed phase liquid chromatography hyphenated to high resolution mass spectrometry. I – optimization of separation conditions. J Chromatogr B 1032:103–111. https://doi.org/10.1016/j.jchromb.2016.06.048

31. Sorensen M, Harmes DC, Stoll DR, Staples GO, Fekete S, Guillarme D, Beck A (2016) Comparison of originator and biosimilar therapeutic monoclonal antibodies using comprehensive two-dimensional liquid chromatography coupled with time-of-flight mass spectrometry. MAbs 8:1224–1234. https://doi.org/10.1080/19420862.2016.1203497
32. Stoll DR, Harmes DC, Danforth J, Wagner E, Guillarme D, Fekete S, Beck A (2015) Direct identification of rituximab main isoforms and subunit analysis by online selective comprehensive two-dimensional liquid chromatography--mass spectrometry. Anal Chem 87:8307–8315. https://doi.org/10.1021/acs.analchem.5b01578
33. Stoll DR, Harmes DC, Staples GO, Potter OG, Dammann CT, Guillarme D, Beck A (2018) Development of comprehensive online two-dimensional liquid chromatography/mass spectrometry using hydrophilic interaction and reversed-phase separations for rapid and deep profiling of therapeutic antibodies. Anal Chem 90:5923–5929. https://doi.org/10.1021/acs.analchem.8b00776
34. Periat A, Fekete S, Cusumano A, Veuthey J-L, Beck A, Lauber M, Guillarme D (2016) Potential of hydrophilic interaction chromatography for the analytical characterization of protein biopharmaceuticals. J Chromatogr A 1448:81–92. https://doi.org/10.1016/j.chroma.2016.04.056
35. D'Atri V, Fekete S, Beck A, Lauber M, Guillarme D (2017) Hydrophilic interaction chromatography hyphenated with mass spectrometry: a powerful analytical tool for the comparison of originator and biosimilar therapeutic monoclonal antibodies at the middle-up level of analysis. Anal Chem 89:2086–2092. https://doi.org/10.1021/acs.analchem.6b04726
36. D'Atri V, Dumont E, Vandenheede I, Guillarme D, Sandra P, Sandra K (2017) Hydrophilic interaction chromatography for the characterization of therapeutic monoclonal antibodies at protein, peptide, and glycan levels. LCGC Europe 30:424–434
37. Domínguez-Vega E, Tengattini S, Peintner C, van Angeren J, Temporini C, Haselberg R, Massolini G, Somsen GW (2018) High-resolution glycoform profiling of intact therapeutic proteins by hydrophilic interaction chromatography-mass spectrometry. Talanta 184:375–381. https://doi.org/10.1016/j.talanta.2018.03.015
38. D'Atri V, Fekete S, Stoll D, Lauber M, Beck A, Guillarme D (2018) Characterization of an antibody-drug conjugate by hydrophilic interaction chromatography coupled to mass spectrometry. J Chromatogr B 1080:37–41. https://doi.org/10.1016/j.jchromb.2018.02.026
39. Chapel S, Rouvière F, Heinisch S Unpublished results
40. Vanhoenacker G, Vandenheede I, David F, Sandra P, Sandra K (2015) Comprehensive two-dimensional liquid chromatography of therapeutic monoclonal antibody digests. Anal Bioanal Chem 407:355–366. https://doi.org/10.1007/s00216-014-8299-1

Chapter 12

Drug Loading and Distribution of ADCs After Reduction or IdeS Digestion and Reduction

Elsa Wagner-Rousset, Olivier Colas, Yannis-Nicolas François, Sabine Heinisch, Davy Guillarme, Sarah Cianférani, and Alain Beck

Abstract

High-resolution native mass spectrometry (MS) provides accurate mass measurements (within 30 ppm) of intact ADCs and can also yield drug load distribution (DLD) and average drug to antibody ratio (DAR) in parallel with hydrophobic interaction chromatography (HIC). Native MS is furthermore unique in its ability to simultaneously detect covalent and noncovalent species in a mixture and for HIC peak identity assessment offline or online.

As an orthogonal method described in this chapter, LC-MS following ADC reduction or IdeS (Fabricator) digestion and reduction can also be used to measure the DLD of light chain and Fd fragments for hinge native cysteine residues such as brentuximab vedotin. Both methods allow also the measurement of average DAR for both monomeric and multimeric species. In addition, the Fc fragments can be analyzed in the same run, providing a complete glycoprofile and the demonstration or absence of additional conjugation of this subdomain involved in FcRn and Fc-gammaR binding.

Key words Brentuximab vedotin, DAR, DLD, Fabricator, HIC, IdeS, Mass spectrometry

1 Introduction

The development and optimization of antibody drug conjugates (ADCs) rely on improving their analytical and bioanalytical characterization, by assessing critical quality attributes (CQAs). Among the CQAs, the glycoprofile, drug load distribution (DLD), the amount of unconjugated antibody (D0), the average drug-to-antibody ratio (DAR), the drug conjugation sites and the residual drug-linker and related product proportions (small-molecule-drugs, SMDs) in addition to high and low molecular weight species (H/LMWS), and charge variants are the most important ones [1].

Even if structural insights can be obtained for intact ADCs by native MS and Ion Mobility-MS (IM-MS) [2], the higher mass accuracy provided by the more straightforward RP-HPLC-MS analysis of their subunits remains valuable for example for Quality

L. Nathan Tumey (ed.), *Antibody-Drug Conjugates: Methods and Protocols*, Methods in Molecular Biology, vol. 2078,
https://doi.org/10.1007/978-1-4939-9929-3_12,

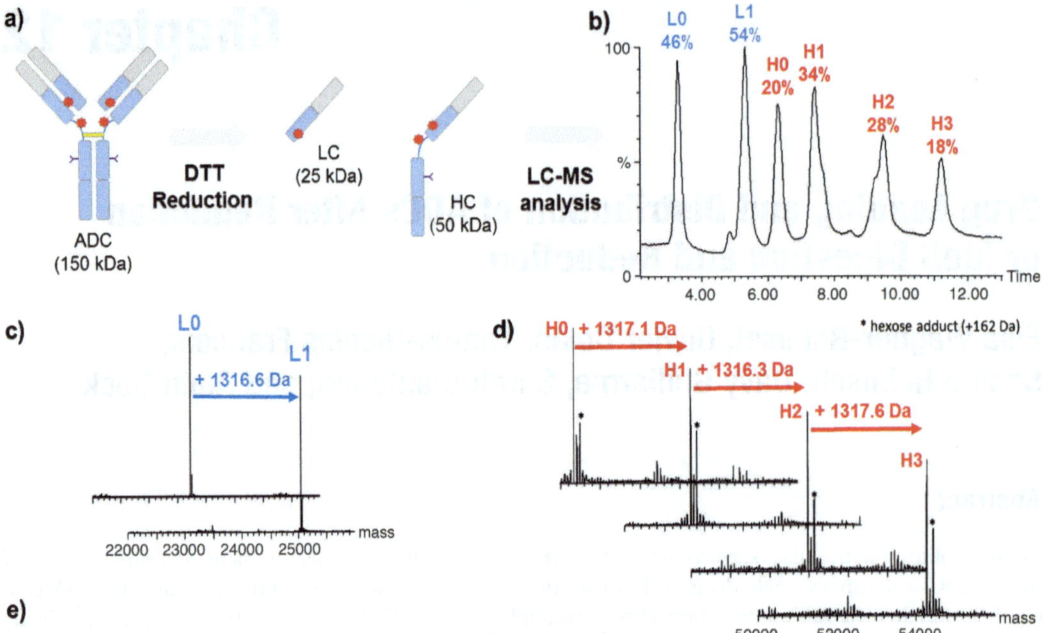

e)

Species	Theoretical mass (Da)	Experimental mass (Da)	Delta (Da)	Retention time (min)	Distribution (%)	Average DAR
L0	23728.3	23727.5	0.8	3.32	46	
L1	25044.1	25044.1	0.0	5.33	54	
H0	50328.6	50327.0	1.6	6.33	20	4.0
H1	51644.4	51644.1	0.3	7.42	34	
H2	52960.2	52960.4	0.2	9.48	28	
H3	54276.0	54278.0	2.0	11.22	18	

Fig. 1 Middle-level characterization of brentuximab vedotin (BV) after reduction. (**a**) Schematic representation of the middle-level workflow. (**b**) rpHPLC chromatogram of BV fragments obtained after DTT reduction and IAA alkylation. Deconvoluted mass spectra of BV LC (**c**) and HC (**d**) fragments. (**d**) Table summarizing masses and proportions of the different BV fragments and the average DAR measured from peak areas

Control Labs. As for unconjugated mAbs, ADC profiles can be simplified by reduction (yielding the light and heavy chains at ~25 and ~50 kDa, respectively) as illustrated in Fig. 1 or by enzymatic treatments, such as *N*-deglycosylation (IgGZERO® or PNGase-F) [3], carboxypeptidase B digestion [4], or glutaminyl–peptide cyclotransferase treatment [5]. Smaller mAb fragments can also be generated by papain digestion (producing ~50 kDa Fab/Fc fragments) or IdeS digestion (Fabricator®, the immunoglobulin degrading enzyme of *Streptococcus pyogenes*) followed by reduction with dithiothreitol (DTT, for Fc/2, LC, and Fd fragments of ~25 kDa), as illustrated in Fig. 2. This approach has the advantages of being fast (requiring less than 2 h for the entire analysis, including digestion and RP-HPLC-MS analysis), informative, and inexpensive in terms of materials. Reduction experiments leading to individual light and heavy chains or IdeS treatment are also used for middle up and down mass spectrometry sequencing of IgGs [6].

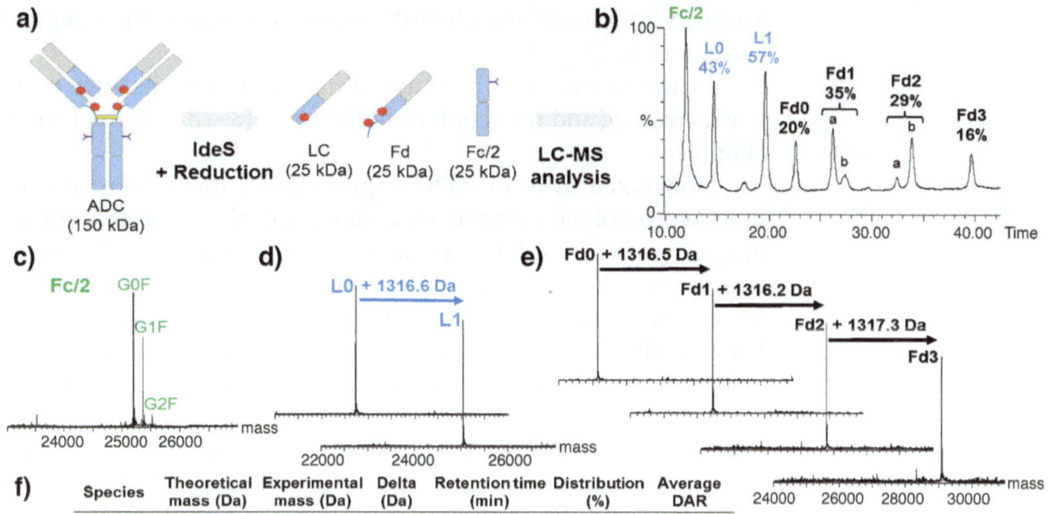

f)

Species	Theoretical mass (Da)	Experimental mass (Da)	Delta (Da)	Retention time (min)	Distribution (%)	Average DAR
Fc/2 (G0F)	25203.6	25203.9	0.3	11.93	-	
Fc/2 (G1F)	25365.8	25365.9	0.1	11.93	-	
Fc/2 (G2F)	25528.0	25528.1	0.1	11.93	-	
L0	23728.3	23727.8	0.5	14.62	43	
L1	25044.1	25044.4	0.3	19.55	57	
Fd0	25142.3	25141.8	0.5	22.53	20	4.0
Fd1a	26459.1	26458.3	0.8	26.15	35	
Fd1b	26459.1	26458.3	0.8	27.40		
Fd2a	27774.9	27774.5	0.4	32.43	29	
Fd2b	27774.9	27774.6	0.3	33.85		
Fd3	29091.7	29091.9	0.2	39.57	16	

Fig. 2 Middle-level characterization of brentuximab vedotin (BV) after IdeS digestion and reduction. (**a**) Schematic representation of the middle-level workflow. (**b**) rpHPLC chromatogram of BV fragments obtained after IdeS cleavage and DTT reduction. Deconvoluted mass spectra of BV LC (**c**), Fc/2 (**d**) and Fd (**e**) fragments. (**f**) Table summarizing masses and proportions of the different BV fragments and the average DAR measured from peak areas

Characterization of brentuximab vedotin subunits under denaturing and reducing conditions (middle-level, 23–54 kDa fragments) (Fig. 1).

Reducing treatments are a routine way to divide the analysis of mAbs and ADCs into more manageable pieces. The drug-loading profile and average DAR can then be obtained by RP-HPLC with MS, as an orthogonal method to HIC [7]—as for the latter, RP-HPLC relies on differences in hydrophobicity. This middle-up strategy can be implemented on any current HPLC-MS instrumentation and is therefore available in most labs. Treatment of cysteine-linked ADCs with DTT or tris(2-carboxyethyl) phosphine (TCEP) fully reduces the remaining inter-chain disulfides and yields six species: light chains with zero or one drug molecule attached (L0 and L1), and heavy chains with zero, one, two, or three drug molecules attached (H0, H1, H2, and H3). These species are stable in the denaturing organic solvent and can be successfully separated on a reversed phase column. The percentage peak area from integration of the light chain and heavy chain peaks, combined with the assigned drug load for each peak, is used to calculate the weighted average DAR (Fig. 1).

Characterization of brentuximab vedotin subunits after enzymatic cleavage and reduction (middle-level, 23–28 kDa fragments) (Fig. 2).

Downsized mAb or ADC fragments can also be obtained by limited proteolytic cleavage under nondenaturing conditions in the hinge region of the heavy chain, yielding Fab or (Fab′)2, and Fc fragments, whose reduction (with DTT) produces even smaller fragments of approximately 25 kDa: the light chain and the two halves of the heavy chain (Fc/2 and Fd). Formerly conducted with proteases with a limited specificity, such as papain, pepsin, and endoprotease Lys-C, the enzymatic cleavage for middle-level analyses is mostly conducted using IdeS, a bacterial protease that specifically cleaves IgGs under the hinge region [8, 9]. The potency of IdeS has been demonstrated for cysteine-linked ADCs on an antibody–fluorophore conjugate [3]. This rapid IdeS- and RP-HPLCMS-based workflow was also employed by Firth et al. for the characterization of two auristatin-based ADCs [10] as well as by Rouse et al. [11, 12]. With IdeS, a complete middle-level characterization can be completed within a few hours, providing the primary sequence and the glycoprofiles of the Fab and Fc fragments. The data can also be used for biosimilar comparability studies and Fc-fusion protein studies. More recently, IdeS digestion has been shown to be preferable to DTT treatment for the characterization of BV, the LC fragments being better separated in the subsequent RP-HPLC-MS analysis, allowing the identification of positional isomers [13]. In addition to the seven expected major peaks (from the Fc/2, L0, L1, Fd0, Fd1, Fd2, and Fd3 fragments), two minor satellite peaks with identical masses are observed close to those from Fd1 and Fd2 (Fig. 2) and tentatively assigned to positional isomers. This was confirmed by peptide mapping with nanoLC-MS/MS following the digestion with endoprotease Lys-C of isolated fragments.

This IdeS and reduction workflow can also be followed by HILIC-MS and orthogonal method as recently reported by Guillarme et al. for brentuximab vedotin [14], followed by CE-MS as highlighted by François et al. [15]. This middle-up approach was also successfully used to characterize 3G-ADCs, by Cianférani et al. [16, 17].

2 Materials

2.1 Chemicals

Ultrapure water produced from a Milli-Q Water System™ (Millipore). All chemicals were of analytical grade. References are given as information and may be replaced by equivalent reagents.

1. Acetic acid 90% (VWR, ref.: 20109.295).
2. Acetonitrile (Carlo Erba, ref.: 412342).
3. Cesium Iodide (CsI, Merck, ref.: 102861).
4. Dithiothreitol (DTT, Aldrich, ref.: 150460).
5. FabRICATOR 2000 units (IdeS, Genovis, ref.: A0-FR1-020).
6. Ethylenediamine tetraacetic acid (EDTA, ref.: ED2SS).
7. Guanidine hydrochloride 99% (Aldrich, ref.: 177253).
8. Trifluoroacetic Acid (TFA, Fluka, ref.: 91699).
9. Tris–HCl (Trizma Base, Sigma, ref.: T6066).

2.2 ADC

Brentuximab vedotin was purchased from Takeda Pharma (Danemark).

2.3 Ultra Performance Liquid Chromatography

1. LC equipment. Acquity™ UPLC system consisting in a Binary solvent manager, a sample manager, and a TUV detector (Waters).
2. PLRP-s column 1000 Å, 2.1 × 150 mm, 8 μm (Agilent PL1912–3802).
3. Mobile phases. Eluting solution A: MilliQ water +0.05% TFA. Eluting solution B: Acetonitrile +0.05% TFA.

2.4 Mass Analysis

LCT Premier™ Waters mass spectrometer equipped with an electrospray (ESI) source and a time-of-flight (TOF) analyzer. MS analysis is performed in the W-positive ion mode.

Calibration and Lock Spray CsI solution: dissolve CsI in water/isopropanol, 50/50 (v/v) to have a 2 mg/mL solution for daily use.

After instrument conditioning with a mixture of eluting solutions A/B 50/50 (v/v) at 0.2 mL/min, calibrate the LCT Premier™ by infusing the CsI calibration solution. CsI forms 12 charged clusters from 900 to 4000 *m/z*.

2.5 Reagents Preparation

1. 0.5 mL Eppendorf tubes.
2. Pipets and corresponding tips.
3. Thermomixer + block tube 0.5 mL.
4. Reduction buffer. 6 M guanidine buffer pH 8 containing 2 mM EDTA and 0.1 M Tris–HCl. For 10 mL: dissolve 0.121 g Tris–HCl, 7.4 mg EDTA, 5.730 g guanidine HCl, solubilize in 9 mL MilliQ water, adjust the pH at 8.0 with 6 N HCl, and complete to 10 mL with MilliQ water.
5. Reducing reagent. Dissolve DTT in MilliQ water to have a 500 mM solution (77 mg/mL) for extemporaneous use.

3 Methods

3.1 General Principle

The ADC is either:

- Reduced into two chains (light chain and heavy chain) which may carry payloads: up to one for the light chain and up to three for the heavy chain and which are designed respectively as L0, L1, H0, H1, H2, and H3.

  or,

- IdeS digested and reduced into three fragments (Fc/2, Fd, LC) which may carry payloads: up to one for the light chain and up to three for the Fd and which are designed respectively as L0, L1, Fd0, Fd1, Fd2, and Fd3.

These ADC fragments are adsorbed on the reversed phase column thanks to hydrophobic interactions. They are then eluted by increasing the amount of eluting solution B during the chromatographic gradient.

UV detection at 210 nm of the separated ADC fragments results in the drug load profile which is used for the average DAR calculation. MS detection is achieved in parallel to check the identity of each fragment.

3.2 Sample Preparation

3.2.1 Reduction

1. Add 25 μg of the ADC sample into an Eppendorf tube.
2. Dilute with reduction buffer to reach a volume of 23.5 μL.
3. Add 1.5 μL of 500 mM DTT. The final concentration of ADC is 1 mg/mL and DTT concentration is 30 mM.
4. Incubate for 45 min in the thermomixer at 56 °C under agitation (750 rpm).
5. Quench the reaction by adding 1 μL acetic acid.

3.2.2 IdeS Digestion and Reduction

1. Add 25 μg of the ADC sample into an Eppendorf tube.
2. Add 1.25 μL of FabRICATOR (IdeS, *see* **Note 4**) (1 unit of IdeS/μg of sample).
3. Complete to 10 μL with MilliQ Water.
4. Incubate for 30 min in the thermomixer at 37 °C under agitation (750 tr/min).
5. Dilute with reduction buffer to reach a volume of 23.5 μL.
6. Add 1.5 μL of 500 mM DTT. The final concentration of ADC is 1 mg/mL and DTT concentration is 30 mM.
7. Incubate for 45 min in the thermomixer at 56 °C under agitation (750 tr/min).
8. Quench the reaction by adding 1 μL acetic acid.

9. Equilibrate the column by running through 70% solvent A at a flow rate of 0.5 mL/min for 10 min.
10. Set up the mass spectrometer and check the stable spray with elution buffer. The voltage applied to the capillary cap was set to 3000 V. The mass spectrometer transmission parameters were optimized for high *m/z* set optimal around 3000 V. Ions are scanned over a *m/z* range of 1000–5000. Source and desolvation temperatures are set to 150 and 300 °C, respectively. Cone and aperture voltages are set to 120 and 40 V, respectively. Nitrogen gas flow rates are set at 50 L/h for the cone and 800 L/h for desolvation.
11. Inject the ADC sample preparation (8 μL) onto the column and simultaneously start both the chromatography gradient and the mass spectrometer data collection.
12. The analytical column is eluted typically at a flow rate of 0.5 mL/min by a three-step linear gradient: (1) 30%B to 45% B in 13 min. (2) 45%B to 95%B of solvent B in 2 min. (3) 95%B to 30%B in 2 min followed by a 10 min equilibration step at 30%B.

3.3 Data Analysis

3.3.1 MS Data Treatment

1. Using Masslynx™, open the Total Ion Chromatogram.
2. The lock mass correction factor is calculated from the MS signal of CsI solution infused within the lockspray (*m/z*: 1691.765) (*see* **Note 1**).
3. Combine spectra of each chromatographically separated peak.
4. Smooth and perform spectrum deconvolution using Maxent-1™.

3.3.2 UV Data Treatment

1. Display the UV chromatogram at 210 nm in Masslynx™.
2. Integrate each chromatographic peak:
   (a) L0, L1, H0, H1, H2, and H3 (Reduced ADC).
   (b) L0, L1, Fd0, Fd1, Fd2, and Fd3 (IdeS digested and reduced ADC).
3. From the result of integration (peak surfaces), calculate the percentage of each loaded fragment: (1) for the light chain and for the heavy chain or (2) for the light chain and for the Fd. This would result in a typical payload distribution (*see* **Note 2**).
4. From the payload distribution, perform the average DAR calculation as follows (*see* **Note 3**):
   - DAR(L) $= \Sigma[n\mathrm{AL}n/\Sigma\mathrm{AL}]$ (in principle from $n = 0$ to $n = 1$).
   - DAR(H) $= \Sigma[n\mathrm{AH}n/\Sigma\mathrm{AH}]$ (in principle from $n = 0$ to $n = 3$).
   - Av.DAR $= 2 \times$ [DAR(L) + DAR(H)].

4 Notes

1. After lock mass correction, measured masses should be within ±5 Da around theoretical masses calculated from the amino acid sequence.
2. The payload distribution (i.e., % of each fragment) calculated from the LC-UV chromatogram should be within ±5 around following values: L0 = 45%; L1 = 55%; H0 = 18%; H1 = 32%; H2 = 30%; H3 = 20%.
3. The calculated average DAR of the control ADC brentuximab vedotin should be 4 ± 0.5.
4. FabRICATOR (IdeS) is a cysteine protease that digests antibodies at a specific site below the hinge, generating a homogenous pool of F(ab′)2 and Fc/2 fragments for Human IgG1–4, IgG from monkey, rat, rabbit, and sheep.

References

1. Beck A, D'Atri V, Ehkirch A et al (2019) Cutting-edge multi-level analytical and structural characterization of antibody-drug conjugates: present and future. Expert Rev Proteomics 16:337–362. https://doi.org/10.1080/14789450.2019.1578215
2. Beck A, Terral G, Debaene F et al (2016) Cutting-edge mass spectrometry methods for the multi-level structural characterization of antibody-drug conjugates. Expert Rev Proteomics 13:157–183. https://doi.org/10.1586/14789450.2016.1132167
3. Wagner-Rousset E, Janin-Bussat M-C, Colas O et al (2014) Antibody-drug conjugate model fast characterization by LC-MS following IdeS proteolytic digestion. MAbs 6:273–285. https://doi.org/10.4161/mabs.26773
4. Beck A, Bussat M-C, Zorn N et al (2005) Characterization by liquid chromatography combined with mass spectrometry of monoclonal anti-IGF-1 receptor antibodies produced in CHO and NS0 cells. J Chromatogr B Analyt Technol Biomed Life Sci 819:203–218. https://doi.org/10.1016/j.jchromb.2004.06.052
5. Xu W, Peng Y, Wang F et al (2013) Method to convert N-terminal glutamine to pyroglutamate for characterization of recombinant monoclonal antibodies. Anal Biochem 436:10–12. https://doi.org/10.1016/j.ab.2013.01.017
6. Srzentić K, Nagornov KO, Fornelli L et al (2018) Multiplexed middle-down mass spectrometry as a method for revealing light and heavy chain connectivity in a monoclonal antibody. Anal Chem 90:12527–12535. https://doi.org/10.1021/acs.analchem.8b02398
7. Basa L (2013) Drug-to-antibody ratio (DAR) and drug load distribution by LC-ESI-MS. In: Ducry L (ed) Antibody-drug conjugates. Humana Press, Totowa, NJ, pp 285–293
8. Chevreux G, Tilly N, Bihoreau N (2011) Fast analysis of recombinant monoclonal antibodies using IdeS proteolytic digestion and electrospray mass spectrometry. Anal Biochem 415:212–214. https://doi.org/10.1016/j.ab.2011.04.030
9. Sjögren J, Olsson F, Beck A (2016) Rapid and improved characterization of therapeutic antibodies and antibody related products using IdeS digestion and subunit analysis. Analyst 141:3114–3125. https://doi.org/10.1039/C6AN00071A
10. Firth D, Bell L, Squires M et al (2015) A rapid approach for characterization of thiol-conjugated antibody–drug conjugates and calculation of drug–antibody ratio by liquid chromatography mass spectrometry. Anal Biochem 485:34–42. https://doi.org/10.1016/j.ab.2015.06.001
11. Friese OV, Smith JN, Brown PW, Rouse JC (2018) Practical approaches for overcoming challenges in heightened characterization of antibody-drug conjugates with new methodologies and ultrahigh-resolution mass spectrometry. MAbs 10:335–345. https://doi.org/10.1080/19420862.2018.1433973

12. Lin TJ, Beal KM, Brown PW et al (2019) Evolution of a comprehensive, orthogonal approach to sequence variant analysis for biotherapeutics. mAbs 11:1–12. https://doi.org/10.1080/19420862.2018.1531965
13. Janin-Bussat M-C, Dillenbourg M, Corvaia N et al (2015) Characterization of antibody drug conjugate positional isomers at cysteine residues by peptide mapping LC–MS analysis. J Chromatogr B 981–982:9–13. https://doi.org/10.1016/j.jchromb.2014.12.017
14. D'Atri V, Fekete S, Stoll D et al (2018) Characterization of an antibody-drug conjugate by hydrophilic interaction chromatography coupled to mass spectrometry. J Chromatogr B 1080:37–41. https://doi.org/10.1016/j.jchromb.2018.02.026
15. Said N, Gahoual R, Kuhn L et al (2016) Structural characterization of antibody drug conjugate by a combination of intact, middle-up and bottom-up techniques using sheathless capillary electrophoresis—tandem mass spectrometry as nanoESI infusion platform and separation method. Anal Chim Acta 918:50–59. https://doi.org/10.1016/j.aca.2016.03.006
16. Beck A, Goetsch L, Dumontet C, Corvaïa N (2017) Strategies and challenges for the next generation of antibody–drug conjugates. Nat Rev Drug Discov 16:315–337. https://doi.org/10.1038/nrd.2016.268
17. Botzanowski T, Erb S, Hernandez-Alba O et al (2017) Insights from native mass spectrometry approaches for top- and middle-level characterization of site-specific antibody-drug conjugates. mAbs 9:801–811. https://doi.org/10.1080/19420862.2017.1316914

Chapter 13

Analysis of ADCs by Native Mass Spectrometry

Oscar Hernandez-Alba, Anthony Ehkirch, Alain Beck, and Sarah Cianférani

Abstract

Mass spectrometry performed in nondenaturing conditions (native MS) has proven its utility for the quantitative and qualitative analysis of antibody-drug conjugates (ADCs), especially when ADCs' subunits involve noncovalent interactions (i.e., cysteine-conjugated ADCs). Its hyphenation to ion mobility spectrometry (IM-MS) allows differentiation of gas-phase ions based on their rotationally averaged collision cross section providing an additional dimension of conformational characterization of ADCs. More recently, size exclusion chromatography (SEC) appeared as an interesting technique to perform online buffer exchange in an automated way prior to native MS/IM-MS analysis. Online SEC-native MS/IM-MS allows the global structural characterization of ADCs and the assessment of some critical quality attributes (CQAs) required for ADC release on the market, such as drug load distribution (DLD), drug-to-antibody ratio (DAR), the average DAR (DAR*av*), and the relative amount of unconjugated mAb.

Key words Native mass spectrometry, Antibody-drug conjugate, Ion mobility mass spectrometry, Size exclusion chromatography-native mass spectrometry

1 Introduction

ADCs are tripartite molecules designed to improve the therapeutic efficacy of monoclonal antibodies (mAbs) through the covalent addition of a cytotoxic molecule via a linker [1]. The heterogeneity associated to ADCs can vary, depending on the bioconjugation chemistry used to attach the cytotoxic molecules to the mAb structure [2]. Several studies have shown the suitability of native mass spectrometry (MS) for ADC analysis [3–13]. The reduced charge state of the ions under nondenaturing conditions facilitates the identification and quantification of all the different DAR populations that can be potentially formed during the conjugation process. Furthermore, the rotationally averaged collision cross section (CCS) of each individual DAR population can be determined by

Oscar Hernandez-Alba and Anthony Ehkirch contributed equally to this work.

L. Nathan Tumey (ed.), *Antibody-Drug Conjugates: Methods and Protocols*, Methods in Molecular Biology, vol. 2078, https://doi.org/10.1007/978-1-4939-9929-3_13,

using ion mobility coupled to mass spectrometry (IM-MS) to assess the impact of the conjugation process on the overall conformation of the original mAb [6, 7]. However, sample preparation (desalting) is still mostly manual, labor intensive, and time-consuming prior to native IM-MS analysis. SEC-native MS not only allows online buffer exchange within few minutes but also provides separation, identification, and quantification of high/low molecular weight species [9]. Online SEC-native MS can be easily implemented in high-throughput automated environments, thus pushing native MS approaches to the forefront of ADC characterization in R&D laboratories.

2 Materials

All solutions are prepared with ultrapure water.

2.1 Mobile Phase for SEC-Native MS

100 mM $AcONH_4$, pH 6.8: weigh 3.08 g of $AcONH_4$ in a 500 mL volumetric flask. Add 400 mL of milli-Q water with stirring. No pH adjustment is needed.

2.2 Deglycosylated ADCs

ADCs were obtained as European Union pharmaceutical-grade drug product from their respective manufacturers. Deglycosylation was performed by incubating for 30 min at 37 °C one unit of IgGZERO (Genovis) per microgram of ADC.

2.3 Manual Buffer Exchange

1. 150 mM $AcONH_4$, pH 6.8: weigh 578 mg of $AcONH_4$ in a 50 mL falcon. Add 50 mL of milli-Q water with stirring.

2.4 Cesium Iodide Solution for Mass Spectrometer Calibration

Prepare a 2 g/L solution of cesium iodide in 50/50 isopropanol/water (v/v).

1. Synapt G2.
   (a) The automated chip-based nanoelectrospray device (Triversa Nanomate, Advion, Ithaca, USA) is operated in the positive ion mode. Set the capillary voltage and the nitrogen nanoflow at 1.75 kV and 0.60 psi respectively.
   (b) In MassLynx MS Tune windows, set the following parameters:
   (c) Operate the instrument in positive and sensitivity modes with a *m/z* range from 1000 to 10,000.
   (d) Nanoflow+ panel: Sampling Cone: 120 V. Extraction con: 5 V. Source Temperature: 90 °C. The Capillary Voltage and the gas flows are not used in the Nanomate interface setup.
   (e) Instrument: Trap and Transfer Collision Energy are turned off.

(f) Start a 2 min TOF-MS acquisition with a *m/z* range from 1000 to 10,000.

(g) Average the signal over the 2 min in the Chromatogram panel. In the spectrum panel, a Spectrum Smooth with ±10 Smooth window and a number of smooths of 2 with a "Mean" Smoothing method were realized. On the smooth spectrum, the TOF Spectrum Center with a min peak width at half height of 2 and a Centroid top at 80% was selected.

(h) In the Acquity UPLC Console, select "Create Calibration."

(i) In the calibration profile editor, select the right Mass Calibration Profile (CsI in the 1000–10,000 *m/z* range in positive and sensitivity modes).

(j) The Reference Compound (Csi_1000–10,000 positive) with reference masses from 1172.1450 to 7927.2031 Da is used for calibration.

2. Exactive Plus EMR.

(a) Using HESI source and the 500 μL Hamilton™ syringe, deliver cesium iodide solution with a flow rate set to 10 μL/min.

(b) In the MS Tune page manually set the following parameters: Operate the instrument in positive mode with a *m/z* range from 1000 to 20,000. Apply 25 eV and 100 eV for the CID and CE parameters, respectively. The source temperature is set at 250 °C, the capillary voltage is set to 4 kV, and the gas flows are set to 10 a.u. The trapping gas pressure is set to 7 a.u. The ion optics are set to 4 V for injection, inter, and bent flatapoles. Set the nominal resolution at 17,500 and activate the EMR mode.

(c) To perform the calibration, wait for a stable TIC (<12%) then select "Calibrate" and check "EMR MS Mass Calibration (pos)."

2.5 Ion Mobility Calibrants

1. 10 mM $AcONH_4$: weight 38 μg of $AcONH_4$ in 50 mL falcon. Add 50 mL of milli-Q water with stirring.
2. Weigh between 400 and 900 μg of concanavalin A from *canavalia ensiformis*, alcohol dehydrogenase from *saccharomyces cerevisiae*, and pyruvate kinase from rabbit muscle. Dissolve each individual calibrant in 100 μL of 10 mM ammonium acetate to reach a final tetrameric concentration between 30 and 40 μM (*see* **Note 1**).
3. Perform manual buffer exchange using a 50-kDa microconcentrator (*see* Subheading 2.3).

4. Use the nanodrop spectrophotometer to determine the concentration of the calibrant solutions after manual desalting.
5. Add the required volume of 10 mM AcONH4 solution to get a final concentration of 10 μM for each individual calibrant solution.

3 Methods

3.1 ADC Sample Preparation

1. A microconcentrator with an appropriate MWCO (such as Vivaspin 50-kD cutoff for classical ADCs, Sartorius, Göttingen, Germany) is used for manual buffer exchange.
2. Equilibrate the microconcentrator by adding 500 μL of 150 mM $AcONH_4$ at 14,000 g over 2 min and remove the eluate.
3. Repeat **step 3** twice.
4. Load between 25 and 50 μL of sample. Add $AcONH_4$ buffer to get a final volume of 500 μL.
5. Centrifuge for 10 min at 14,000 × *g* to concentrate down to 50 μL and remove the eluate. Add 450 μL of $AcONH_4$ buffer. Repeat the dilution concentration cycle five times.
6. After the last cycle, transfer the 50 μL of sample to an Eppendorf tube. Protein concentration is determined by UV absorbance using a NanoDrop spectrophotometer (Thermo Fisher Scientific, France).

3.2 Mass Spectrometer Calibration

1. Synapt G2.
   (a) The automated chip-based nanoelectrospray device (Triversa Nanomate, Advion, Ithaca, USA) is operated in the positive ion mode. Set the capillary voltage and the nitrogen nanoflow at 1.75 kV and 0.60 psi respectively.
   (b) In MassLynx MS Tune windows, set the following parameters:
   (c) Operate the instrument in positive and sensitivity modes with a m/z range from 1000 to 10,000.
   (d) Nanoflow+ panel: Sampling Cone: 120 V. Extraction con: 5 V. Source Temperature: 90 °C. The Capillary Voltage and the gas flows are not used in the Nanomate interface setup.
   (e) Instrument: Trap and Transfer Collision Energy are turned off.
   (f) Start a 2 min TOF-MS acquisition with a m/z range from 1000 to 10,000.

(g) Average the signal over the 2 min in the Chromatogram panel. In the spectrum panel, a Spectrum Smooth with ±10 Smooth window and a number of smooths of 2 with a "Mean" Smoothing method were realized. On the smooth spectrum, the TOF Spectrum Center with a min peak width at half height of 2 and a Centroid top at 80% was selected.

(h) In the Acquity UPLC Console, select "Create Calibration."

(i) In the calibration profile editor, select the right Mass Calibration Profile (CsI in the 1000–10,000 m/z range in positive and sensitivity modes).

(j) The Reference Compound (Csi_1000–10,000 positive) with reference masses from 1172.1450 to 7927.2031 Da is used for the calibration.

2. Exactive Plus EMR.

(a) Using HESI source and the 500 μL Hamilton™ syringe, deliver cesium iodide solution with a flow rate set to 10 μL/min.

(b) In the MS Tune page manually set the following parameters: Operate the instrument in positive mode with a m/z range from 1000 to 20,000. Apply 25 eV and 100 eV for the CID and CE parameters, respectively. The source temperature is set at 250 °C, the capillary voltage is set to 4 kV, and the gas flows are set to 10 a.u. The trapping gas pressure is set to 7 a.u. The ion optics are set to 4 V for injection, inter, and bent flatapoles. Set the nominal resolution at 17,500 and activate the EMR mode.

(c) To perform the calibration, wait for a stable TIC (<12%) then select "Calibrate" and check "EMR MS Mass Calibration (pos)."

3.3 Direct Infusion on Exactive Plus EMR for Native MS Experiment

1. Mass spectrometry setting for native MS experiment.

(a) Desalt between 100 μg and 150 μg of ADC in 150 mM ammonium acetate.

(b) Determine the concentration of the ADC solution after desalting by UV absorbance using NanoDrop spectrophotometer (Thermo Fisher Scientific, France).

(c) Prior to ADC mass analysis, perform Exactive Plus EMR calibration with 8 μL of cesium iodide solution (*see* Subheading 2.4).

(d) Connect the automated chip-based nanoESI infusion source (Triversa Nanomate, Advion, Ithaca, USA) to the Exactive Plus EMR.

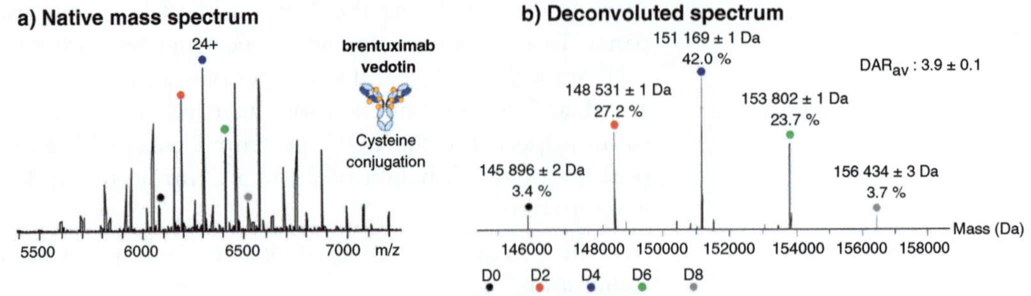

Fig. 1 Native MS analysis of deglycosylated brentuximab vedotin (Cysteine conjugate) on Exactive Plus EMR. (**a**) Native mass spectrum corresponding to brentuximab vedotin. (**b**) Deconvoluted mass spectrum representing the drug load distribution with the average DAR

(e) In the Tune page, set the following parameters: Positive mode with a *m/z* range from 1000 to 14,000. Activate the EMR mode and set the trapping gas pressure at 7 a.u., the ion optics at 8 V, 7 V, 6 V for inter, injection, and bent flatapoles respectively, the S-lens RF voltage at 200 V, the temperature at 250 °C, the fragmentation parameters at 75 eV and 10 eV for CID and CE values, respectively. Select a nominal resolution of 17,500.

(f) Start a 2 min acquisition with a stable TIC. The mass spectrum is presented in Fig. 1a.

2. Data interpretation.

(a) In BioPharma Finder 2.0, select your raw data file and Intact Protein Analysis.

(b) In chromatogram and Source Spectra, select a *m/z* range from 5500 to 7500. In ReSpect Deconvolution Algorithm, set a Model Mass Range from 145,000 to 160,000 with a mass tolerance of 10 ppm. Select a charge state range from 18 to 35. For the Choice of Peak Model, select Raw File Specific for the Resolution at 400 *m/z*.

(c) Process the algorithm in order to have the deconvoluted spectrum presented in Fig. 1b.

(d) For average DAR (DARav), *see* Subheading 3.4.

3.4 Direct Infusion on Synapt G2 for Native MS/IM-MS Experiment

1. Mass spectrometry settings for native MS experiment.

(a) Desalt between 100 and 150 μg of ADC in 150 mM ammonium acetate.

(b) Determine the concentration of the ADC solution after desalting by UV absorbance using NanoDrop spectrophotometer (Thermo Fisher Scientific, France).

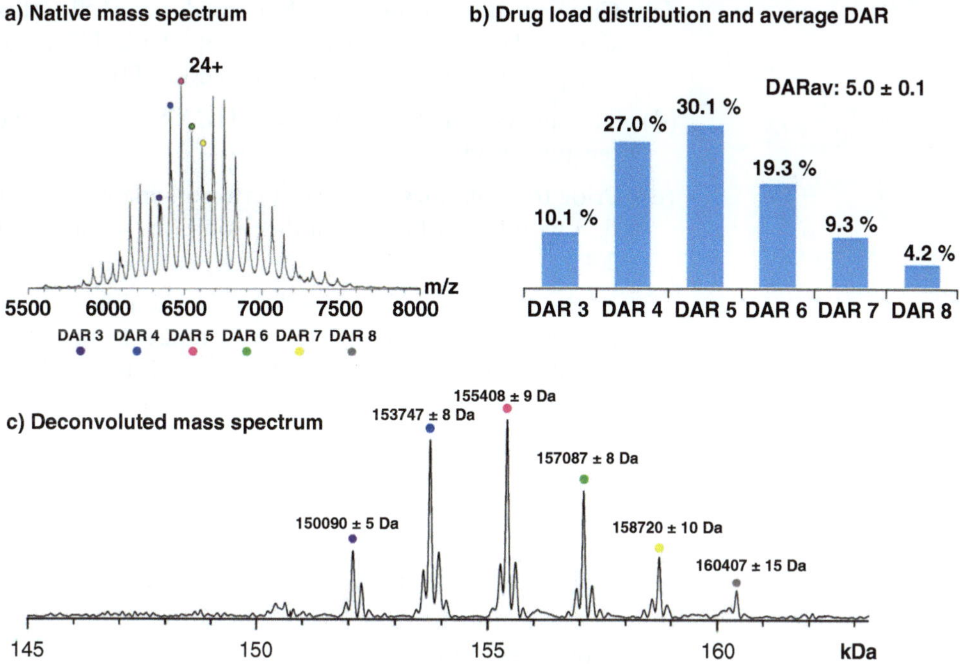

Fig. 2 NanoESI MS analysis in nondenaturing conditions of deglycosylated inotuzumab ozogamicin (IO), a lysine ADC, after direct infusion. (**a**) Full scan native mass spectrum of IO representing the different DAR populations (from DAR 2 to DAR 8). (b) Relative intensities of each individual DAR populations. (c) Deconvoluted mass spectrum of deglycosylated IO

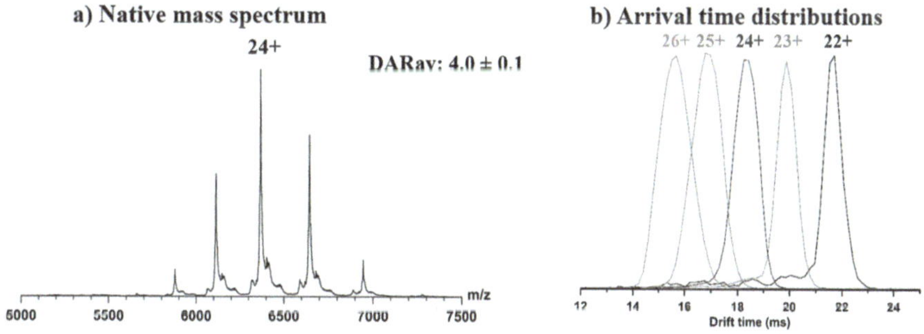

c) Collision cross section and drift times of different DAR4 site specific ADC charge states

Z	22+	23+	24+	25+	26+
$^{TW}CCS_{N2}$ (nm^2)	65.7 ± 0.1	67.6 ± 0.1	69.1 ± 0.1	71.2 ± 0.1	72.8 ± 0.1
Drift time (ms)	21.7 ± 0.1	19.9 ± 0.1	18.4 ± 0.1	17.0 ± 0.1	15.6 ± 0.1

Fig. 3 NanoESI IM-MS analysis in nondenaturing conditions of deglycosylated site-specific DAR4 ADC [8] after direct infusion. (**a**) Native mass spectrum of deglycosylated site-specific DAR4 ADC. (**b**) Arrival time distributions (ATDs) of different DAR 4 charge states observed in the mass spectrum. (**c**) Experimental collision cross section ($^{TW}CCS_{N2}$) and drift times corresponding to the different charge state populations upon ion mobility separation

(c) Connect the automated chip-based nanoESI infusion source (Triversa Nanomate, Advion, Ithaca, USA) to the Synapt G2 HDMS (Waters, Manchester, UK).

(d) The analysis on the Synapt G2 HDMS is performed in sensitive mode.

(e) Prior to ADC mass analysis, perform Synapt G2 calibration with 8 μL of cesium iodide solution (*see* Subheading 2.4).

(f) In the MassLynx Tune windows set the following parameters: Positive ion mode, *m/z* range from 1000 to 10,000, sampling cone: 180 V (*see* **Note 2**), backing pressure: 6 mbar, source offset: 5 V, source temperature: 90 °C, trap collision energy: 10 V, transfer collision energy: 5 V, trap gas: 5 mL/min, scan time: 4 s, and acquisition time: 2 min.

(g) Put between 10–20 μL of ADC solution at 5 μM concentration in the well plate of the Nanomate.

(h) In MaxEnt 1, the ranges are set from 145,000 to 162,000 with a resolution of 1 Da/channel. The width at half height is set to 2 Da for the uniform Gaussian. The deconvoluted spectrum is presented in Fig. 2b.

(i) For the DARav calculation, *see* Subheading 3.4.

2. Data interpretation for native MS experiment.

(a) Open the chromatogram option in MassLynx menu.

(b) Combine the mass signal over the 2 min acquisition time.

(c) Smooth the signal using the following parameters: Smooth window: 10, number of smooths: 2, and smoothing method: Mean (Fig. 2a).

(d) Perform MaxEnt 1 deconvolution with the following parameters: Ranges 145,000–165,000, Resolution: 1.00 Da/channel, Uniform Gaussian width at half height: 5 Da, and minimum intensity ratios: 33% left and 33% right (*see* **Note 3**).

(e) Take the intensities of each individual DAR population to assess the DLD (Fig. 2b) and calculate the DARav (*see* Subheading 3.4).

3. Ion mobility mass spectrometry settings for native IM-MS.

(a) For IM-MS, in the MassLynx Tune windows set the following parameters: Positive ion mode, *m/z* range from 1000 to 10,000, sampling cone: 80 V (*see* **Note 4**), backing pressure: 6 mbar, source offset: 5 V, source temperature: 90 °C, trap collision energy: 4 V, transfer collision energy: 5 V, trap gas: 5 mL/min, scan time: 4 s, and acquisition time: 2 min.

(b) In the ion mobility cell set the following parameters: N_2 flow rate: 45 mL/min, He flow rate: 120 mL/min, IM wave height: 40 V, and IM wave velocity: 923 m/s (*see* **Note 5**).

(c) In the masslynx tune page, activate the Mobility TOF mode in the acquisition mode menu.

(d) Put between 10–20 μL of ADC solution at 5 μM concentration in the well plate of the Nanomate. (*see* **Note 6**).

(e) Record the mass spectrum. Do not forget to activate the option "add drift time function" to record the arrival time distribution of each ion (*see* **Note 7**).

(f) Put between 10–20 μL of each individual solution of IM calibrants in the well plate of the Nanomate.

(g) Record the IM chromatogram of each individual calibrant in triplicate and under identical instrumental conditions as those used for the ADC IM-MS analysis.

4. Data interpretation for native IM-MS experiment.

(a) In the chromatogram menu of MassLynx, open the IM function.

(b) Combine the whole mobilogram signal to extract the mass spectrum (Fig. 3a).

(c) In your mass spectrum, combine the peak of interest at the half-maximum. The chromatogram menu will automatically open, showing the arrival time distribution associated with the ion selected previously (Fig. 3b).

(d) Take the drift time associated with the center of the ATD Gaussian.

5. Calibration curve to convert drift time on collision cross section (CCS).

(a) Proceed as described in Subheading 3.4, **step 4** to obtain the drift time associated with each peak of the calibrant solutions: For concanavalin A take the drift time of the 19+, 20+, and 21+ charge states, for ADH take the 24+, 25+, and 26+ charge states, and finally for PK take the 32+, 33+, and 34+ charge states.

(b) Correct the drift times of all these charge states using the following equation (*see* **Note 8**):

$$t'_d = t_d - \frac{\left(\iota * \sqrt{\frac{m}{z}}\right)}{1000}$$

(c) Calculate the reduced cross section (Ω') of the reference charge states of the calibrant systems reported in the literature with the following equation:

$$\Omega' = \Omega_{\text{literature}} / (z\sqrt{\mu})$$

(d) Make a graph $\ln(t'_d)$ vs $\ln(\Omega')$, fit the data with a linear equation

$$\ln(\Omega') = a + b \ln(t_d')$$

(e) Make the final correction of the drift times from the equation:

$$t''_d = t'^X_d (z|\sqrt{\mu})$$

(f) Build a second graph t''_d vs $\Omega_{\text{literatutre}}$ and fit the data with a linear regression

$$\Omega_{\text{literature}} = b\, t_d''$$

(g) Use the b and X parameters to convert the drift time of the different DAR populations of your ADC sample on CCS values (Fig. 3c) with the following equation:

$$\text{CCS}\ (\text{nm}^2) = \left(t_d - \left(1.57\sqrt{\frac{m}{z}}\right)/1000\right)^X z\left(\sqrt{1/\mu}\right) b$$

3.5 Online SEC-Native MS

1. LC setup for SEC-native MS.

(a) The column used is a BEH SEC column 200 Å, 1.7 μm, 4.6 × 150 mm (*see* **Note 9**). The chromatographic system is an Acquity UPLC H-Class system (Waters, Manchester, UK) comprising a quaternary solvent manager, a sample manager set at 10 °C, a column oven at room temperature, and a TUV detector operating at 280 and 214 nm.

(b) For the analyses of ADC, the elution is performed in isocratic mode with the following flow rate gradient: 0.25 mL/min over 4 min, then 0.1 mL/min over 5.5 min, and finally 0.25 mL/min over 2.5 min (*see* **Notes 10** and **11**).

(c) Load the LC method and equilibrate the LC system with ten column volumes of mobile phase (*see* Subheading 2.1).

2. Native mass spectrometry settings for SEC-native MS experiment.

(a) Prior to ADC mass analysis, perform Synapt G2 calibration with 8 μL of cesium iodide solution (*see* Subheading 2.4).

(b) For the tune page parameters, the Synapt G2 HDMS is operated in sensitive mode with a capillary voltage of 3.0 kV. The sample cone and pressure in the interface region were set to 180 V for lysine conjugate and 120 V for cysteine conjugate (*see* **Note 2**) and 6 mbar, respectively. Source and desolvation temperature were set to 100 and 450 °C, respectively. Desolvation and cone gas flows were set at 750 and 60 L/h, respectively.

(c) The MS file is set up with the following parameters: Start time: 0 min; End time: 12 min; Polarity: Positive; Analyser Mode: Sensitivity; Dynamic Range: Normal; Sensitivity: Normal; Low Mass: 1000 Da; High Mass: 10,000 Da; Scan Time: 1.5 s (Continuum); No Trap or Transfer CE. Events for flow state are created to direct salts to waste: 0 min Flow State directed to Waste, 4 min Flow State directed to LC, 9 min Flow State directed to Waste.

(d) In MassLynx, create a sample list with the MS file, Inlet file, MS tune file. Specify the sample position (Bottle). The injected volume should be between 1 and 10 μL. No manual desalting is needed prior to SEC-native MS experiment due to online desalting provided by SEC.

3. Data interpretation.

(a) Chromatogram (Fig. 4a) and TIC are obtained in the Chromatogram panel.

(b) In MaxEnt 1, the ranges are set from 145,000 to 162,000 with a resolution of 1 Da/channel. The width at half height is set to 2 Da for the uniform Gaussian. The deconvoluted spectrum is presented in Fig. 4b (*see* **Note 12**).

(c) For the DARav calculation, *see* Subheading 3.4.

4. Ion mobility settings for SEC-native IM-MS experiment.

(a) In the MassLynx Tune window set the following parameters: Positive ion mode, m/z range from 1000 to 10,000, sampling cone: 80 V, backing pressure: 6 mbar, source offset: 5 V, source temperature: 100 °C, desolvation temperature: 450 °C, trap collision energy: 4 V, transfer collision energy: 5 V, trap gas: 5 mL/min.

(b) In the ion mobility cell set the following parameters: N_2 flow rate: 45 mL/min, He flow rate: 130 mL/min, IM wave height: 40 V, and IM wave velocity: 923 *m/s*.

(c) The MS file is set up with the following parameters: Start time: 0 min; End time: 12 min; Polarity: Positive; Analyser Mode: Sensitivity; Dynamic Range: Normal; Sensitivity: Normal; Low Mass: 1000 Da; High Mass: 10,000 Da; Scan Time: 1.5 s (Continuum); No Trap or Transfer CE. Check Add Drift Time Function and Maintain Mobility Separation. Events for flow state are created to direct salts to waste: 0 min Flow State directed to Waste, 4 min Flow State directed to LC, 9 min Flow State directed to Waste.

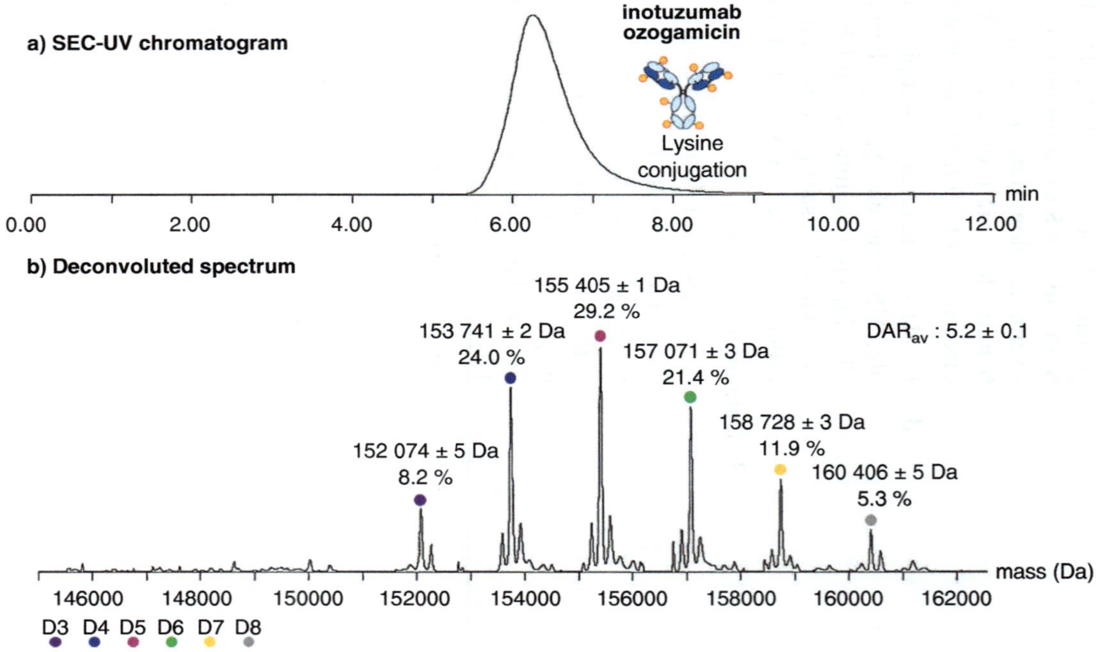

Fig. 4 SEC-native MS analysis of deglycosylated inotuzumab ozogamicin (Lysine conjugate). (**a**) SEC-UV chromatogram corresponding to ADC monomer. (**b**) Deconvoluted mass spectrum representing the drug load distribution with the average DAR

(d) In MassLynx, create a sample list with the MS file, Inlet file, MS tune file. Specify the sample position (Bottle). The injected volume has to be between 1 and 10 μL. Record each IM experiment in triplicate to calculate a more reliable collisional cross section.

(e) Load the SEC column with 1 to 10 μL of each individual solution of IM calibrants (*see* Subheading 2.5, **item 2**).

(f) Record the IM chromatogram of each individual calibrant in triplicate and under identical instrumental conditions as those used for the ADC SEC-native MS analysis.

(g) For data interpretation, *see* Subheading 3.4.4 and 3.4.5.

3.6 Average DAR Calculation and Drug Load Distribution

The average DAR value represents the sum of relative peak intensities in the mass spectrum for each DAR multiplied by its corresponding number of drugs. It was calculated from the relative peak intensities measured from the raw mass spectra, by using the following equation

$$\mathrm{DAR_{av}} = \frac{\sum_{0}^{8} k\, I_k}{\sum_{0}^{8} I_k}$$

where k is the number of drugs and I_k is the relative peak intensity of DAR_k.

4 Notes

1. Ion mobility calibrants have to be chosen depending on the mass and the charge state of the analyzed mAb/ADC. Here we chose to use ion mobility calibrants that range from 100 kDa to 230 kDa and exhibit positive charge states from 15+ to 35+. Usually ADCs are proteins around 150 kDa with 20+ to 28+ positive charges under our experimental conditions.
2. The sampling cone (Vc) voltage is a crucial parameter on Waters instrument. A high voltage (180 V) increases transmission of high m/z ions along with more efficient desolvation [14]. However, high Vc values also favor dissociation of non-covalent assemblies, especially for cysteine-linked ADCs. An intermediate Vc value of 100–120 V is thus usually more adapted. An optimum value has to be found to provide compromise between good ion transmission and desolvation while maintaining ADC integrity.
3. The parameters of the MaxEnt1 deconvolution are protein dependent. In particular, the mass range and the FWHM

have to be optimized for each mAb/ADC. The latter has to be chosen as a function of the resolution of the experimental mass spectrum.

4. The sampling cone voltage applied in the source of the mass spectrometer is an important parameter for native IM-MS experiments. Ion heating can occur as a consequence of the effect of this acceleration voltage and eventually can lead to conformational changes (protein unfolding) on protein structures while ions are transmitted into the mass spectrometer. Be sure that the sampling cone voltage you are using allows the transmission of your molecular ions of interest and does not induce any structural changes. From our experience, 80 V provides a good MS signal (ion transmission and desolvation) without modifying ADCs conformation.
5. These parameters are going to drive the separation of the ions in the ion mobility cell. They have to be carefully optimized to ensure ion focusing (He flow) prior to IM separation and provide the best separation (N_2 flow, wave height, and wave velocity [15]). These parameters are protein dependent.
6. When performing native IM-MS experiments, we slightly increase the concentration of the analyte compared to native MS experiments to compensate the loss of sensitivity due to the activation of the IM device.
7. Record each IM experiment in triplicate to calculate a more reliable collision cross section.
8. The c constant has been determined empirically and it is specific of the Synapt G2 mass spectrometer. For ion signals lower than 5000 m/z, $c = 1.41$. For ion signals above 5000 m/z, $c = 1.57$ [16].
9. Other columns are available for SEC-native MS experiment. For a unique fast desalting goal, shorter column dimension (i.e., BEH SEC 4.6 × 30 mm, 200 Å, Waters) could be used. For a separation goal, longer column dimension (i.e., BEH SEC 4.6 × 150/300 mm, 200 Å, Waters) is preferred.
10. The flow rate gradient provides improved sensitivity on the Synapt G2 HDMS mass spectrometer.
11. The flow rate gradient method is a generic method which can be easily adapted. If the LC method is changed, do not forget to change events in MS file for directing salts to waste.
12. SEC-native MS coupling provides higher MS spectral resolution and mass accuracy due to the more efficient desalting afforded by SEC compared to manual desalting.

References

1. Chari RVJ (2008) Targeted cancer therapy: conferring specificity to cytotoxic drugs. Acc Chem Res 41(1):98–107
2. Carter PJ, Lazar GA (2018) Next generation antibody drugs: pursuit of the 'high-hanging fruit'. Nat Rev Drug Discov 17(3):197–223
3. Valliere-Douglass JF, McFee WA, Salas-Solano O (2012) Native intact mass determination of antibodies conjugated with monomethyl Auristatin E and F at interchain cysteine residues. Anal Chem 84(6):2843–2849
4. Chen J, Yin S, Wu YJ, Ouyang J (2013) Development of a native nanoelectrospray mass spectrometry method for determination of the drug-to-antibody ratio of antibody-drug conjugates. Anal Chem 85(3):1699–1704
5. Hengel SM, Sanderson R, Valliere-Douglass J, Nicholas N, Leiske C, Alley SC (2014) Measurement of in vivo drug load distribution of cysteine-linked antibody-drug conjugates using microscale liquid chromatography mass spectrometry. Anal Chem 86(7):3420–3425
6. Debaene F, Boeuf A, Wagner-Rousset E, Colas O, Ayoub D, Corvaia N, Van Dorsselaer A, Beck A, Cianferani S (2014) Innovative native MS methodologies for antibody drug conjugate characterization: high resolution native MS and IM-MS for average DAR and DAR distribution assessment. Anal Chem 86(21):10674–10683
7. Marcoux J, Champion T, Colas O, Wagner-Rousset E, Corvaïa N, Van Dorsselaer A, Beck A, Cianférani S (2015) Native mass spectrometry and ion mobility characterization of trastuzumab emtansine, a lysine-linked antibody drug conjugate. Protein Sci 24 (8):1210–1223
8. Botzanowski T, Erb S, Hernandez-Alba O, Ehkirch A, Colas O, Wagner-Rousset E, Rabuka D, Beck A, Drake PM, Cianférani S (2017) Insights from native mass spectrometry approaches for top- and middle-level characterization of site-specific antibody-drug conjugates. MAbs 9(5):801–811
9. Ehkirch A, Hernandez-Alba O, Colas O, Beck A, Guillarme D, Cianférani S (2018) Hyphenation of size exclusion chromatography to native ion mobility mass spectrometry for the analytical characterization of therapeutic antibodies and related products. J Chromatogr B 1086:176–183
10. Ehkirch A, Goyon A, Hernandez-Alba O, Rouviere F, D'Atri V, Dreyfus C, Haeuw J-F, Diemer H, Beck A, Heinisch S, Guillarme D, Cianferani S (2018) A novel online four-dimensional SEC×SEC-IM×MS methodology for characterization of monoclonal antibody size variants. Anal Chem 90 (23):13929–13937
11. Ehkirch A, D'Atri V, Rouviere F, Hernandez-Alba O, Goyon A, Colas O, Sarrut M, Beck A, Guillarme D, Heinisch S, Cianferani S (2018) An online four-dimensional HIC×SEC-IM×MS methodology for proof-of-concept characterization of antibody drug conjugates. Anal Chem 90(3):1578–1586
12. D'Atri V, Causon T, Hernandez-Alba O, Mutabazi A, Veuthey JL, Cianferani S, Guillarme D (2018) Adding a new separation dimension to MS and LC–MS: what is the utility of ion mobility spectrometry? J Sep Sci 41(1):20–67
13. Beck A, D'Atri V, Ehkirch A, Fekete S, Hernandez-Alba O, Gahoual R, Leize-Wagner E, François Y, Guillarme D, Cianférani S (2019) Cutting-edge multi-level analytical and structural characterization of antibody-drug conjugates: present and future. Expert Rev Proteomics 16:337–362
14. Ramstrom H, Sanglier S, Leize-Wagner E, Philippe C, Van Dorsselaer A, Haiech J (2003) Properties and regulation of the bifunctional enzyme HPr kinase/phosphatase in Bacillus subtilis. J Biol Chem 278 (2):1174–1185
15. Atmanene C, Petiot-Becard S, Zeyer D, Van Dorsselaer A, Hannah VV, Sanglier-Cianferani S (2012) Exploring key parameters to detect subtle ligand-induced protein conformational changes using traveling wave ion mobility mass spectrometry. Anal Chem 84(11):4703–4710
16. Ruotolo BT, Benesch JLP, Sandercock AM, Hyung S-J, Robinson CV (2008) Ion mobility–mass spectrometry analysis of large protein complexes. Nat Protoc 3:1139

Chapter 14

High-Resolution Characterization of ADCs by Orbitrap LCMS

Jintang He, Surinder Kaur, and Keyang Xu

Abstract

Antibody-drug conjugates (ADCs) have complex molecular structures as they are composed of both small and large molecules, and they often undergo biotransformation over time in circulation. Here we describe a high-resolution Orbitrap MS approach for the characterization of ADC biotransformation and stability. Compared with conventional approach by Q-TOF MS, the method described here significantly improved the mass resolution and enabled more comprehensive characterization of ADC catabolites. It is particularly beneficial for characterizing ADC biotransformations with small mass changes.

Key words Antibody-drug conjugate, Characterization, Biotransformation, High resolution, Orbitrap MS

1 Introduction

Antibody-drug conjugates (ADCs) are a promising class of therapeutics designed to deliver cytotoxic drugs specifically to tumor cells [1, 2]. ADCs are composed of three components: antibody, linker, and drug, resulting in the formation of complex molecular structures. Many ADCs are dosed as a mixture of components with various drug-to-antibody ratios (DARs) and often undergo biotransformations in vivo which further increase the structural complexity of ADCs [3–6]. An affinity capture LC-MS method previously developed in our laboratory has been frequently used to characterize in vivo stability and biotransformations of ADCs [7, 8]. Conventionally, quadrupole time-of-flight (Q-TOF) MS is used successfully in this approach for detection of intact ADCs with high molecular weights. However, for the ADC undergoing biotransformations that result in small mass changes, the resolution of TOF MS was found not sufficient [3, 8]. Recent advancement in the Orbitrap technology provides new opportunities for characterizing intact therapeutics with greater resolution [9, 10].

In this chapter, we describe a high-resolution Orbitrap MS approach for the characterization of both intact and reduced

L. Nathan Tumey (ed.), *Antibody-Drug Conjugates: Methods and Protocols*, Methods in Molecular Biology, vol. 2078, https://doi.org/10.1007/978-1-4939-9929-3_14,

ADCs. This method is suitable for ADCs with site-specific cysteine conjugations or random lysine conjugations. Thereby, we recently characterized multiple THIOMAB™ antibody-drug conjugates (TDCs) [11] and a lysine-linked ADC—Kadcyla [12]. Compared with the conventional Q-TOF MS approach, high-resolution Orbitrap MS enabled more comprehensive investigation of changes to ADCs in vivo, specially modifications with small mass shifts (Fig. 1).

2 Materials

2.1 Affinity Capture

1. KingFisher 96 magnetic particle processor is purchased from Thermo Fisher Scientific.
2. Dynabeads M-280 Streptavidin is purchased from Invitrogen.
3. HBS-EP buffer: 10 mM Hepes (pH 7.4), 150 mM NaCl, 3.4 mM ethylenediaminetetraacetic acid (EDTA), 0.005% Surfactant P20.
4. N-Glycanase is purchased from Prozyme.
5. Elution buffer: 30% acetonitrile, 1% formic acid.
6. Beckman Coulter Allegra X-14R centrifuge.

2.2 Reversed Phase Liquid Chromatography

1. nanoACQUITY UPLC® system is purchased from Waters Corporation.
2. PS-DVB monolithic column (500 μm i.d. × 5 cm) is purchased from Thermo Fisher Scientific.
3. PS-DVB monolithic column (200 μm i.d. × 25 cm) is purchased from Thermo Fisher Scientific.
4. Mobile phase A: 0.1% formic acid.
5. Mobile phase B: acetonitrile, 0.1% formic acid.
6. Tris(2-carboxyethyl)phosphine (TCEP) is purchased from Sigma-Aldrich.

2.3 High-Resolution Orbitrap MS

1. Q Exactive Plus mass spectrometer is purchased from Thermo Fisher Scientific.
2. Protein Deconvolution 4.0 software is purchased from Thermo Fisher Scientific.

3 Methods

3.1 Affinity Capture

ADCs are selectively extracted from plasma samples by affinity capture as described previously [7, 11, 12]. A KingFisher 96 magnetic particle processor is used to mix, wash, gather, and transfer the paramagnetic beads in the following steps (*see* **Note 1**).

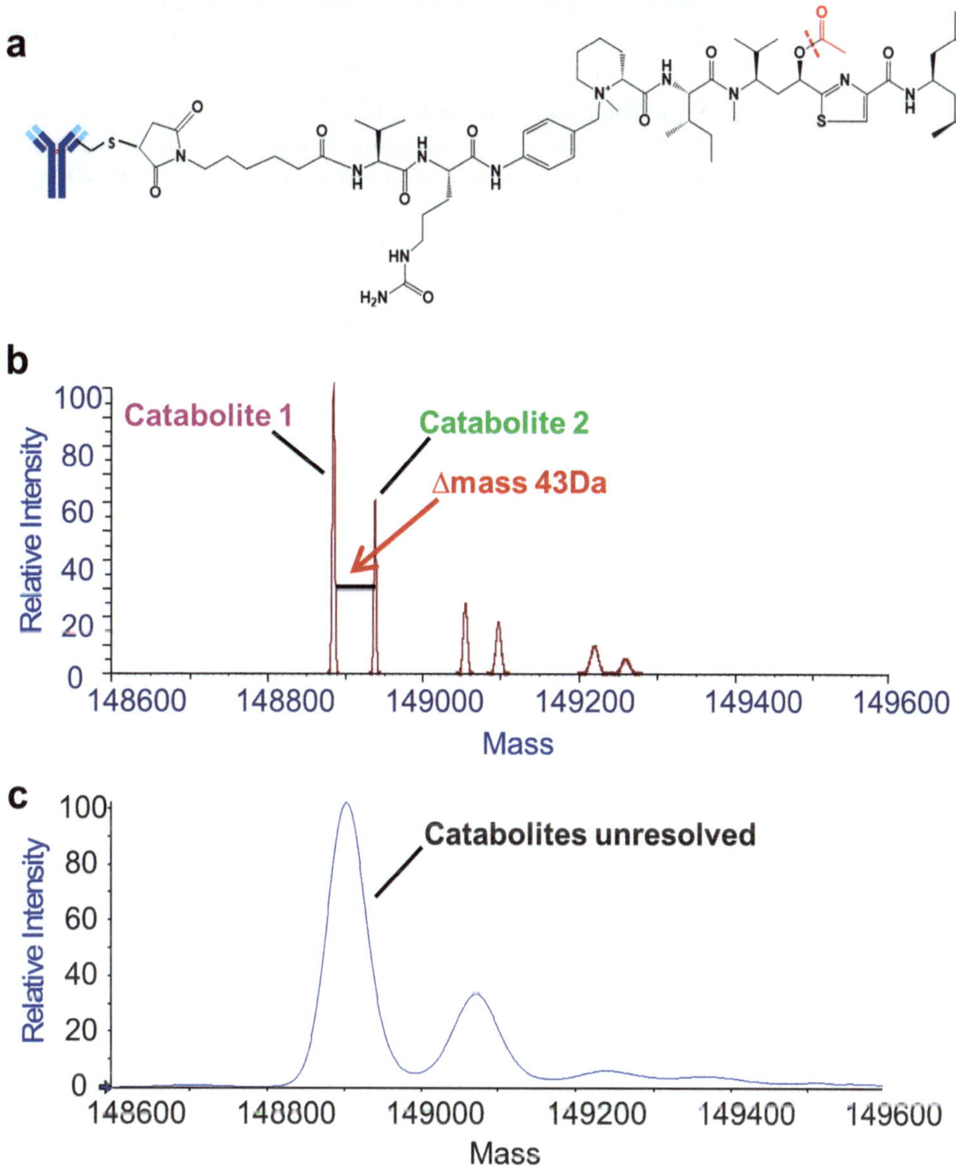

Fig. 1 Characterization of an anti-CD22 MC-vc-PAB Tubulysin M TDC. SCID mice were dosed intravenously with 1 mg/kg of anti-CD22 MC-vc-PAB Tubulysin M TDC (**a**). Plasma samples were harvested at 1 day post dose and the conjugate was analyzed by affinity capture LCMS on both Q-TOF and Orbitrap instruments. Two catabolites of the TDC with a mass difference of 43 Da were baseline resolved by Orbitrap MS (**b**) but not resolved by TOF MS (**c**). Due to the enhanced mass resolution, many more TDC catabolites were characterized by Orbitrap MS than by TOF MS (**b**, **c**). (Reproduced from ref. 11 with permission from American Chemical Society)

1. Incubate biotinylated antigen extracellular domain (ECD) (*see* **Note 2**) with Dynabeads M-280 Streptavidin in a 96-well plate for 1 h to immobilize ECD onto beads.

2. Wash the beads twice with HBS-EP buffer, and then use the ECD coupled beads to capture ADCs by incubating with plasma samples containing ADCs for 2 h at room temperature.
3. Wash the beads twice with HBS-EP buffer, and then digest the captured ADCs on beads using N-Glycanase (10 mU per sample) at 37 °C overnight with moderate shaking (200–400 rpm) (*see* **Note 3**).
4. Wash the beads extensively with HBS-EP buffer (twice), water (twice), and 10% acetonitrile (*see* **Note 4**), and then elute ADCs using 50 μL of elution buffer (*see* **Note 5**).
5. Centrifuge the eluents in the 96-well plate using a Beckman Coulter Allegra X-14R centrifuge at 3700 × *g* for 10 min at RT.
6. Place the 96-well plate onto a magnet, and transfer 60 μL of supernatant to a new 96-well plate (*see* **Note 6**).
7. Centrifuge the 96-well plate at 3700 × *g* for 10 min at RT. The supernatant is subsequently injected onto LC-MS for analysis.

3.2 Separation of Intact ADCs by Reversed Phase Liquid Chromatography

Chromatographic desalting and separation of ADCs are performed on a Waters nanoACQUITY UPLC® system.

1. Inject 5 μL intact ADC analyte using an autosampler, and load it onto a PS-DVB monolithic column (500 μm i.d. × 5 cm) with mobile phase A.
2. Perform chromatographic separation at 60 °C with a gradient of mobile phase A and mobile phase B at a flow rate of 15 μL/min (*see* **Note 7**). The gradient is as follows:

   0% B (0–4 min)

   0–40% B (4–8 min)

   40% B (8–11 min) (*see* **Note 8**)

   40–100% B (11–12.5 min)

   100% B (12.5–13.5 min)

   100–0% B (13.5–14.2 min)

   0% B (14.2–15 min).

3.3 Separation of Reduced ADCs by Reversed Phase Liquid Chromatography

1. Following affinity capture, reduce ADCs by adding 10 mM tris (2-carboxyethyl)phosphine (TCEP) in the elution buffer and incubate at 37 °C for 40 min.
2. Inject 5 μL reduced ADC analyte using an autosampler, and load it onto a PS-DVB monolithic column (200 μm i.d. × 25 cm) (Thermo Fisher Scientific, Waltham, MA) with mobile phase A.
3. Perform chromatographic separation of the ADC light chain and heavy chain at 65 °C with a gradient of mobile phase A and

mobile phase B at a flow rate of 3 μL/min (*see* **Note 9**). The gradient is as follows (*see* **Note 10**):

0% B (0–4 min)

0–25% B (4–4.1 min)

25% B (4.1–7 min)

25–35% B (7–29 min)

35–60% B (29–32 min)

60–100% B (32–32.1 min)

100% B (32.1–34 min)

100–0% B (34–34.1 min)

0% B (34.1–40 min).

3.4 ADC Analysis by High-Resolution Orbitrap MS

Both intact and reduced ADCs are analyzed on a Q Exactive Plus mass spectrometer.

1. Operate Q Exactive Plus with an Ion Max API source.
2. Acquire mass spectra using a full MS method at a resolution setting of 17,500 (*see* **Note 11**).
3. Set the key parameters as follows: spray voltage, 3.2 kV; sheath gas flow rate, 8; S-lens RF level, 100; in-source CID, 100 ev (*see* **Note 12**); AGC target, 3×10^6; maximum injection time, 150 ms; microscans, 10.
4. Extract full MS spectra from the total ion chromatograms (TICs) and perform deconvolution using the ReSpect™ algorithm incorporated in Protein Deconvolution 4.0 software. Set the mass tolerance as 25 ppm.
5. Characterize ADC biotransformation and drug-to-antibody ratio (DAR) distribution based on the mass of different DAR species (*see* **Note 13**).

4 Notes

1. Affinity capture can also be conducted manually. However, it is highly recommended to use a KingFisher 96 magnetic particle processor because it enables higher throughput and greater consistency.
2. If ECD is not available, biotinylated anti-human IgG will also work for nonclinical samples.
3. To ensure efficient deglycosylation, it is recommended to conduct N-Glycanase treatment with moderate shaking.
4. It is important to wash the beads extensively with HBS-EP, water, and 10% acetonitrile before the elution step. This will remove most of nonspecific binding molecules and salts.

5. The elution buffer contains 30% acetonitrile and 1% formic acid, which will denature ADCs. Therefore, this method is not intended to be used for analysis of intact ADCs where the linker-drug is conjugated to the antibody via reduced interchain disulfide bonds.
6. This step will remove most of residual beads from each sample. This will prevent clogging the LC system by beads.
7. Microflow LC is highly recommended. Compared with analytical flow LC, microflow LC allows more sensitive detection of ADCs.
8. Intact ADCs typically elute at ~9–10 min under these conditions.
9. A longer column and a lower flow rate are used here to ensure efficient separation of light and heavy chain species.
10. Depending on the structure of ADCs, reduction could result in multiple light chain or heavy chain species which carry different number of drugs. The retention time of these reduced species is typically different under these separation conditions.
11. A resolution setting of 17,500 is typically used for analysis of intact ADCs and heavy chain species. When specifically analyzing light chain species, a higher resolution setting such as 70,000 or 140,000 can be used.
12. In-source CID is applied to enhance the desolvation of intact ADC molecules. However, in-source CID might also result in fragmentation of certain linkers or drugs. Therefore, it is recommended to carefully monitor any potential in-source fragmentation of linker-drug when high in-source CID energy is used.
13. ADC biotransformations are typically characterized based on the mass differences between the newly formed and the original DAR species. Average DAR of the ADC can be calculated based on the relative abundance of different DAR species.

Acknowledgments

We would like to thank Carl Ng, Dian Su, and Luna Liu for their help with method development.

References

1. Jaracz S, Chen J, Kuznetsova LV, Ojima I (2005) Recent advances in tumor-targeting anticancer drug conjugates. Bioorg Med

Chem 13(17):5043–5054. https://doi.org/10.1016/j.bmc.2005.04.084

2. Polakis P (2016) Antibody drug conjugates for cancer therapy. Pharmacol Rev 68(1):3–19. https://doi.org/10.1124/pr.114.009373
3. Kaur S, Xu K, Saad OM, Dere RC, Carrasco-Triguero M (2013) Bioanalytical assay strategies for the development of antibody-drug conjugate biotherapeutics. Bioanalysis 5 (2):201–226. https://doi.org/10.4155/bio.12.299
4. Tumey LN, Rago B, Han X (2015) In vivo biotransformations of antibody-drug conjugates. Bioanalysis 7(13):1649–1664. https://doi.org/10.4155/bio.15.84
5. Shen BQ, Xu K, Liu L, Raab H, Bhakta S, Kenrick M, Parsons-Reponte KL, Tien J, Yu SF, Mai E, Li D, Tibbitts J, Baudys J, Saad OM, Scales SJ, McDonald PJ, Hass PE, Eigenbrot C, Nguyen T, Solis WA, Fuji RN, Flagella KM, Patel D, Spencer SD, Khawli LA, Ebens A, Wong WL, Vandlen R, Kaur S, Sliwkowski MX, Scheller RH, Polakis P, Junutula JR (2012) Conjugation site modulates the in vivo stability and therapeutic activity of antibody-drug conjugates. Nat Biotechnol 30 (2):184–189. https://doi.org/10.1038/nbt.2108
6. Doronina SO, Toki BE, Torgov MY, Mendelsohn BA, Cerveny CG, Chace DF, DeBlanc RL, Gearing RP, Bovee TD, Siegall CB, Francisco JA, Wahl AF, Meyer DL, Senter PD (2003) Development of potent monoclonal antibody auristatin conjugates for cancer therapy. Nat Biotechnol 21(7):778–784. https://doi.org/10.1038/nbt832
7. Xu K, Liu L, Saad OM, Baudys J, Williams L, Leipold D, Shen B, Raab H, Junutula JR, Kim A, Kaur S (2011) Characterization of intact antibody-drug conjugates from plasma/serum in vivo by affinity capture capillary liquid chromatography-mass spectrometry. Anal Biochem 412(1):56–66. https://doi.org/10.1016/j.ab.2011.01.004
8. Xu K, Liu L, Dere R, Mai E, Erickson R, Hendricks A, Lin K, Junutula JR, Kaur S (2013) Characterization of the drug-to-antibody ratio distribution for antibody-drug conjugates in plasma/serum. Bioanalysis 5 (9):1057–1071. https://doi.org/10.4155/bio.13.66
9. Rosati S, Rose RJ, Thompson NJ, van Duijn E, Damoc E, Denisov E, Makarov A, Heck AJ (2012) Exploring an orbitrap analyzer for the characterization of intact antibodies by native mass spectrometry. Angew Chem Int Ed Engl 51(52):12992–12996. https://doi.org/10.1002/anie.201206745
10. Debaene F, Boeuf A, Wagner-Rousset E, Colas O, Ayoub D, Corvaia N, Van Dorsselaer A, Beck A, Cianferani S (2014) Innovative native MS methodologies for antibody drug conjugate characterization: high resolution native MS and IM-MS for average DAR and DAR distribution assessment. Anal Chem 86(21):10674–10683. https://doi.org/10.1021/ac502593n
11. He J, Su D, Ng C, Liu L, Yu SF, Pillow TH, Del Rosario G, Darwish M, Lee BC, Ohri R, Zhou H, Wang X, Lu J, Kaur S, Xu K (2017) High-resolution accurate-mass mass spectrometry enabling in-depth characterization of in vivo biotransformations for intact antibody-drug conjugates. Anal Chem 89 (10):5476–5483. https://doi.org/10.1021/acs.analchem.7b00408
12. He J, Yu SF, Yee S, Kaur S, Xu K (2018) Characterization of in vivo biotransformations for trastuzumab emtansine by high-resolution accurate-mass mass spectrometry. MAbs 10 (7):960–967. https://doi.org/10.1080/19420862.2018.1494487

Chapter 15

Conjugation Site Analysis by MS/MS Protein Sequencing

Linjie Han, Yanqun Zhao, and Qunying Zhang

Abstract

In-depth knowledge about the site of drug-linker conjugation is important for the understanding of the conjugation efficiency and the exact locations of payloads for antibody-drug conjugates (ADCs). Here we describe a peptide mapping-based protocol, covering sample preparation procedure, LC-MS/MS setup, and data processing (auto and manual), to determine the locations of drug-linker attachment on mAbs. In comparison with classical mAb peptide mapping, some improvements will be highlighted for maintaining hydrophobic drug-loaded peptides in solution, enabling efficient chromatographic separation and mass spectrometric detection, and allowing for their unambiguous identification in LC-MS/MS map by using diagnostic fragmentation ions of the payload.

Key words Peptide mapping, Enzymatic digestion, LC-MS/MS, Cysteine-conjugated ADC, Hydrophobic drug-linker

1 Introduction

In-depth knowledge of drug-linker conjugation site is very important for antibody-drug conjugate (ADC) structural elucidation at both drug discovery and development stages. The locations typically used for conjugation are the amino groups of lysine residues or the sulfhydryl groups of the interchain cysteine residues, constituting lysine- and cysteine-based conjugation systems, respectively, resulting in heterogeneous mixtures of ADCs bearing various numbers of drugs attached to different positions on the monoclonal antibody (mAb). Recent efforts have focused on site-specific conjugation and produced more homogeneous ADCs, for example, by using engineered cysteines [1]. Many studies have demonstrated that the conjugation site modulates ADC linker stability [2], pharmacokinetics [3], and payload metabolism [4], and therefore impacts the overall efficacy and safety of the ADC. As to lysine-based ADCs, any lysine residue in the complementarity-determining regions (CDRs) that is accessible for conjugation will raise concerns about modulating antigen binding affinity

L. Nathan Tumey (ed.), *Antibody-Drug Conjugates: Methods and Protocols*, Methods in Molecular Biology, vol. 2078, https://doi.org/10.1007/978-1-4939-9929-3_15,

[5]. Therefore, understanding the conjugation site profile will help to design conjugates with improved therapeutic index. Additionally, conjugation site analysis will provide deep insight into conjugation selectivity and kinetics thus enhancing the process understanding and development [6].

Peptide mapping has proven itself an effective tool for determination of conjugation sites. It can be considered as a "bottom-up" analysis of a protein on the peptide level. Peptide mapping is achieved by site-specific protein cleavage with a proteolytic enzyme followed by gradient elution of the resulting peptides through reverse phase liquid chromatography (RPLC). Other separation techniques such as capillary electrophoresis (CE) have also been increasingly applied to peptide mapping as a complementary tool to HPLC due to the different separation mechanisms in CE from HPLC [7]. When coupled with high-resolution mass spectrometry, HPLC can be used for characterizing protein modifications, for example, analyzing sequence deviations, post-translational modifications, and disulfide scrambling for mAbs and ADCs. In addition, recent literature has suggested that peptide mapping approaches can be employed to locate the conjugation sites for lysine, native cysteine, and engineered cysteine conjugates [5, 8–13]. In contrast to bottom-up MS strategy, top-down and middle-down analysis has gained more attention for mAb characterization in the past decade due to advances in instrumentation and methodology [14]. Without the need of time-consuming sample preparation, the intact mAb or the ~25 kDa subunits that are derived from mAb IdeS digestion and chemical reduction can be introduced directly into the mass spectrometer and fragmented with the proper technique, such as higher-energy collisional dissociation (HCD), electron transfer dissociation (ETD), electron capture dissociation (ECD), and ultraviolet photodissociation (UVPD). The application of such middle-down approaches has been recently extended to provide conjugation site information for cysteine and lysine ADC modalities.

In this chapter, we will focus on introducing the peptide mapping protocol to identify ADC drug-linker conjugation sites for targeting broader audience. The improvements will be highlighted compared with classical mAb peptide mapping to address the challenges for not only maximizing digest efficiency and diminishing modification artifacts that might occur on mAb, but also retaining the structure of conjugated drug-linkers during sample preparation when they have been found to be structurally sensitive to pH, light, or temperature. Moreover, the protocol will also highlight ways to maintain the drug-linker loaded peptides in solution prior to MS electrospray given the challenge that the drug-linker moiety is sometimes highly hydrophobic. This approach has been demonstrated to work successfully for interchain cysteinyl-linked ADCs [8, 9]. In the data analysis section, identification of linker-drug loaded peptides via software searching algorithm and manual data processing will both be presented. Specially, a quick and easy approach will be discussed by employing the characteristic fragmentation ions of the payload.

2 Materials

Prepare all solutions using purified water and analytical grade reagents (unless indicated otherwise).

1. 100 mM tromethamine hydrochloride (Tris–HCl), pH 7.8 buffer. Add 2.127 g Tris–HCl and 0.7877 g Tris base to an appropriate container. Add 180 mL purified water using graduated cylinder. Mix the solution until homogeneous by stirring on a stir plate. Adjust the solution to pH 7.8 ± 0.02 by drop-wise addition of 1 mol/L hydrochloric acid with a calibrated pH meter. Transfer the solution to 200 mL volumetric flask and bring to volume with purified water. Mix well by inversion. Filter the solution through a 0.22 μm cellulose acetate membrane and store at 2 °C to 8 °C until use.
2. Denaturing Buffer: 8 M urea in 100 mM Tris–HCl, pH 7.8 buffer. Add 4.804 g urea to a 10 mL volumetric flask and fill the volumetric flask to 10.0 mL mark with 100 mM Tris–HCl, pH 7.8 solution. Filter the solution through a 0.22 μm cellulose acetate membrane and store at 2 °C to 8 °C until use.
3. 500 mM dithiothreitol (DTT). Centrifuge the tube containing 7.7 mg DTT (pre-weighed by manufacturer; Pierce No-Weigh Format DTT Cat #20291) briefly to bring all materials to the bottom. Add 100 μL of purified water to the tube and mix the contents of the tube well. The DTT solution should be prepared freshly for each experiment.
4. 500 mM iodoacetamide (IAM). Centrifuge the tube containing 56 mg IAM (pre-weighed by manufacturer; Sigma pre-weighed vials, Cat #A3221) briefly to bring all materials to the bottom. Add 600 μL of purified water to the tube and mix the contents of the tube well. The IAM solution should be prepared freshly for each experiment, and kept protected from light.
5. Mobile phase A: LC-MS grade water with 0.085% formic acid (FA), 0.015% trifluoroacetic acid (TFA). Add 850 μL FA and 150 μL TFA to 1000 mL LC-MS grade water and mix well.
6. Mobile phase B: LC-MS grade acetonitrile with 0.085% formic acid (FA), 0.015% trifluoroacetic acid (TFA). Add 850 μL FA and 150 μL TFA to 1000 mL LC-MS grade acetonitrile and mix well.

3 Methods

Before use, allow samples and reagents to reach room temperature. Vortex each sample gently. Carry out all procedures at room temperature unless otherwise specified.

3.1 Denaturation

Dilute the sample to 1 mg/mL in 500 μL of Denaturation Buffer (8 M urea in 100 mM Tris–HCl, pH 7.8 solution) (*see* **Note 1**).

For example, if the sample concentration is 10 mg/mL, add 50 μL of 10 mg/mL sample to 450 μL denaturing buffer in a polypropylene tube.

3.2 Reduction

1. Add 5 μL of 500 mM DTT to the tube to obtain a final concentration of ~5 mM DTT in the sample solution. Mix the contents of the tube gently (*see* **Note 2**).
2. Incubate the tube at 37 °C for 30 min in the dark (*see* **Note 3**).
3. Cool down the tube to room temperature.

3.3 Alkylation

1. Add 10.2 μL of 500 mM IAM to the tube to obtain a final concentration of ~10 mM. Mix the contents of the tube gently (*see* **Note 4**).
2. Incubate the tube at room temperature for 30 min in the dark.

3.4 Buffer Exchange

1. Prepare Thermo Scientific Zeba Spin Desalting Columns (0.5 mL, 7 K MWCO, P/N 89882) for buffer exchange according to the manufacturer's specifications (*see* **Note 5**).
2. Place the column in a new 1.5 mL polypropylene tube after the column is exchanged to 100 mM Tris–HCl, pH 7.8 solution, and remove cap.
3. Add 100 μL of the reduced and alkylated sample to the center of the column bed without disturbing the bed with the pipet tip.
4. Centrifuge the column according to the manufacturer's specifications to collect the sample which is then in 100 mM Tris–HCl, pH 7.8 solution.

3.5 Digestion

1. Measure the protein concentration of the buffer-exchanged sample by UV-VIS at 280 nm. Use 100 mM Tris–HCl, pH 7.8 solution as blank for baseline correction (*see* **Note 6**).
2. Calculate the volume needed for 50 μg of buffer-exchanged sample and transfer this volume to a new polypropylene tube.

   For example, after buffer exchange, if the resulting concentration is measured at 2 mg/mL or 2 μg/μL, then the volume needed is: 50 μg ÷ 2 μg/μL = 25 μL.

3. Add acetonitrile to the sample to a final concentration of 10% (v/v), and mix the contents of the tube gently (*see* **Note 7**).
4. Dissolve the lyophilized trypsin in water to a final concentration of 1 mg/mL (*see* **Note 8**).
5. Add certain volume of fresh-made 1 mg/mL trypsin to the 50 μg aliquot of the sample which has been added with 10% acetonitrile to achieve an enzyme:substrate (E:S) ratio (w/w) of 1:25–1:18. Mix the contents of the tube gently and incubate the sample at 37 °C for 1–2 h in the dark (*see* **Note 9**).

   For example, if the targeted E:S ratio is 1:20, the volume of 1 mg/mL trypsin needed is 50 μg ÷ 20 ÷ 1 μg/μL = 2.5 μL.
6. Add isopropanol to the sample to a final concentration of 40% (v/v), and mix the contents of the tube gently (*see* **Note 10**).
7. The resulting sample is ready for analysis. Store the digested sample at −80 °C until analysis if necessary (*see* **Note 11**).

3.6 Separation

Reversed-phase liquid chromatography (RPLC) is routinely used for separation of digested peptides. A typical RPLC method condition is introduced below as the starting conditions for peptide mapping. It is of note that method optimization is needed to obtain the highest quality reproducible chromatogram.

1. Chromatographic system: Ultra High Performance Liquid Chromatography (UHPLC) (*see* **Note 12**).
2. Column: Octadecylsilane (C18) column with 300 Å or smaller pores and particle size of 2–3 μm or less (*see* **Note 13**).
3. Mobile phase: LC-MS grade water with 0.085% FA, 0.015% TFA as mobile phase A (MPA), LC-MS grade acetonitrile with 0.085% FA, 0.015% TFA as mobile phase B (MPB) (*see* **Note 14**). Percent for mobile phase mentioned here is volume to volume.
4. Column temperature: Follow manufacturer's recommendations (*see* **Note 15**).
5. Flow rate: It mainly depends on particle size, inner diameter (I.D.), and length of the column being used. Typical flow rate is 0.1–0.2 mL/min.
6. Gradient: 0% MPB for 4 min, 0–65% MPB for 60 min, 65–100% MPB for 10 min, 100% B for 5 min, 100–0% B for 1 min, 0% B for 10 min (*see* **Note 16**).
7. Ultraviolet (UV) detection wavelength: 214 nm and the λ_{max} of the drug-linker (*see* **Note 17**).

3.7 MS Detection

Time of flight (TOF) and Orbitrap-based MS are the two most commonly used platforms to perform peptide mapping for conjugation site analysis. Some important steps are highlighted below to enable the MS detection and identification of digested peptides, including drug-linker loaded peptides. It is of note that the instrumentation of different models or from different vendors may have special requirements and operation practices.

1. Ionization and desolvation: Electrospray ionization (ESI) source operated in positive mode is used to introduce positively charged peptide ions. Capillary voltage, cone voltage, desolvation and source temperatures, and dry gas flow rate are typical tuning parameters used to optimize ion signal while minimizing in-source fragmentation.
2. MS calibration: Follow manufacturer's recommendations.
3. Scan mode: Acquire the MS scan with mass/charge (m/z) range of 50–2500, followed by MS/MS (tandem MS) scans of precursor ions (*see* **Note 18**).

3.8 Data Analysis

3.8.1 Software Searching Algorithm

Input the experimental data, and light chain and heavy chain sequence in the searching engine software, set enzyme as trypsin, select the fragmentation type (e.g., CID), and input the common PTMs (N-linked glycosylation, deamidation (Asn, Gln), oxidation (Met, Trp, Cys), N-terminal pyroglutamate formation, or C-terminal Lysine truncations) and also the mass shift caused by drug-linker conjugation as modifiers. Set the mass tolerance for precursor ions and fragment ions (typically ±5 ppm) and the intensity threshold as filters. Once completed, search algorithm identification for drug-linker loaded peptides can be performed (*see* **Note 19**).

3.8.2 Manual Data Review

1. For interchain cysteine-conjugated ADCs (native or engineered), calculate the expected mass of all the putative, uncleaved tryptic peptides that incorporate the reduced interchain cysteine (LC peptide [GEC], HC peptide [SCDK] at the arm or HC peptide [xxxCPPCxxxxxxx] at the hinge for most IgG1-based ADCs) with a mass increase of drug-linker. Then search in the LC-MS profile for these masses by plotting extracted ion chromatograms (EICs) (*see* **Note 20**).
2. Use the characteristic MS/MS fragment ions originating from the payload as signature ions for quick identification of conjugation sites without ambiguity (for example, m/z 718.51, 686.49, 506.36, 411.26, 321.21, 170.11, 152.10, and 134.09 are observed in all MS/MS spectra of molecules containing monomethyl auristatin E (MMAE) [8–10]; m/z 435.18, 485.22, and 547.22 are diagnostic ions for derivative of maytansine (DM1)-attached peptides upon CID fragmentation [11–13]).

   For example, for drug-linker conjugated peptides assigned by software, screen out any false positive due to the absence of signature ions. On the other hand, extract MS/MS spectra using the signature ions to identify the drug-linker conjugated peptides that are not identified by the software.

3. In addition to signature ions, the chromatogram by UV detection at the λ_{max} can help to identify conjugated peptides (for example, UV 252 nm profile can be used to identify the emtansine-conjugated peptides [11]).

4 Notes

1. 8 M urea is preferred over 6 M guanidine chloride (GndHCl) as the denaturing buffer because 8 M urea provides a stronger denaturing condition which enables proteolytically resistant proteins to be digested more efficiently. In addition, the trypsin activity can be significantly reduced even by residual level of GndHCl present. (A small amount of the GdnHCl is typically carried through during buffer exchange into the digestion buffer.) This is due to the fact that the guanidine group is energetically favorable to form a hydrogen bond/salt bridge with the carboxyl group of Asp189, which is in the active region of trypsin [15], therefore preventing the interaction between trypsin and the target protein. In contrast, the trypsin digestion condition is tolerable with up to 1 M urea in the digestion buffer as this concentration is not sufficiently high to detrimentally inhibit digestion via denaturation of the enzyme [16].

   Additionally, alcohols and acetonitrile are not suitable as chaotropes for protein denaturation because high concentrations (>30%) of organic solvents often lead to irreversible protein precipitation.

2. DTT is preferred over tris(2-carboxyethyl)phosphine (TCEP) as the reducing agent because TCEP can reduce oxidized methionine residues if already present on the molecule prior to digestion [17]. The reducing conditions described here provide a 20- to 25-fold molar excess of DTT over cysteine which is necessary for complete reduction. If the IgG is reduced at a higher concentration, the concentration of DTT must be increased proportionally.

3. As urea is used to denature proteins, this allows the reducing agent access to disulfide bonds at a lower temperature. The recommended temperature condition to perform reduction is 37 °C. This can prevent protein carbamylation which occurs in urea solutions at high temperatures (>60 °C) [18].

   On the condition that the drug-linker of the ADC sample is found to be thermally unstable, the reduction can be performed at room temperature for 60 min in the dark.

4. IAM is preferred over iodoacetic acid (IAA) as the alkylating agent due to its faster reaction time, and unlike IAA it does not introduce a negative charge to the derivatized peptide. Since any remaining DTT competes with the sulfhydryl group for the alkylating agent, IAM is typically used in excess of the reducing agent to ensure complete alkylation. However, using too high a concentration runs the risk of overalkylation of the protein, including alkylation on residues other than cysteine [19].

   The reaction of N-Ethylmaleimide (NEM) with thiols is even faster than IAM or IAA and less dependent on pH. However, NEM may be less specific than iodo derivatives. At alkaline pH, NEM also reacts with the side chains of lysine and histidine [20].

5. Although the efficiency of salt removal is comparable for columns from different manufacturers (>95%), Thermo Scientific Zeba Spin Desalting columns typically offer higher levels of protein recovery and lower rates of sample dilution over a wider range of sample sizes and sample concentrations compared to the other desalting products.

   During the centrifuge step for column preparation, the cap should be kept loosened (do not remove cap).

6. Concentration determination is important because it helps to not only evaluate the recovery percentage of the spin column, but also determine the volume needed for enzymatically digesting 50 μg of buffer-exchanged sample (*see* Subheading 3.5, **step 2**). It is strongly recommended to use NanoDrop microvolume spectrophotometer so that the majority of the sample remains untouched from the auto-pipette and cuvette to avoid sample contamination and degradation.

7. In order to maintain hydrophobic drug-linker loaded peptides in solution such that all the conjugated peptides can be identified on the LC-MS chromatogram, 10% acetonitrile is suggested to be added to the sample prior to digestion. There is one more step after digestion to keep hydrophobic drug-linker loaded peptides soluble (*see* Subheading 3.5, **step 6**).

8. Trypsin is the first-choice enzyme for peptide mapping analysis of mAbs and ADCs, which specifically cleaves at the carboxylic side of lysine and arginine residues. It is available from many vendors. Among them, Promega Sequencing Grade Modified Trypsin (Cat # V5111) is porcine trypsin modified by reductive methylation, which causes it to be resistant to proteolytic digestion. It is also resistant to mild denaturing conditions such as 0.1% SDS, 1 M urea, or 10% acetonitrile.

9. The enzyme is suggested to be added more than conventional use (E:S ratio of 1:50) in order to shorten the digestion time to minimize the mAb in-digestion modification (asparagine

deamidation or N-terminal glutamine cyclization) given that the pH value of digestion buffer is 7.8.

If the drug-linker is thermally unstable, the incubation can be conducted at room temperature for 4 h in the dark.

10. To keep the hydrophobic drug-linker loaded peptides in solution after enzymatic digestion, it is suggested that 10% acetonitrile should be added to the sample before digestion and 40% isopropanol after digestion. This approach has been proven effective to successfully identify drug-linker loaded peptides for interchain cysteinyl-linked ADCs [8, 9].
11. It is strongly recommended to make fresh digested peptide sample right before the LC-MS experiment for the concern of stability and solubility of drug-linker loaded peptide.
12. UHPLC system is recommended, as it significantly enhances the efficiency of LC by using the columns with sub-2-μm particle size and UHPLC systems with low dead volume and tolerance of up to 15,000 psi. UHPLC has also been used to reduce run time of existing methods by higher flow rate and mobile phase consumption.
13. With the column development in surface chemistry and particle technology, there are a wider range of choices for the columns from different vendors to accomplish higher separation performance. For example, the high surface area and dense C18 bonding provide Phenomenex Luna Omega column with excellent retention for small and more polar peptides. The positively charged functional group is modified on the surface for the columns (e.g., Waters CSH column and Phenomenex Luna Omega PS column) to minimize tailing effects and render mobile phase more MS-friendly. Compared with commonly used porous sub-2-μm columns on UHPLC system, superficially porous columns (e.g., Agilent AdvanceBio column) can provide equivalent or better performance during very fast run times (two to three times faster than with fully porous HPLC columns) and low system pressures. Furthermore, the introduction of sub-2-μm superficially porous columns (e.g., Phenomenex Aeris column) demonstrates improved efficiency over fully porous media of the same particle size.
14. The most common mobile phase B composition for RPLC separation of peptides is acetonitrile. However other organic solvent such as methanol and isopropanol can be employed as well. Solvents such as isopropanol may be useful for separating samples that contain many highly hydrophobic peptides, but it should be noted that hydrophilic or small peptides may elute in the column void volume.

Mobile phase additives such as acids are generally needed to produce good chromatographic separations of peptides. The most common mobile phase additive has been TFA with typical concentrations of 0.05%–0.2% being employed. While TFA has a significant positive impact on the quality of peptide separation, sensitivity with mass spectrometer detection can suffer with TFA due to ion suppression. To overcome this, formic acid, acetic acid, or combinations of these with TFA (e.g., 0.1% formic acid with <0.02% TFA) can be used to increase mass spectrometer sensitivity by reducing ion suppression.

15. If there is no recommendation from the vendor for column temperature, 40 °C is ideal starting temperature. The column temperature may be used to optimize peptide separation or improve the retention or elution of certain peptides since the resolution of the peptides typically increases with column temperature for a reversed-phase column.
16. Gradient needs to be tuned to increase resolution. Given the hydrophobic property of drug-linker loaded peptide, it is sometimes needed to elute them by using higher percentage of mobile phase B.
17. The most common detection method is UV light absorption at 214 nm. The peptides resulting from protein digestion may not contain amino acids with aromatic side chains that absorb light at higher wavelengths (e.g., 280 nm) so detection at 214 nm (i.e., wavelength where peptide bonds absorb light) is essential to ensure sequence coverage of the protein while minimizing background due to the mobile phase.

    Dual wavelength detection is recommended by including the λ_{max} of the drug-linker as the second UV channel. For example, 252 nm is set for emtansine-based drug-linker [11]. This helps to readily identify the peaks of the drug-linker loaded peptides in UV chromatogram during data analysis (*see* Subheading 3.8.2, **step 3**).
18. MS/MS scan of the peptide fragmentation ions is important for characterization of drug-linker loaded peptides. Firstly, MS/MS spectra associated with drug-linker loaded peptides are usually populated by fragments originating from the drug, which can be used to recognize conjugated peptides in LC-MS/MS map (*see* Subheading 3.8.2, **step 2**). Secondly, MS/MS spectra may allow for identification of conjugation sites without ambiguity even in the situation where multiple modification sites are present in a single digest peptide. This can happen to lysine-conjugated peptides [12, 13] or cysteine-conjugated peptides at hinge region with "CPPC" motif [8]. Thirdly, peptide identification is always based on both peptide mass measurement and fragmentation products using

MS/MS spectra in order to enable unambiguous characterization.

To perform MS/MS, collision-induced dissociation (CID) is the most commonly used fragmentation approach.

19. Peptide identification by searching engine is in principle based on both peptide mass measurement and fragmentation products using MS/MS spectra in order to enable unambiguous characterization. However, MS/MS scan of the drug-linker loaded peptides via CID fragmentation in some cases produces poor peptide backbone fragmentation. Relying on only MS1 data may lead to false positives or missing data, as is limited by software filter setting. To address this, manual data review is needed to confirm the assignment (*see* Subheading 3.8.2, **step 2**).

    On the other hand, other fragmentation techniques, if available, can be used to provide more fragment ion information, such as higher-energy collisional dissociation (HCD) which provides multiple fragmentations [13], and electron transfer dissociation (ETD) or electron capture dissociation (ECD) which offers different fragmentation mechanisms [21]. Additionally, trap-type instruments can be used for low-abundance ion enrichment.

20. This approach can help quickly confirm the characterization of the expected drug-linker loaded peptides linked to the interchain cysteine of the HC and LC. However it cannot work very efficiently for lysine-conjugated ADCs as lysine conjugation process is believed to be a nonspecific process, and all the lysine residues in the mAb molecules are candidates for drug-linker conjugation.

    Even for cysteine conjugation, possibilities cannot be ruled out with regard to the nonspecific cysteine attachment (e.g., sulfhydryl groups of the intrachain cysteine) and lysine attachment (due to the chemistry reactivity of drug-linker). Under such circumstance, manual data review is needed to identify the unexpected, nonspecific drug-linker conjugation sites (*see* Subheading 3.8.2, **step 2**).

References

1. Chudasama V, Maruani A, Caddick S (2016) Recent advances in the construction of antibody-drug conjugates. Nat Chem 8 (2):114–119. https://doi.org/10.1038/nchem.2415
2. Shen BQ, Xu K, Liu L, Raab H, Bhakta S, Kenrick M, Parsons-Reponte KL, Tien J, Yu SF, Mai E, Li D, Tibbitts J, Baudys J, Saad OM, Scales SJ, McDonald PJ, Hass PE, Eigenbrot C, Nguyen T, Solis WA, Fuji RN, Flagella KM, Patel D, Spencer SD, Khawli LA, Ebens A, Wong WL, Vandlen R, Kaur S, Sliwkowski MX, Scheller RH, Polakis P, Junutula JR (2012) Conjugation site modulates the in vivo stability and therapeutic activity of antibody-drug conjugates. Nat Biotechnol 30 (2):184–189. https://doi.org/10.1038/nbt.2108
3. Strop P, Liu SH, Dorywalska M, Delaria K, Dushin RG, Tran TT, Ho WH, Farias S,

Casas MG, Abdiche Y, Zhou D, Chandrasekaran R, Samain C, Loo C, Rossi A, Rickert M, Krimm S, Wong T, Chin SM, Yu J, Dilley J, Chaparro-Riggers J, Filzen GF, O'Donnell CJ, Wang F, Myers JS, Pons J, Shelton DL, Rajpal A (2013) Location matters: site of conjugation modulates stability and pharmacokinetics of antibody drug conjugates. Chem Biol 20(2):161–167. https://doi.org/10.1016/j.chembiol.2013.01.010

4. Su D, Kozak KR, Sadowsky J, Yu SF, Fourie-O'Donohue A, Nelson C, Vandlen R, Ohri R, Liu L, Ng C, He J, Davis H, Lau J, Del Rosario G, Cosino E, Cruz-Chuh JD, Ma Y, Zhang D, Darwish M, Cai W, Chen C, Zhou H, Lu J, Liu Y, Kaur S, Xu K, Pillow TH (2018) Modulating Antibody-Drug Conjugate Payload Metabolism by Conjugation Site and Linker Modification. Bioconjug Chem 29(4):1155–1167. https://doi.org/10.1021/acs.bioconjchem.7b00785
5. Wang L, Amphlett G, Blattler WA, Lambert JM, Zhang W (2005) Structural characterization of the maytansinoid-monoclonal antibody immunoconjugate, huN901-DM1, by mass spectrometry. Protein Sci 14(9):2436–2446. https://doi.org/10.1110/ps.051478705
6. Liu-Shin L, Fung A, Malhotra A, Ratnaswamy G (2018) Influence of disulfide bond isoforms on drug conjugation sites in cysteine-linked IgG2 antibody-drug conjugates. MAbs 10 (4):583–595. https://doi.org/10.1080/19420862.2018.1440165
7. Whitmore CD, Gennaro LA (2012) Capillary electrophoresis-mass spectrometry methods for tryptic peptide mapping of therapeutic antibodies. Electrophoresis 33(11):1550–1556. https://doi.org/10.1002/elps.201200066
8. Janin-Bussat MC, Dillenbourg M, Corvaia N, Beck A, Klinguer-Hamour C (2015) Characterization of antibody drug conjugate positional isomers at cysteine residues by peptide mapping LC-MS analysis. J Chromatogr B Analyt Technol Biomed Life Sci 981–982:9–13. https://doi.org/10.1016/j.jchromb.2014.12.017
9. Said N, Gahoual R, Kuhn L, Beck A, Francois YN, Leize-Wagner E (2016) Structural characterization of antibody drug conjugate by a combination of intact, middle-up and bottom-up techniques using sheathless capillary electrophoresis - Tandem mass spectrometry as nanoESI infusion platform and separation method. Anal Chim Acta 918:50–59. https://doi.org/10.1016/j.aca.2016.03.006
10. Junutula JR, Raab H, Clark S, Bhakta S, Leipold DD, Weir S, Chen Y, Simpson M, Tsai SP, Dennis MS, Lu Y, Meng YG, Ng C, Yang J, Lee CC, Duenas E, Gorrell J, Katta V, Kim A, McDorman K, Flagella K, Venook R, Ross S, Spencer SD, Lee Wong W, Lowman HB, Vandlen R, Sliwkowski MX, Scheller RH, Polakis P, Mallet W (2008) Site-specific conjugation of a cytotoxic drug to an antibody improves the therapeutic index. Nat Biotechnol 26(8):925–932. https://doi.org/10.1038/nbt.1480
11. Sandra K, Vanhoenacker G, Vandenheede I, Steenbeke M, Joseph M, Sandra P (2016) Multiple heart-cutting and comprehensive two-dimensional liquid chromatography hyphenated to mass spectrometry for the characterization of the antibody-drug conjugate ado-trastuzumab emtansine. J Chromatogr B Analyt Technol Biomed Life Sci 1032:119–130. https://doi.org/10.1016/j.jchromb.2016.04.040
12. Sang H, Lu G, Liu Y, Hu Q, Xing W, Cui D, Zhou F, Zhang J, Hao H, Wang G, Ye H (2017) Conjugation site analysis of antibody-drug-conjugates (ADCs) by signature ion fingerprinting and normalized area quantitation approach using nano-liquid chromatography coupled to high resolution mass spectrometry. Anal Chim Acta 955:67–78. https://doi.org/10.1016/j.aca.2016.11.073
13. Luo Q, Chung HH, Borths C, Janson M, Wen J, Joubert MK, Wypych J (2016) Structural Characterization of a Monoclonal Antibody-Maytansinoid Immunoconjugate. Anal Chem 88(1):695–702. https://doi.org/10.1021/acs.analchem.5b03709
14. Hada V, Bagdi A, Bihari Z, Timari SB, Fizil A, Szantay C Jr (2018) Recent advancements, challenges, and practical considerations in the mass spectrometry-based analytics of protein biotherapeutics: a viewpoint from the biosimilar industry. J Pharm Biomed Anal 161:214–238. https://doi.org/10.1016/j.jpba.2018.08.024
15. Ren D, Pipes GD, Liu D, Shih LY, Nichols AC, Treuheit MJ, Brems DN, Bondarenko PV (2009) An improved trypsin digestion method minimizes digestion-induced modifications on proteins. Anal Biochem 392(1):12–21. https://doi.org/10.1016/j.ab.2009.05.018
16. Mouchahoir T, Schiel JE (2018) Development of an LC-MS/MS peptide mapping protocol for the NISTmAb. Anal Bioanal Chem 410 (8):2111–2126. https://doi.org/10.1007/s00216-018-0848-6
17. Lundell N, Schreitmuller T (1999) Sample preparation for peptide mapping—A pharmaceutical quality-control perspective. Anal

Biochem 266(1):31–47. https://doi.org/10.1006/abio.1998.2919

18. Cole EG, Mecham DK (1966) Cyanate formation and electrophoretic behavior of proteins in gels containing urea. Anal Biochem 14 (2):215–222
19. Boja ES, Fales HM (2001) Overalkylation of a protein digest with iodoacetamide. Anal Chem 73(15):3576–3582
20. Ying J, Clavreul N, Sethuraman M, Adachi T, Cohen RA (2007) Thiol oxidation in signaling and response to stress: detection and quantification of physiological and pathophysiological thiol modifications. Free Radic Biol Med 43 (8):1099–1108. https://doi.org/10.1016/j.freeradbiomed.2007.07.014
21. Coon JJ, Syka JE, Shabanowitz J, Hunt DFJB (2005) Tandem mass spectrometry for peptide and protein sequence analysis. Biotechniques 38(4):519–523

Chapter 16

Conjugation Site Analysis of Lysine-Conjugated ADCs

Hua Sang, Ning Wan, Gaoyuan Lu, Yang Tian, Guangji Wang, and Hui Ye

Abstract

Lysine-conjugated antibody-drug conjugates (ADCs) are formed by attaching cytotoxic drugs to reactive lysine residues of monoclonal antibodies (mAbs) through chemical linkers. During production, the payloads are conjugated nonspecifically to lysine residues in mAbs, resulting in a heterogeneous mixture of ADCs with both different number and conjugation sites of drug payloads per mAb. On account of the drug conjugation sites and levels that both have significant influences on physical and pharmaceutical properties of ADCs, a reliable and straightforward approach for conjugation site analysis for ADCs is highly demanded. Herein, we used a lysine-conjugated ADC, Trastuzumab-MCC-DM1 (T-DM1), as a model ADC, and described an integrative strategy that combines the signature ion fingerprinting method for rapid and reliable filtering of DM1-conjugated peptides, and the normalized area quantitation approach for accurately gauging the conjugation levels for each identified site. This approach is believed to be readily applicable to other maytansinoid derivatives-modified ADCs, and more importantly, universally applicable to lysine-conjugated ADCs for both the recognition of conjugation sites and the measurement of conjugation levels.

Key words ADC, Conjugation site analysis, Conjugation level, Lysine conjugation, T-DM1, Signature ion fingerprinting, Normalized area quantitation

1 Introduction

Antibody drug conjugates (ADCs) is embracing its emerging advancements in the past decade as the most promising therapeutic agents for targeted cancer treatment [1, 2]. ADCs are monoclonal antibodies (mAbs) attached to cytotoxic drugs as payloads. The drug-conjugated antibodies carry the payloads to targeted antigens that are often overexpressed on the surface of tumor cells, become internalized into cells, are transported to lysosomes, undergo degradation, and ultimately release cytotoxic drugs to kill cells, resulting in increased antitumor specificity and reduced toxicity compared to nontargeted chemotherapy [3].

Lysine-conjugated ADCs, a major class of ADCs, are manufactured by covalently attaching drugs to reactive lysine residues through linkers, with acylation chemistry being most commonly

L. Nathan Tumey (ed.), *Antibody-Drug Conjugates: Methods and Protocols*, Methods in Molecular Biology, vol. 2078, https://doi.org/10.1007/978-1-4939-9929-3_16,

used [4]. Intriguingly, unlike cysteine-conjugated ADCs, lysine-conjugated ADCs have more available sites for conjugation. In the case of Trastuzumab, the heavy and light chains contain a total of 90 lysine residues. All the lysine-conjugated protein therapeutics including those currently on the market (Mylotarg and Kadcyla) and ADCs still in clinical trials (IMGN289 [5] and AMG595 [6]) are thus viewed as mAbs conjugated with payloads in a nonspecific manner. This characteristic leads to the production of heterogeneous lysine-conjugated ADC mixtures that exhibit a great degree of complexity with varying number of drugs attached at different positions on the naked mAbs.

Expectedly, the structural complexity of lysine-conjugated ADCs results in variant physical and pharmaceutical properties [7]. Extensive studies have demonstrated the impact of differences in conjugation sites on the final products of ADCs. A representative study by Shen et al. demonstrated that, through site-specific engineered conjugation sites, in vivo stability, toxicity, and therapeutic efficacy of ADCs were all influenced [8]. Boswell et al. and Junutula et al. also found that the interchain disulfide cysteine-modified ADCs displayed different in vivo pharmacokinetic (PK) profiles and therapeutic index compared with engineered conjugation that modified cysteines located in the constant domain of the Fab region of mAbs [9, 10]. Specifically, drug conjugation on residues in the complementarity determining regions (CDRs) of mAbs significantly affected the ADCs' binding capacity to target antigens and thereby the pharmacological responses [11]. This is in line with Wang's study that reported similar binding affinity of ADCs to the naked antibody when the lysine residues in the CDRs of huN901 remained unmodified [12]. These evidences thus collectively indicate that the precise control of payload-conjugated sites and the extent of conjugation are crucial to ensure consistent delivery and release of payload, which warrants reliable and reproducible therapeutic efficacy and PK behavior.

Since the task to identify drug conjugation site from ADCs is straightforward, it has been accomplished by peptide mapping for lysine-conjugated ADCs in previous literature [12, 13]. Nevertheless, few analytical approaches have been reported to appraise the degree of conjugation at each identified site after the assignment of conjugation sites has been made [14, 15]. A reliable and convenient approach to analyze conjugation site and level is thus highly demanded for researchers aiming to dissect the roles of position, drug, and linker and thereby to achieve optimal therapeutic index of ADCs. Previously, Luo et al. quantified the decreased abundance of peptides that remain unmodified between the naked mAb and T-DM1 samples, respectively, and inferred the conjugation levels at each site [15]. Nevertheless, this approach probes the drug occupancy at each conjugation site only in an indirect way. Meanwhile, it requires the quantitative analysis of targeted peptides to be

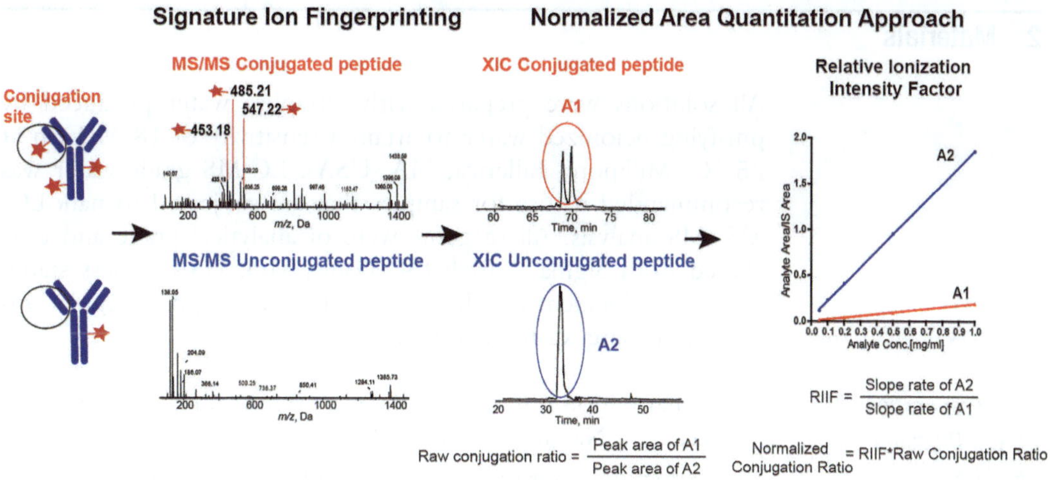

Fig. 1 General scheme of an integrative strategy that combines the signature ion fingerprinting method for rapid and reliable filtering of drug-conjugated peptides, and the normalized area quantitation approach for accurately gauging the conjugation levels for each identified site

performed between two samples, which potentially suffer from inaccuracy induced by inconsistent digestion across batches and instrumental fluctuations.

The current chapter describes a more straightforward approach that directly measures the occupancy level of each drug-conjugated site by analyzing single ADC sample. Consequently, additional interferences with conjugation site analysis results due to inconsistency in protein digestion and other processing steps are avoided using our approach. Specifically, we used Trastuzumab-MCC-DM1 (TDM1) as a model ADC to showcase this strategy for conjugation level analysis in this chapter (Scheme shown in Fig. 1). We first used the signature MS/MS ions of DM1 as fingerprints to eliminate false positive hits of DM1-adducted peptides. Using the same set of data, we extracted the chromatograms of DM1-conjugated peptides and its unconjugated counterpart, and quantified raw conjugation ratio for each identified site. Interestingly, we noticed generally suppressed ionization efficiencies of peptides after DM1-conjugation, and thus quantified normalized conjugation ratio by performing additional MRM experiment to calculate "relative ionization intensity factor" (RIIF) for each peptide. RIIF is used to normalize the discrepancy of observed raw conjugation ratio from actual occupancy level due to signal suppression. The summed-up values of normalized conjugation ratio for all identified conjugation sites should be in agreement with the drug-antibody ratio (DAR) of ADCs, which is readily obtained by intact mass measurement. In general, this integrative approach for conjugation site analysis can be adapted to other maytansinoid analogs-modified ADCs and is universally applicable to other lysine-conjugated ADCs with slight modifications.

2 Materials

All solutions were prepared with ultrapure water produced by purifying deionized water to attain a sensitivity of 18 MΩ-cm at 25 °C (Millipore, Billerica, MA, USA). LC-MS grade water was recommended to use for samples that are subjected to nanoLC-MS/MS analysis. All reagents were of analytical grade and purchased from Sigma-Aldrich (St. Louis, MO, USA) unless stated otherwise. Diligently follow all local waste disposal regulations when disposing waste materials.

2.1 Preparation of ADC Digested Peptides

1. Denaturation buffer: 8 M urea in 50 mM NH_4CO_3 (Nanjing Reagent, Nanjing, China) buffer.
2. Reduction solution: 0.5 M Dithiothreitol (DTT) in 50 mM NH_4CO_3 buffer.
3. Alkylation solution: 0.4 M Iodoacetamide (IAA) (Aladdin, Shanghai, China) in 50 mM NH_4CO_3 buffer.
4. Chymotrypsin (Promega, Madison, WI, USA) at 20 μg/mL dissolved in 50 mM acetic acid.
5. 10% formic acid (FA) (Acros Organics, Belgium).
6. ZipTip™ with 0.2 μL resin (Millipore, Billerica, MA, USA) and C_{18} HLB SPE columns (Waters, Milford, MA, USA) for micro-scale- and regular scale-peptide desalting.
7. Activation solution for desalting: ACN with 0.1% FA.
8. Equilibrium solution for desalting: ultrapure water with 0.1% FA.
9. Eluent solution for desalting: ACN-water (1:1, v/v) with 0.1% FA.
10. Pressure blowing concentrator: Scdeall VX-II (Scdeall, Beijing, China) or vacuum concentrator (SpeedVac, Thermo Savant, NY, USA).
11. Original T-DM1 (Roche, Basel, Switzerland) and generic T-DM1 (Hengrui, Shanghai, China) freeze-dried powder injection.

2.2 LC-MS/MS Analysis for Identification of Lysine Conjugation Sites

1. Solvent A: LC-MS grade water with 0.1% FA.
2. Solvent B: LC-MS grade ACN with 0.1% FA.
3. A nano-scale liquid chromatography (nanoLC) system: Prominence Nano-flow liquid chromatography system (Shimadzu, Kyoto, Japan).
4. A reversed-phase C_{18} nano-column (75 μm × 150 mm, 3 μm particle size) (Eksigent, Dublin, CA, USA) for peptide separation.

5. Mass spectrometry: TripleTOF 5600 system (AB SCIEX, Framingham, MA, USA).

2.3 LC-MS/MS for Quantitative Analysis of Lysine Conjugation Levels

1. LC-MS/MS Solvent A: ultrapure water with 0.1% FA.
2. LC-MS/MS Solvent B: ACN (Merck, Darmstadt, Germany) with 0.1% FA.
3. Liquid chromatography system: LC-20 AD HPLC system (Shimadzu).
4. A Sepax Bio-C_{18} column (2.1 × 150 mm, 5 μm, 300 Å) for peptide separation (Sepax, Delaware, USA).
5. Mass spectrometry instrument: 5500 QTRAP system (AB SCIEX).
6. DM1 and lys-MCC-DM1 (HengRui, Shanghai, China) dissolved in MeOH (Merck, Darmstadt, Germany) at 1 mg/mL.
7. High speed freezing centrifuge: SORVALL Stratos (Thermo Fisher, MA, USA).

3 Methods

3.1 Identify Drug-Conjugated Lysine by Signature Ion Fingerprinting

3.1.1 Acquire Signature Fragment Ions of Drug Payloads

1. Prepare pure standard of drug payloads, DM1 of T-DM1 in our case, in sampling vials.
2. Direct the sample into a high resolution mass spectrometer to acquire the accurate *m/z*, and subsequently select it as the precursor ion and perform MS/MS experiments. Collisional-induced dissociation (CID) mode or higher-energy collisional dissociation (HCD) is recommended.

As shown in Fig. 2, signature fragment ions of DM1 and the proposed substructures were produced upon MS/MS fragmentation, including ions at *m/z* 435.18, 485.22, and 547.22. The presence of these signature fragment ions (SFIs) at relatively high abundance was thus employed to manually eliminate false positive identifications, which needs to be taken care with caution in post-translational modification (PTM) studies. Although our study only showcased the SFIs of DM1, this strategy can be adopted with any drug payloads that can generate SFIs during MS/MS events.

3.1.2 Preparation of Antibody-Drug-Conjugates for LC-MS/MS Analysis

1. Dissolve the T-DM1 freeze-dried powder injection in ultrapure water to prepare the ADC sample solution (~10 mg/mL) for digestion.
2. Transfer 10 μL of ADC sample solution to 100 μL of 8 M urea and briefly vortex the mixture. Add 2 μL of 0.5 M DTT and incubate the solution in 56 °C water bath for 30 min. A 10 μL of 0.4 M IAA was then added followed by incubation in the dark at 37 °C for another 30 min. Subsequently, add 2 μL of

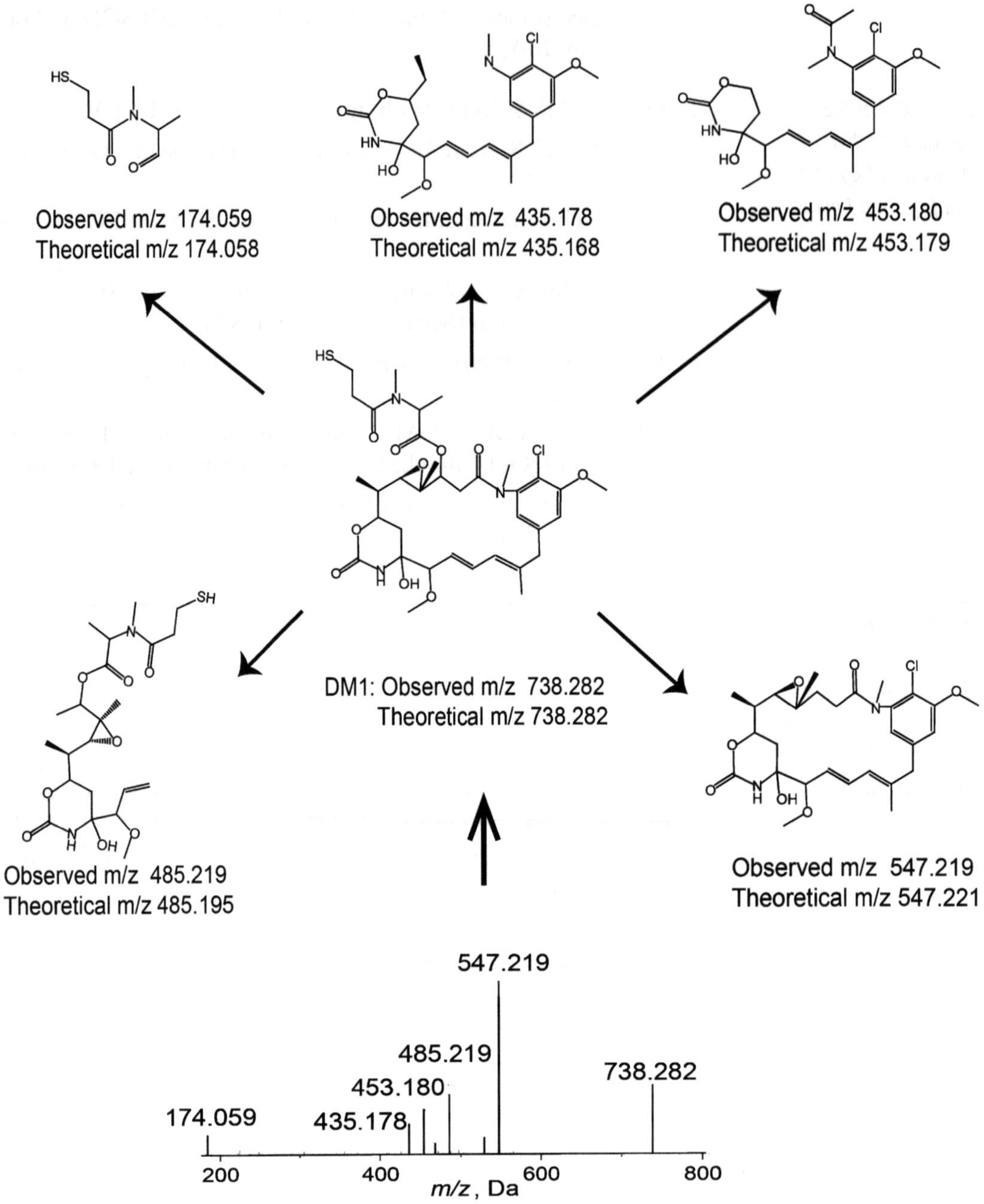

Fig. 2 The collisional-induced dissociation fragmentation spectrum of DM1 and the proposed structures of these ions. (Reprinted from Analytica Chimica Acta, Vol 955, Sang H, Lu GY, Liu YZ et al., Conjugation site analysis of antibody-drug-conjugates (ADCs) by signature ion fingerprinting and normalized area quantitation approach using nano-liquid chromatography coupled to high resolution mass spectrometry, Pages No. 67–78, Copyright (2017), with permission from Elsevier)

0.5 M DTT and incubate at room temperature for 15 min (*see* **Note 1**).

3. Prepare ~50 mM NH_4CO_3 solution at pH 7.4. Add chymotrypsin to the T-DM1 sample at a ratio of 1:50 for overnight digestion at room temperature.
4. Add 10% FA to acidify the digested peptide sample to 0.1% FA.
5. Activate C_{18} Ziptip by rinsing the tip with 10 μL 0.1% FA in ACN for five times. Then equilibrate the tips by rinsing with 10 μL 0.1% FA in water. Load the digested peptide sample onto the tip followed by washing with 10 μL 0.1% FA in water three times. Elute the desalted peptides by 10 μL 0.1% FA in ACN-water (1:1, v/v) (*see* **Note 2**), and collect the eluted fraction in a tube.
6. Dry the eluted peptides using a pressure blowing concentrator with N_2. Store the peptide samples at −80 °C until use.

3.1.3 LC-MS/MS Analysis for Identification of Conjugation Sites

1. Redissolve the ADC digestion samples with 20 μL 0.1% FA in LC-MS grade water.
2. Centrifuge samples at 18,000 × *g* for 10 min at 4 °C.
3. Transfer 15 μL supernatant to sampling vials for nanoLC-MS/MS analysis coupled to TripleTOF 5600 (AB SCIEX).
4. Set up the elution gradient by using solvent (A) 0.1% (v/v) FA in water and solvent (B) 0.1% (v/v) FA in ACN. We used a 100-min gradient as follows: 5% B for 4 min, 5–60% B for 56 min, 60–95% B for 15 min, 95% B for 10 min, 95–5% B for 5 min, and 5% B for 10 min equilibration. Flow rate: 300 nL/min. The gradient should be modified based on different LC systems.
5. Set up analysis parameters for nanoESI-MS/MS. The nanoESI source conditions were set as follows: Ion Source Gas 1 (GS1) as 10, Ion Source Gas 2 (GS2) as 0, Curtain gas (CUR) as 30, Interface Heater temperature 150 °C, Ion Spray Voltage Floating (ISVF) 2300 V in the positive mode. The Mass spectrometer (Triple TOF 5600) conditions were set as follows: Collision gas N_2, Q1 vacuum gauge 2.4×10^{-5} torr, TOF vacuum 0.369×10^{-6} torr. The information-dependent acquisition (IDA) mode was employed for peptide mapping and subsequent identification of drug-conjugated lysine. The scan parameters under IDA mode were set as follows: the *m/z* range of 350–1500 Da for TOF MS scan, the *m/z* range of 100–2500 for product ion scan, declustering potential (DP) as 100 V. Select unit resolution for precursor ion selection, and determine collision energy (CE) according to a set of scripted equations, $|CE| = (\text{slope}) \times (m/z) + (\text{intercept})$ (*see* **Note 3**). Set IDA parameters as follows: charge state 2 to

4, intensity threshold 150 cps, exclude isotopes within 4 Da, mass tolerance 50 mDa, and maximum number of candidate ions as 10. Set the accumulation time for TOF-MS scan and MS/MS scan at 0.25 and 0.05 s, respectively. The “exclude former target ions” function should be enabled and the exclusion window was set as 9 s after 1 occurrence (*see* **Note 4**).

3.1.4 Analysis of Drug-Conjugated Sites

1. A proprietary software ProteinPilot (AB SCIEX, Framingham, MA, USA) was used for peptide mapping and DM1-conjugated site identification (*see* **Note 5**).
2. Input the heavy chain (HC) and light chain (LC) sequences of the antibody, trastuzumab in our case, to a .fasta file and import the sequence file to ProteinPilot.
3. To identify lysine that carries the drug payload, the drug-induced modification must be set as a variable PTM. We thus used the DM1 conjugation as an exemplary PTM in this chapter. The conjugation of DM1 to lysine delivers a mass difference of 956.36 Da (a DM1 molecule plus linker, formula $C_{47}H_{61}ClN_4O_{13}S$). All the precursors and specific fragment ions of lysine-containing peptides carrying an appropriate mass shift are thus assigned as DM1-conjugated peptides (*see* **Note 6**). To perform this search, we need to first include the DM1 modification to ProteinPilot (*see* **Note 7**). Specifically, add DM1 modification code under “MODIFICATION SETS” to the “ParameterTranslation” file. Under “<!--WORKUP MODIFICATION SETS-USE SET NUMBERS IN RANGE 1-10-->”, add “<MOD_FEATURE mod=“DM1”><OCCURRENCE target=“Lysine” prob=“0.03″/>”.
4. In the “ProteinPilot.DataDictionary” file, a DM1 modification code must also be added. Under “<!-- BIOLOGICAL MODIFICATIONS SECTION -->”, add “<Mod rKey=“0”> <Nme>DM1</Nme><TLC>DM1</TLC><Tgt>Lysine </Tgt><TS>255</TS><Fma>C47H61ClN4O13S</Fma> <RpF></RpF><NLF></NLF> <IIF></IIF><Chg>0 </Chg></Mod>”.
5. Open the ProteinPilot software, and select the “LC” option of “Identify Proteins” under the “Workflow Tasks”. Edit the “Paragon Method” and set the searching parameters as follows: select “Identification” under “Sample Type”, “Iodoacetic acid” under “Cys Alkylation”, “Chymotrypsin” under “Digestion”, “Urea denaturation” under “Special Factors”, and “None” under “Species”. Select the protein sequence of targeted ADCs, trastuzumab as an example in this chapter, under “database”. Choose “Thorough ID” under “Search Effort”, and set “Detected Protein Threshold” as 0.05. Check “Run

False Discovery Rate Analysis". Save the identification method as "mAb" for future use. Click "Add" to load the acquired .wiff data file and click "OK" to perform the database search.

3.1.5 Conjugated Peptide Screening by Signature Ion Fingerprinting

1. Summarize all the lysine-containing peptides that exhibited a mass shift corresponding to DM1 conjugation, and are spectrally matched to the antibody sequence produced by database search described in Subheading 3.1.4.
2. Examine the SFIs of DM1 (collected in Subheading 3.1.1) at *m/z* 435.18, 485.22, and 547.22 from the MS/MS spectra of potential DM1-conjugated peptides summarized in **step 1** (Fig. 3a, c). Exclude peptides as false positive hits due to the absence of DM1 SFIs in MS/MS spectra (Fig. 3b).
3. For conjugated peptides which possess multiple available sites for DM1 conjugation, carefully examine and compare (if available) the acquired CID MS/MS spectra. This allows for the differentiation of peptide isomers that possess multiple lysine residues yet carrying DM1 conjugation at distinct sites (Fig. 4a–c). The conjugation of stereoisomeric maleimide linker to ADCs makes the conjugated peptides diastereomers, thus it is common to observe a pair of peaks in XIC chromatograms when the *m/z* of conjugated peptides are extracted (Fig. 4d). K4, K7, and K10 refer to the fourth, seventh, and tenth lysine of this peptide counting from the N-terminal, respectively.
4. Prepare multiple samples for LC-MS/MS injections to increase the collected LC-MS/MS spectra for improved coverage of drug-conjugated peptides.

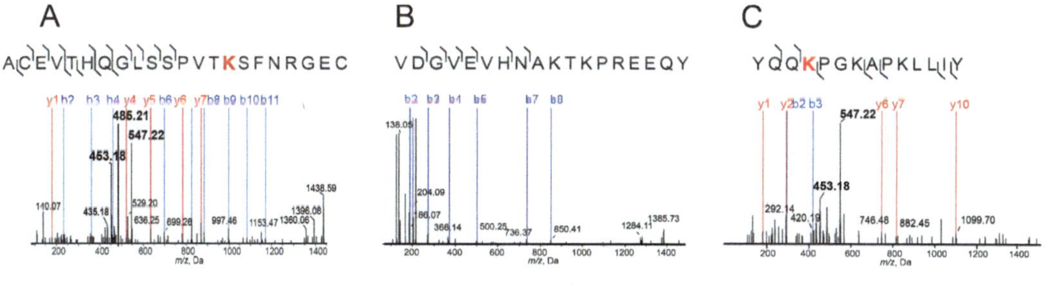

Fig. 3 Illustrated examples of how signature fragment ions of drug payloads are used for rapid screening of false positive hits of drug-conjugated peptides. (**a**) The DM1-conjugated peptide produced the signature fragment ions of DM1. The peptide shown in (**b**) was designated as a false positive hit due to the absence of the signature ions of DM1 in its MS/MS spectrum, whereas the peptide in (**c**) was identified as DM1-attached due to the presence of the DM1-specific ions despite the relatively low score assigned by the search engine. (Reprinted from Analytica Chimica Acta, Vol 955, Sang H, Lu GY, Liu YZ et al., Conjugation site analysis of antibody-drug-conjugates (ADCs) by signature ion fingerprinting and normalized area quantitation approach using nano-liquid chromatography coupled to high resolution mass spectrometry, Pages No. 67–78, Copyright (2017), with permission from Elsevier)

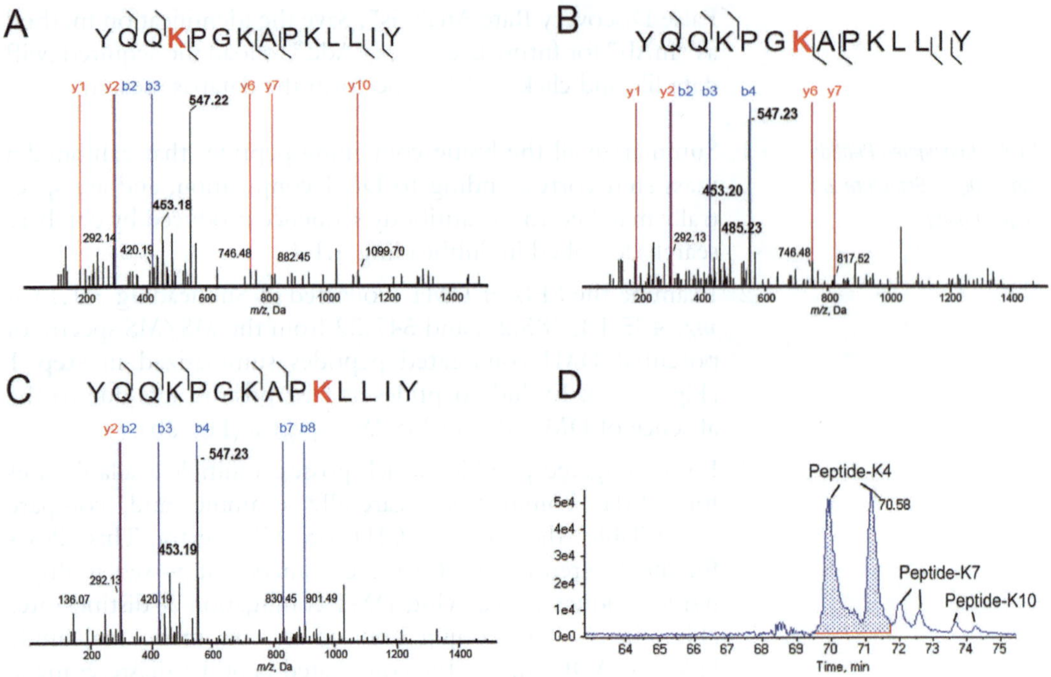

Fig. 4 MS/MS information aids in assigning different drug-conjugated lysine residues from peptides of identical sequence. (**a–c**) MS/MS spectra of the peptide YQQKPGKAPKLLIY conjugated at different lysine residues (K4, K7, and K10). (**d**) XIC of the three paired DM1-conjugated peptide isomers. (Reprinted from Analytica Chimica Acta, Vol 955, Sang H, Lu GY, Liu YZ et al., Conjugation site analysis of antibody-drug-conjugates (ADCs) by signature ion fingerprinting and normalized area quantitation approach using nano-liquid chromatography coupled to high resolution mass spectrometry, Pages No. 67–78, Copyright (2017), with permission from Elsevier)

3.2 Quantify Conjugation Levels of Identified Lysine Residues by Normalized Area Quantitation Approach

3.2.1 Sample Preparation for Conjugation Level Analysis

1. Digest TDM1 as described in Subheading 3.1.2, and desalt the digested peptides with HLB C_{18} SPE columns (*see* **Note 8**) using a protocol similar to Ziptip desalting.
2. Reconstitute the digested samples in aqueous 0.1% FA buffer to a concentration of approximately 1 mg/mL.
3. Aliquot the sample and dilute the aliquots to 2.5-, 5-, 10-, and 25-fold. Designate the original concentration as $Conc_0$, which makes the serial concentrations of peptide digests from lowest to highest as $0.04 \times Conc_0$, $0.1 \times Conc_0$, $0.2 \times Conc_0$, $0.4 \times Conc_0$ and $Conc_0$. A minimum of five concentrations are required to calculate the relative ionization intensity factor (RIIF) for identified DM1-conjugated and unconjugated peptides. A minimum of three replicates for ADC digests of each concentration are needed for following statistical analysis.
4. A peptide standard delivering stable signal intensity at *m/z* not interfering with targeted transitions was spiked into each sample and serves as internal standard (IS) for following quantitative analysis.

5. Centrifuge serially diluted samples at 30,000 × *g* for 5 min at 4 °C and transfer the supernatant of 5 μL to sampling vials for following analysis on a LC system (LC-20 AD, Shimadzu) coupled to QTRAP 5500 (AB SCIEX).

3.2.2 MRM Analysis to Obtain RIIF for Normalized Conjugation Level Analysis

1. To calculate the normalized conjugation ratio, make a list of pseudo-multiple reaction monitoring (MRM) transitions by monitoring the *m/z* of targeted peptides as both the precursor and fragment ions. All the DM1-conjugated and unconjugated peptides identified in Subheading 3.1 are included as targeted peptides (*see* **Note 9**).
2. Set up analysis parameters for LC separation. Solvent (A) we used is 0.1% (v/v) formic acid in water, and solvent (B) is 0.1% (v/v) formic acid in ACN. A 60-min gradient was used as follows: 5% B for 1 min, 5–65% B for 42 min, 65–90% B for 2 min, 90% B for 7 min, 90–5% B for 2 min, 5% B for 6 min on a HPLC column (Sepax). Flow rate was set at 0.2 mL/min.
3. Set up the ESI source conditions as follows: Ion Source Gas 1 (GS1) as 40, Ion Source Gas 2 (GS2) as 60, Curtain Gas (CUR) as 40, Collision Gas (CAD) as Medium, Temperature 550 °C, Ion Spray Voltage (ISV) 5000 V in the positive mode.
4. Set up the mass spectrometer parameters for MRM transitions: Collision gas N_2, Q1 vacuum gauge 2.1×10^{-5} torr. Set DP and CE as 100 and 5 V for each MRM transition. Set dwell time and pause time as 20 and 5 ms, respectively (*see* **Note 10**). Subsequently, MRM analysis was performed for peptide digest samples that have been diluted to different concentrations.
5. Record the MRM responses for each monitored peptide and quantify the corresponding peak area values collected from samples of serial concentrations. Make the concentration-response curves for all the conjugated and unconjugated peptides by plotting the peak areas of each conjugated peptide and its unconjugated counterpart, respectively, against the five different concentrations, ranging from $0.04 \times Conc_0$, $0.1 \times Conc_0$, $0.2 \times Conc_0$, $0.4 \times Conc_0$ to C_0.
6. Calculate the corresponding slope rates. These two steps (**5** and **6**) can be automatically performed by Analyst TF 1.6.1 (AB SCIEX).

3.2.3 Data Analysis to Process Normalized Conjugation Levels of Lysine

1. Before we can calculate the normalized conjugation level for each DM1-modified lysine, the raw conjugation ratio of each identified DM1-modified lysine should be calculated based on the same set of nanoLC-MS/MS data used for identification of DM1-conjugation sites (data acquired in Subheading 3.1.3). The raw conjugation ratio for each conjugation site is acquired by dividing the peak area under the extracted ion

chromatogram (XIC) of the peptide carrying DM1-conjugated lysine by the peak area of the peptide of identical sequence yet in its unconjugated form (Eq. 1). The peak areas under XICs were integrated by MultiQuant (AB SCIEX) and extracted from the data (*see* **Note 11**). The raw conjugation ratio of each peptide was averaged from at least three replicates with standard error of the mean (SEM) calculated by Excel (Microsoft, Redmond, USA).

$$\text{Raw conjugation ratio}_i = \frac{\text{Peak area peptide(DM1)}_i}{\text{Peak area peptide}_i} \times 100\% \quad (1)$$

2. The raw conjugation ratio cannot indicate the extent of DM1 conjugation on identified conjugation site due to the distinct ionization efficiencies between conjugated and unconjugated peptides. To make such corrections, one should obtain the relative ionization intensity factor (RIIF) for each unconjugated-conjugated peptide pair. The RIIF for each peptide pair was calculated by dividing the slope rate of the unconjugated peptides by the conjugated counterpart using the concentration-response curves prepared from serially diluted ADC digests as detailed in Subheading 3.2.1 using Eq. 2.

$$\text{RIIF} = \frac{\text{Slope rate of peptide}_i}{\text{Slope rate of peptide (DM1)}_i} \quad (2)$$

As shown in Fig. 5a–c, the RIIF of the conjugated peptide SKLTVDK(DM1) SRWQQGNVF that carries a conjugation site at HC K417 and the unconjugated form SKLTVDKSRWQ QGNVF (*see* **Note 12**) is 1.84/0.182 = 10.11. Moreover, another two peptide pairs (Fig. 5d, e) also suggest the significantly suppressed ionization efficiency of peptides upon DM1 conjugation, highlighting the necessity of correcting the raw conjugation ratios.

3. Calculate the normalized conjugation ratios by applying RIIF using Eq. 3.

$$\text{Normalized conjugation ratio} = \text{RIIF} \times \text{Raw conjugation ratio} \times 100\% \quad (3)$$

Specifically, for HC K^{417}, the normalized conjugation ratio = 10.11 × 1.32 × 100% = 13.35%.

4. The conjugation level for each site is thereby determined using Eq. 4:

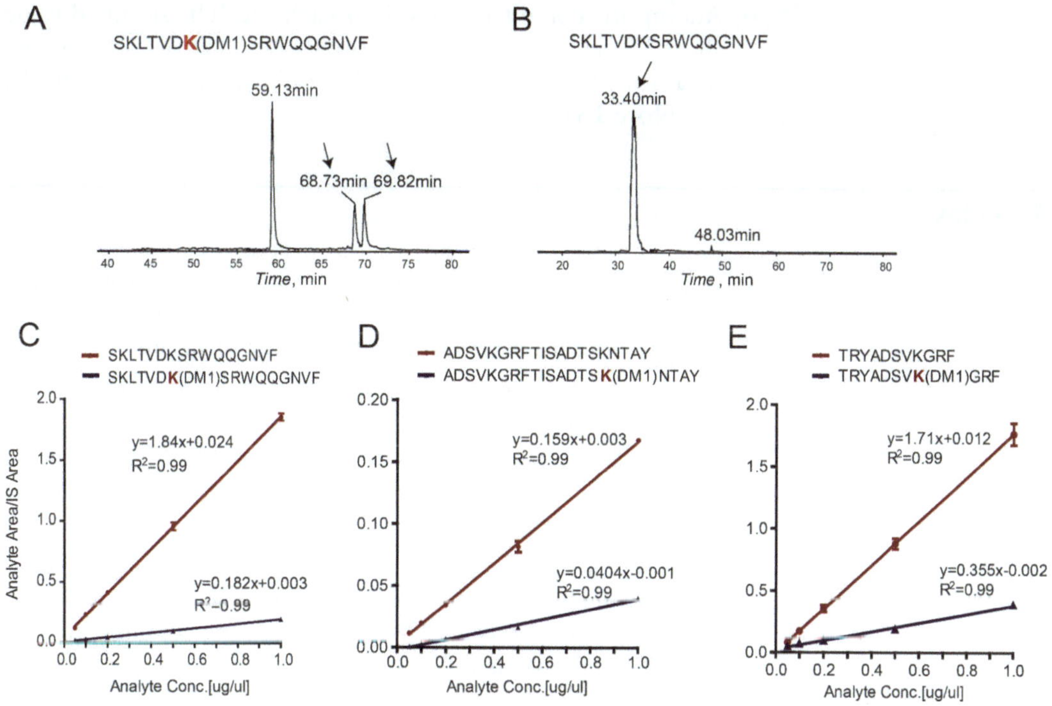

Fig. 5 Conjugation level analysis was first performed by calculating the raw conjugation ratio for each conjugation site. The retention time of the extracted ion chromatograms of (**a**) the ion of *m/z* 713.10 detected at 68.73 and 69.82 min and (**b**) the ion of *m/z* 474.00 observed at 33.40 min (all denoted by arrows), which correspond to the conjugated peptide SKLTVDK(DM1)SRWQQGNVF and its unconjugated form SKLTVDKSRWQQGNVF. The peak areas of the peak pairs were quantified, respectively. The peak area of DM1 modified peptide was divided by the peak area of unmodified peptide to obtain the raw conjugation ratio. The raw conjugation ratio was then converted to the normalized conjugation ratio by applying the correction of relative ionization intensity factor (RIIF). (**c**–**e**) The RIIF was determined by dividing the slope rate of unconjugated peptides by that of the conjugated peptides in ADC digests prepared at serial concentrations. (**c**) The RIIF of SKLTVDKSRWQQGNVF/SKLTVDK(DM1)SRWQQGNVF is 10.11. (**d**) The RIIF of ADSVKGRFTISADTSKNTAY/ADSVKGRFTISADTSK(DM1)NTAY is 3.94. (**e**) The RIIF of TRYADSVKGRF/TRYADSVK(DM1)GRF is 4.82 (inserted to Subheading 3.2.3). (Reprinted from Analytica Chimica Acta, Vol 955, Sang H, Lu GY, Liu YZ et al., Conjugation site analysis of antibody-drug-conjugates (ADCs) by signature ion fingerprinting and normalized area quantitation approach using nano-liquid chromatography coupled to high resolution mass spectrometry, Pages No. 67–78, Copyright (2017), with permission from Elsevier)

$$\text{Conjugation level}_i = \frac{\text{Normalized conjugation ratio}_i}{\text{Normalized conjugation ratio}_i + 1} \times 100\% \quad (4)$$

For instance, the conjugation level of HC K^{417} = 13.35%/(13.35% + 1) = 11.77%.

5. Perform **steps 1–4** for all the identified DM1 conjugation peptides to obtain the conjugation level of each modified lysine residue.

6. Add up the conjugation level for each site. The summed value should be close to the drug-antibody ratio (DAR) acquired by measuring the intact masses of the conjugated and naked mAbs (*see* **Note 13**).

4 Notes

1. DTT and IAA should be freshly prepared. IAA must be kept away from light. Adding DTT to samples after IAA incubation is for removal of excess IAA to avoid side reactions.
2. The times of applying activation, equilibration, washing, and elution buffers to Ziptips and SPE columns can be modified for improved desalting and enrichment performance. The percentage of ACN in elution buffer should be optimized based on the properties of drug payload.
3. CE is set based on charge and m/z values of detected peptides. The parameters must be optimized based on different instruments. The most recent IDA CE parameters recommended by SCIEX are shown as follows:

Charge	Slope	Intercept
Unknown	0.049	−1
1	0.05	5
2	0.049	−1
3	0.048	−2
4	0.05	−2
5	0.05	−2

4. The optimal setting of “exclude former target ions” must be optimized and we used an estimated duration corresponding to the full-width at half-maximum (FWHM) of a typical chromatographic peak.
5. Other open-source software, i.e., Maxquant software (http://www.biochem.mpg.de/5111795/maxquant), PEAKS (Bioinformatics Solutions, Waterloo, ON, Canada), or ProteomeDiscover (Thermo Scientific, USA), are all reliable alternatives.
6. The conjugation of cytotoxic drugs to antibodies leads to incremental masses of precursors and fragment ions corresponding to DM1 conjugation for peptides that carry such modification. Drug conjugation also results in the generation of SFIs of the drug payload present at relatively high abundances in MS/MS spectra. Therefore, we used these SFIs as a golden standard to exclude the false positive hits

from the database search results. However, the SFIs vary by the nature of the drug payload and must be customized case by case as we described in Subheading 3.1.1.

7. A detailed guide can be found in the manual of ProteinPilot. The probability of the presence of drug conjugation should be optimized for best coverage with minimal false positive hits.
8. We chose the SPE columns for desalting since the acquisition of RIIF was performed on a QTRAP coupled to a regular ESI source. A microscale desalting device, such as Ziptip or Stage-tip, is recommended if a nanoESI source is coupled to the mass spectrometer on which quantitative analysis of peptides is carried out.
9. Peptides have multiple charges and thus multiple *m/z* values. We made the transition list by importing the IDA.wiff data into SKYLINE (MacCoss, University of Washington, Seattle, WA) to determine the charged form that delivers highest MS responses as parent ions. The charges of conjugated and unconjugated peptides we chose to monitor for MRM analysis are identical.
10. These parameters can be optimized based on different gradients and the number of peptide transitions that need to be monitored.
11. Make sure the *m/z* (among different charge states)values of unconjugated and conjugated peptide pairs one choose for raw conjugation ratio calculation is the same as those one choose for normalized conjugation ratio calculation.
12. HC K^{417} refers to the lysine residue located at the 417th residue from the N-terminal in the heavy chain of ADCs.
13. How to perform intact mass measurement for DAR calculation has been reported in previous literature including our publication [14, 16, 17].

Acknowledgments

This study was financially supported by the National Natural Science Foundation of China (No. 81872838), the Natural Science Foundation of Jiangsu Province (BK20180079), National Key R&D Program of China (2018YFD0901101), Double First-rate Project (CPU2018GY09, CPU2018GF09), the Project of State Key Laboratory of Natural Medicines in China Pharmaceutical University (SKLNMZZCX201817), and the Project for Major New Drugs Innovation and Development (2018ZX09711001-002-003). The authors also appreciated useful discussions with Prof. Lingjun Li at the University of Wisconsin-Madison.

References

1. Lambert JM, Berkenblit A (2018) Antibody-drug conjugates for cancer treatment. Annu Rev Med 69:191–207
2. Chalouni C, Doll S (2018) Fate of antibody-drug conjugates in cancer cells. J Exp Clin Cancer Res 37(1):20–31
3. Kraynov E, Kamath AV, Walles M et al (2016) Current approaches for absorption, distribution, metabolism, and excretion characterization of antibody-drug conjugates: an industry white paper. Drug Metab Dispos 44 (5):617–623
4. Strop P, Liu SH, Dorywalska M et al (2013) Location matters: site of conjugation modulates stability and pharmacokinetics of antibody drug conjugates. Chem Biol 20(2):161–167
5. Setiady YY, Park PU, Ponte JF et al (2013) Development of a novel antibody-maytansinoid conjugate, IMGN289, for the treatment of EGFR-expressing solid tumors. Cancer Res 73(8). https://doi.org/10.1158/1538-7445.AM2013-5463
6. Hamblett KJ, Kozlosky CJ, Siu S et al (2015) AMG 595, an anti-EGFRvIII antibody-drug conjugate, induces potent antitumor activity against EGFRvIII-expressing glioblastoma. Mol Cancer Ther 14(7):1614–1624
7. Wagh A, Song H, Zeng M et al (2018) Challenges and new frontiers in analytical characterization of antibody-drug conjugates. MAbs 10 (2):222–243
8. Shen BQ, Xu K, Liu L et al (2012) Conjugation site modulates the in vivo stability and therapeutic activity of antibody-drug conjugates. Nat Biotechnol 30(2):184–189
9. Boswell CA, Mundo EE, Zhang C et al (2011) Impact of drug conjugation on pharmacokinetics and tissue distribution of anti-STEAP1 antibody-drug conjugates in rats. Bioconjug Chem 22(10):1994–2004
10. Junutula JR, Raab H, Clark S et al (2008) Site-specific conjugation of a cytotoxic drug to an antibody improves the therapeutic index. Nat Biotechnol 26(8):925–932
11. Wakankar A, Chen Y, Gokarn Y et al (2011) Analytical methods for physicochemical characterization of antibody drug conjugates. MAbs 3(2):161–172
12. Wang L, Amphlett G, Blattler WA et al (2005) Structural characterization of the maytansinoid-monoclonal antibody immunoconjugate, huN901-DM1, by mass spectrometry. Protein Sci 14(9):2436–2446
13. Sandra K, Vanhoenacker G, Vandenheede I et al (2016) Multiple heart-cutting and comprehensive two-dimensional liquid chromatography hyphenated to mass spectrometry for the characterization of the antibody-drug conjugate ado-trastuzumab emtansine. J Chromatogr B 1032:119–130
14. Kim MT, Chen Y, Marhoul J et al (2014) Statistical modeling of the drug load distribution on trastuzumab emtansine (Kadcyla), a lysine-linked antibody drug conjugate. Bioconjug Chem 25(7):1223–1232
15. Luo Q, Chung HH, Borths C et al (2016) Structural characterization of a monoclonal antibody-maytansinoid immunoconjugate. Anal Chem 88(1):695–702
16. Huang RY, Deyanova EG, Passmore D et al (2015) Utility of ion mobility mass spectrometry for drug-to-antibody ratio measurements in antibody-drug conjugates. J Am Soc Mass Spectrom 26(10):1791–1794
17. Marcoux J, Champion T, Colas O et al (2015) Native mass spectrometry and ion mobility characterization of trastuzumab emtansine, a lysine-linked antibody drug conjugate. Protein Sci 24(8):1210–1223

Chapter 17

Characterization of ADCs by Capillary Electrophoresis

Wenjing Ning and Yanqun Zhao

Abstract

Capillary electrophoresis (CE) is a highly efficient separation technique that resolves ions based on their electrophoretic mobility in the presence of an applied voltage. It has been broadly applied for characterizing biotherapeutics including ADCs. In this chapter, step-by-step procedures for characterizing ADCs using CE will be described with focus placed on reduced and non-reduced capillary electrophoresis sodium dodecyl sulfate (CE-SDS) for purity determination and imaged capillary isoelectric focusing (iCIEF) for charge heterogeneity analysis.

Key words Antibody-drug conjugates, CE, Reduced and non-reduced CE-SDS, iCIEF, Charge heterogeneity

1 Introduction

Antibody-drug conjugates (ADCs) are a new class of highly potent biopharmaceutical drugs, which consist of antibodies conjugated to cytotoxic compounds or payloads via chemical linkers [1, 2]. ADCs can be designed using different types of antibodies, linkers, and payloads through different conjugation sites or chemistry [3]. When the cysteine residues are used as the conjugation sites, whether it is a native IgG or an engineered IgG, it can be referred as cysteine-conjugated ADCs [4–7]. In this chapter, discussions are focused on the characterization of cysteine-conjugated ADCs using capillary electrophoresis (CE) based techniques.

CE has been widely used for the characterization of biotherapeutics including ADCs [8–10]. Several operation modes of CE, including CE-SDS, capillary zone electrophoresis (CZE), capillary isoelectric focusing (CIEF), and imaged capillary isoelectric focusing (iCIEF), have been utilized in the characterization of ADCs for purity, identification, and charge variants determination [11]. In addition, CE-MS has also become a promising platform to analyze biotherapeutics such as obtaining primary structure information for intact ADCs [12, 13]. Among all the CE-based techniques,

L. Nathan Tumey (ed.), *Antibody-Drug Conjugates: Methods and Protocols*, Methods in Molecular Biology, vol. 2078, https://doi.org/10.1007/978-1-4939-9929-3_17,

CE-SDS and iCIEF are most commonly used for ADC analysis and quality control.

CE-SDS can be performed in reduced and non-reduced modes. SDS is employed for denaturation to dissociate protein components linked by noncovalent interactions for better separations. The migration of protein components is driven by the surface charge induced by SDS binding, which is proportional to the protein components' molecular weight [11, 14]. CE-SDS, reduced and non-reduced, has been used for purity determination for ADCs [8]. In addition to purity, charge heterogeneity is also a critical attribute that needs to be monitored for ADCs. Compared to other techniques for characterizing the charge variants such as ion-exchange chromatography, CZE, and CIEF, iCIEF has been used widely due to its easy method development, short run time, and ease of use. In this chapter, we will focus on the CE-SDS method for ADC purity determination and iCIEF method for charge heterogeneity analysis.

2 Materials

2.1 CE-SDS, Reduced and Non-reduced, for ADC Purity Analysis

2.1.1 Equipment

1. CE instrument, Beckman Coulter PA800 *plus* with 32 Karat software or equivalent.
2. Detector, Ultraviolet or Photodiode Array.
3. Capillary, 50 μm I.D. bare-fused silica.
4. Beckman capillary cartridge, 100 × 200 μm aperture, approximate length 30.2 cm total (20 cm effective), or equivalent.
5. Microcentrifuge.
6. Water bath or heat block (up to 70 °C).

2.1.2 Chemicals and Solutions

1. SDS MW Analysis kit or IgG Purity and Heterogeneity Assay kit from AB Sciex (*see* **Note 1**) or equivalent that contains reagents as listed below.
   (a) SDS-MW Gel Buffer: proprietary formulation, pH 8, 0.2% SDS.
   (b) SDS-MW Sample Buffer: 100 mM Tris–HCl, pH 9.0, 1% SDS.
   (c) Acidic Wash Solution: 0.1 M HCl.
   (d) Basic Wash Solution: 0.1 M NaOH.
2. Purified water.
3. 2-Mercaptoethanol.
4. Iodoacetamide, single use ampule of 56 mg from Sigma-Aldrich, or equivalent.
5. 0.5 M iodoacetamide solution preparation: add 606 μL of purified water to one ampule of iodoacetamide above and mix thoroughly.

2.2 iCIEF for ADC Charge Heterogeneity Analysis

2.2.1 Equipment

1. iCE3 analyzer with PrinCE MicroInjector and iCE3.0 CFR Software, ProteinSimple or equivalent. cIEF cartridge: 50 mm, 100 μm I.D. fluorocarbon-coated capillary with built-in electrolyte tanks (*see* **Note 2**).
2. Microcentrifuge.

2.2.2 Chemicals and Solutions

1. Purified water.
2. 8 M Urea from Sigma-Aldrich (after reconstitution with 16 mL of purified water) (*see* **Note 3**).
3. pH 5–8 Pharmalytes from GE Healthcare or equivalent.
4. pH 8–10.5 Pharmalytes from GE Healthcare or equivalent.
5. pH 3–10 Pharmalytes from GE Healthcare or equivalent.

And the following from ProteinSimple:

6. 1% Methyl Cellulose Kit.
7. 0.5% Methyl Cellulose Kit.
8. pI 7.05 Marker and pI 9.77 Marker (*see* **Note 4**).
9. Electrolyte Kit, contains Anolyte (0.1 M sodium hydroxide in 0.1% methyl cellulose) and Catholyte (0.08 M phosphoric acid in 0.1% methyl cellulose).
10. Time Transfer Measurement (TTM) Solution Kit or equivalent containing 8% pH 3–10 Pharmalytes in 0.35% methyl cellulose.

3 Methods

3.1 CE-SDS, Reduced and Non-reduced, for ADC Purity Analysis

1. Preparation of the CE Instrument
   Follow the manufacture procedures to set up PA 800 *plus* instrument. Install a 50 μm I.D. bare-fused silica capillary into a cartridge for a total capillary length of 30.2 cm with 20 cm effective length.
2. Preparation of reduced ADC sample (*see* **Note 5**)
   (a) Dilute the ADC sample to 2 mg/mL with water (for ADC sample with concentration lower than 2 mg/mL, no dilution is needed). Pipette 100 μL of diluted ADC sample into a 0.5 mL microcentrifuge tube.
   (b) Add 100 μL of SDS-MW Sample Buffer and 10 μL of 2-mercaptoethanol into the microcentrifuge tube containing diluted ADC sample.
   (c) Vortex the microcentrifuge tube for 10 s, heat the mixture at 70 °C for 10 min, and cool the mixture to room temperature. The final protein concentration is about 1 mg/mL (*see* **Note 6**).

3. Preparation of non-reduced ADC sample (*see* **Note 5**)
   (a) Dilute the ADC sample to 2 mg/mL with water (for ADC sample with concentration lower than 2 mg/mL, no dilution is needed). Pipette 100 μL of the diluted ADC sample into a 0.5 mL microcentrifuge tube.
   (b) Add 100 μL of SDS-MW Sample Buffer and 10 μL of 0.5 M iodoacetamide into the microcentrifuge tube containing diluted ADC sample (*see* **Note 7**).
   (c) Vortex the microcentrifuge tube for 10 s, heat the mixture at 55 °C for 10 min, and cool the solution to room temperature. The final protein concentration is about 1 mg/mL (*see* **Note 6**).
4. Blank preparation
   Replace the sample with the formulation buffer. Follow **steps 2** and **3** for reduced and non-reduced CE-SDS Blank preparations, respectively.
5. Centrifuge blank samples and ADC samples (reduced and non-reduced) at 10,000 rpm (9500 × *g*) for 2 min.
6. Transfer 100 μL of all samples and blanks from **step 5** into autosampler vials and place vials into the autosampler trays (*see* **Note 8**). The autosampler temperature is typically set at 10 °C.
7. Fill the Universal Vials with Basic Wash Solution, Acidic Wash Solution, SDS-MW Gel Buffer, and purified water. Cap the Universal Vials and place them into system inlet (left) and outlet (right) buffer trays.
8. Launch 32 Karat software and select the "SDS MW" icon.
9. Instrument methods
   (a) Conditioning method:
   If a new capillary or a used capillary that has been stored for a long period of time will be used, conditioning of the capillary must be performed before starting CE separation for best performance. The capillary can be conditioned by rinsing with Basic Wash Solution, Acidic Wash Solution, and SDS-MW Gel Buffer with example conditions as shown below.

Event	Value	Duration	Solution
Rinse pressure	20 psi	10 min	Basic wash solution
Rinse pressure	20 psi	5 min	Acidic wash solution
Rinse pressure	20 psi	2 min	Water
Rinse pressure	70 psi	10 min	SDS-gel buffer
Separate voltage	15 KV	10 min	SDS-gel buffer

(b) Separation method:
The separation method can be set up as below. The UV detection is set at 214 nm, capillary temperature is controlled at 25 °C, and autosampler temperature is set at 10 °C (*see* **Note 9**). Set up sequence and run the Blank, SDS-MW Working Standard, reduced and non-reduced ADC samples (*see* **Note 10**).

Event	Value	Duration	Solution
Rinse pressure	70 psi	3 min	Basic wash solution
Rinse pressure	70 psi	1 min	Acidic wash solution
Rinse pressure	70 psi	1 min	Water
Rinse pressure	70 psi	10 min	SDS-gel buffer
Wait		0 min	Water
Wait		0 min	Water
Injection voltage	5 KV	20 s	Sample
Wait		0 min	Water
Separate voltage	15 KV	40 min	SDS-gel buffer
Autozero			

(c) Shutdown method:
At the end of analysis, use a shutdown method shown below to rinse the capillary and switch off the lamp.

Event	Value	Duration	Solution
Rinse pressure	70 psi	10 min	Basic wash solution
Rinse pressure	50 psi	5 min	Acidic wash solution
Rinse pressure	50 psi	2 min	Water
Rinse pressure	70 psi	10 min	SDS-gel buffer
Separate voltage	15 KV	10 min	SDS-gel buffer
Wait		0 min	Water
Lamp-off		10 min	Water

10. Data analysis
For reduced CE-SDS analysis of cysteine-linked ADCs, two major peaks are typically expected: light chain (LC) and heavy chain (HC). The LC or HC with and without drugs is generally not separated or only partially separated. The profile of non-reduced CE-SDS analysis of cysteine-linked ADCs with broad DAR distribution contains more fragments under the

Table 1
IgG1 ADC positional isomers and corresponding expected fragments in non-reduced CE-SDS analysis

DAR	IgG1 ADC positional isomers with expected fragments[a] in non-reduced CE-SDS
0	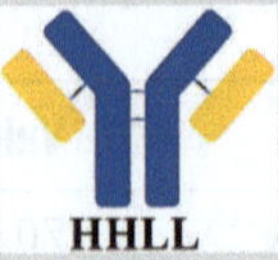
2	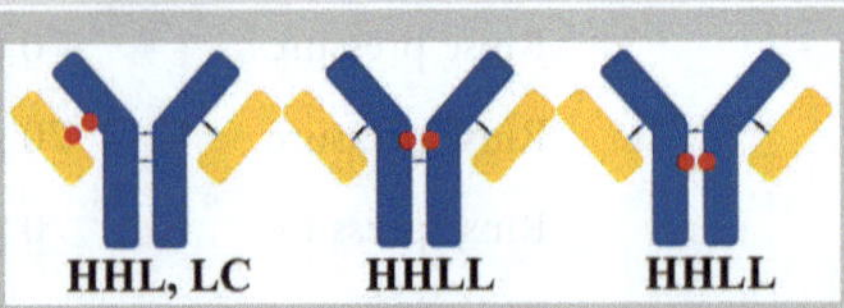
4	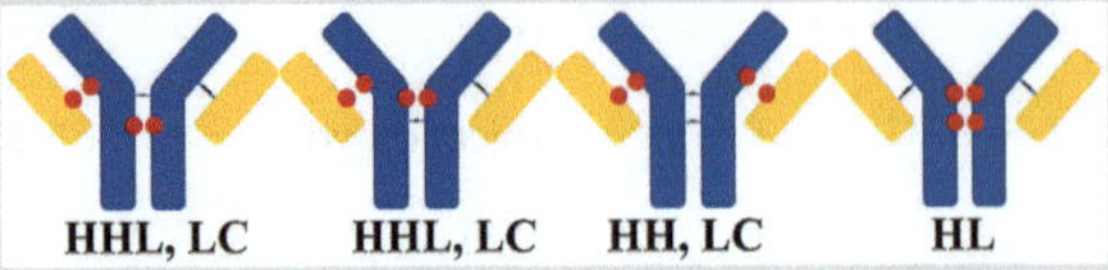
6	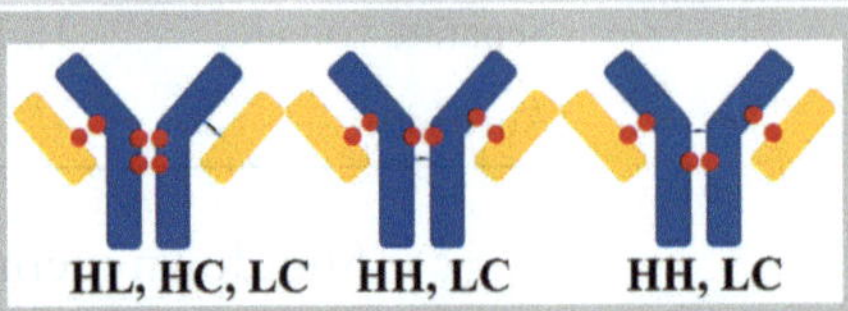
8	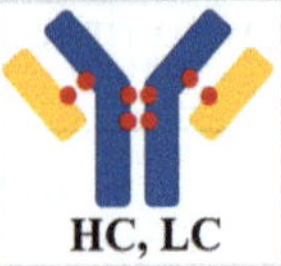

Red dot - drug; *HC* - heavy chain; *LC* - light chain; *HH* - two heavy chains linked by disulfide bond; *HL* - heavy chain and light chain linked by disulfide bond; *HHL* - two heavy chains and one light chain linked by disulfide bonds; *HHLL* - intact mAb or ADC
[a]No differentiation on the number of drugs on the fragments

denatured conditions due to the reduction of the intra-disulfide bond as a result of the conjugation. The expected fragments include LC, HC, heavy-light (HL), heavy-heavy (HH), heavy-heavy-light (HHL), and the intact mAb or ADC (HHLL). An illustration of the expected fragments of positional isomers from cysteine-conjugated IgG1 ADCs is shown in Table 1.

Example electropherograms from reduced and non-reduced CE-SDS of cysteine-linked ADCs are shown in Fig. 1a, b respectively. In Fig. 1a, in addition to the expected profiles of two major peaks corresponding to heavy chain (HC) and light chain (LC), partial separation of LC without

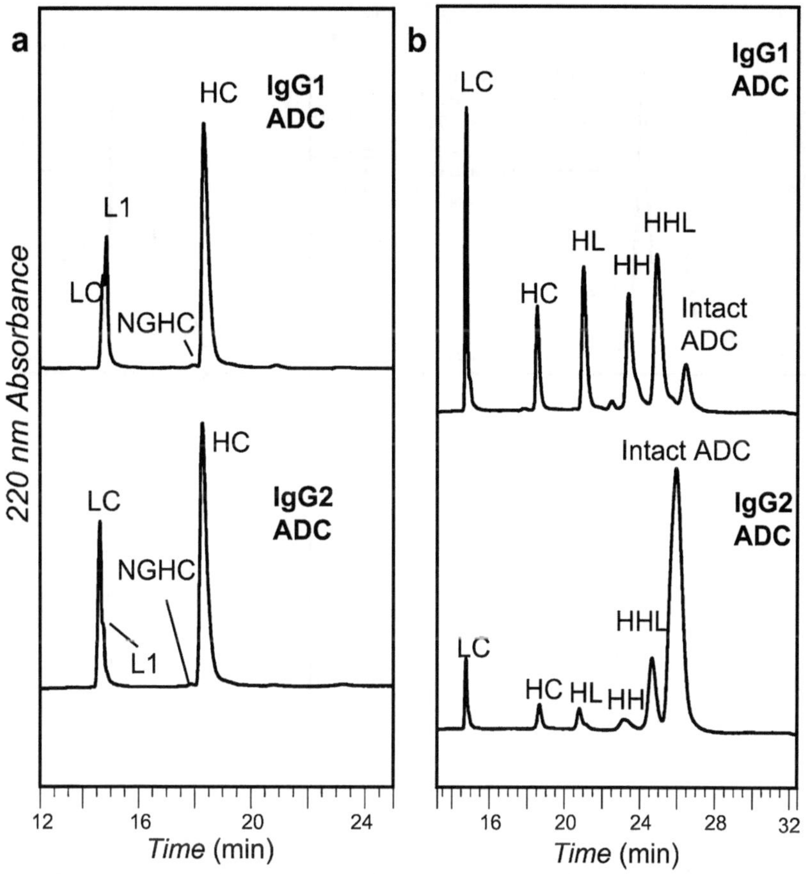

Fig. 1 Representative reduced (**a**) and non-reduced (**b**) CE-SDS electropherograms of cysteine-linked IgG1 and IgG2 ADCs. NGHC is nonglycosylated heavy chain. (Reprinted from ref. 14 with permission)

drug (L0) and LC with one drug (L1) is also observed (*see* **Note 11**). Under non-reduced conditions, as shown in Fig. 1b, both IgG1 and IgG2 ADCs show a distribution of LC, HC, HL, HH, HHL, and intact ADC (HHLL).

The purity of ADCs by reduced CE-SDS can be expressed as the sum of the percent areas of light and heavy chain. And the percent purity determination of ADC by non-reduced CE-SDS depends on the ADC conjugation sites and its drug to antibody ratio. The percent purity will be the sum of peak area of expected fragment species over the total peak area (*see* **Note 12**).

3.2 iCIEF for ADC Charge Heterogeneity Analysis

1. Preparation of TTM solution
   Transfer 200 μL of the TTM Solution into a microcentrifuge tube and centrifuge at approximately 10,000 rpm (9500 × *g*) for at least 5 min.
2. Preparation of Pharmalyte Mix
   Pharmalyte Mix solution needs to be freshly prepared before each run and the preparation can be scaled accordingly based

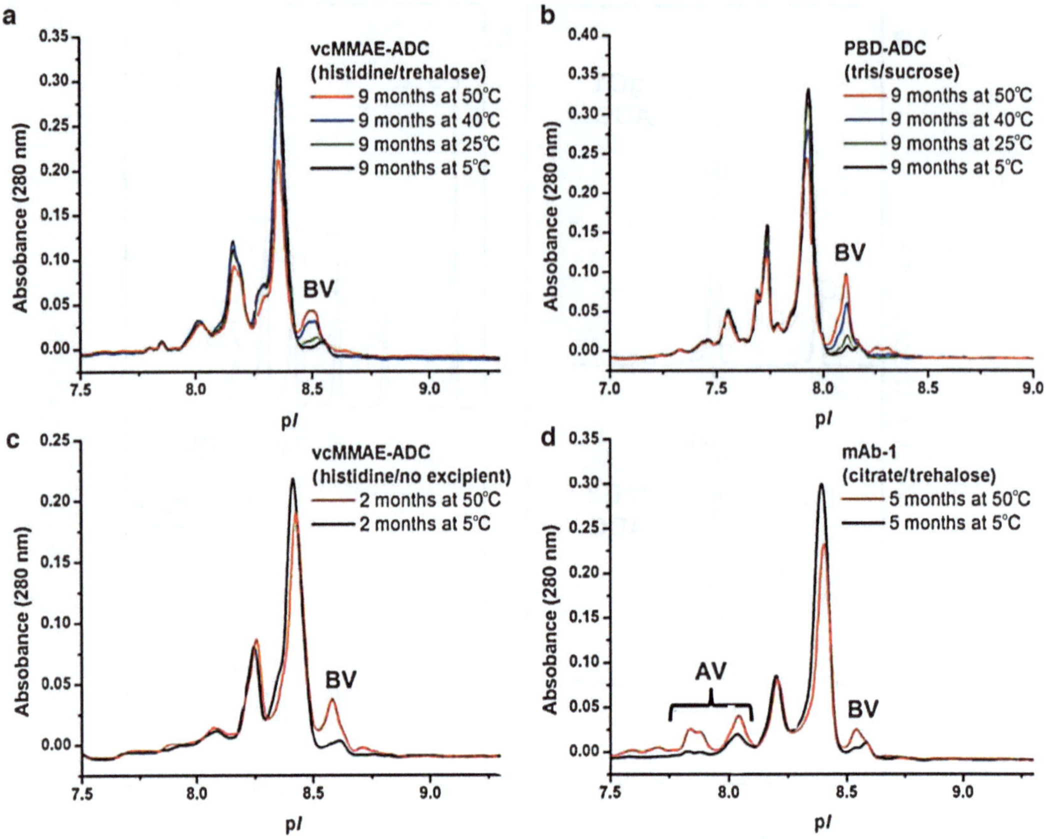

Fig. 2 iCIEF electropherograms for lyophilized-stressed mAbs and ADCs in various formulations. vcMMAE–ADC 9 month stability sample stressed at 5, 25, 40, and 50 °C (**a**), PBD–ADC 9 month stability samples stressed at 5, 25, 40, and 50 °C (**b**), vcMMAE–ADC 2 month stability sample stressed at 5 and 50 °C (**c**), and mAb-1 5 month stability sample stressed at 5 and 50 °C (**d**). Temperature-induced increases in acidic variant (AV) and basic variant (BV) populations are indicated. (Reprinted from ref. 15 with permission)

on the number of samples. For example, mixing 880 μL of 1% methyl cellulose, 50 μL of pH 5–8 Pharmalytes, 50 μL of pH 8–10.5 Pharmalytes, 10 μL of pI 7.05 Marker, and 10 μL of pI 9.77 Marker (*see* **Note 13**).

3. Preparation of ADC sample and Blank
   (a) Dilute ADC sample to 0.5 mg/mL with water.
   (b) Add 50 μL of 8 M urea and 100 μL of Pharmalyte Mix to 100 μL of diluted ADC sample and mix well (*see* **Note 14**). The resulting sample is in the final composition of 0.35% methyl cellulose, 2% pH 5–8 Pharmalytes, 2% pH 8–10.5 Pharmalytes, 0.4% pI 7.05 Marker, 0.4% pI 9.77 Marker, 1.6 M urea, and 0.2 mg/mL ADC (*see* **Note 15**).
   (c) Prepare a Blank by mixing 100 μL of formulation buffer, 50 μL of 8 M urea, and 100 μL of Pharmalyte Mix.

(d) Centrifuge the sample and Blank solutions at approximately 10,000 rpm (9500 × *g*) for at least 5 min, transfer approximately 200 μL of the supernatant to an autosampler vial for analysis (*see* **Note 16**).

4. Perform the cartridge installation, system startup. Set up all the solutions including 0.5% Methyl Cellulose, TTM solution, electrolytes, Blank, and samples. Conduct light intensity check following the step-by-step instruction in the software and instrument manual.
5. Determine the sample transfer time prior to analysis. The start of the plateau should not be greater than 60 s. The height of the plateau should not be lower than 5 μA.
6. Set up a run sequence for Blank and sample in the iCE software.
7. Isoelectric focusing method parameters were set as pre-focusing at 1500 V for 1 min, and focusing at 3000 V for 10 min, sample transfer time as 60 seconds, and the autosampler tray temperature is typically set to 10 °C (*see* **Note 17**).
8. Data Analysis

(a) After the completion of the run, process the images in the iCE software by identifying the lower and upper pI markers and calibrate the pI scale in all electropherograms following the user's manual.

(b) Export all the processed electropherograms to *.cdf format from the iCE CFR software.

(c) Open the exported file with ChromPerfect (ProteinSimple) or other appropriate software to review and integrate all the electropherograms. Report the PA% of acidic, main, and basic species. Example iCIEF electropherograms of lyophilized-stressed mAbs and ADCs in various formulations are shown in Fig. 2. Typically, acidic species are the peaks eluting to the left (lower pI) and basic species are to the right (higher pI) of the main.

4 Notes

1. The application guide for SDS-MW Analysis Kit and IgG Purity and Heterogeneity Assay kit can be found on SCIEX website. SDS-MW Size Standard in the SDS-MW Analysis Kit and IgG Control Standard in the IgG Purity and Heterogeneity Assay kit can be used to estimate the molecular weight and identify different ADC fragments during the early method development when the reference material may not be available.
2. iCE280 and Maurice (ProteinSimple) can also be used for iCIEF analysis. For iCIEF analysis on Maurice instrument,

Maurice cIEF Cartridge needs to be used instead. The same sample preparation procedure can be used for UV detection.

3. Urea solution needs to be prepared freshly and kept away from heat to avoid thermal degradation. One of the thermal degradation products of urea, isocyanic acid, could react rapidly with amine groups and lead to artificial increase of the level of acidic species.
4. pI markers should be selected based on the pI of ADCs. All peaks of interest from ADC samples should be bracketed by the pI markers. Two pI markers are needed for calibration of the pI scale of the electropherogram.
5. The ADC reference materials can be prepared following the sample preparation procedures.
6. The total protein concentration in the final solution for CE-SDS analysis should be within the range of 0.2 mg/mL to 2 mg/mL. High protein concentration can result in broad peaks and poor resolution, while low protein concentration can result in low signal. For best results, the recommended protein concentration is 1 mg/mL. However, this could be varied and optimized depending on the properties of ADC samples. The incubation temperature could be optimized for the actual sample as well.
7. For non-reducing conditions, iodoacetamide was added to the sample buffer as an alkylating agent.
8. Make sure no bubbles in the sample solution during preparation and transfer. If bubbles exist, centrifuge the micro vials and repeat if necessary.
9. The UV detection can be set at other wavelength depending on the maximum UV absorbance of ADC samples. The capillary temperature can also be optimized.
10. When both non-reduced and reduced preparations are analyzed in one sequence, begin the sequence with the non-reduced preparations first.
11. The example is for cysteine-linked ADC. For lysine-linked or other types of ADCs, different fragments would be expected. The separation of L0 and L1 depends on the size and properties of payloads and antibodies.
12. All peak areas used in calculations are corrected area.
13. For ADCs with different pI values, the pI range of the carrier ampholytes can be varied to improve the resolution. The ADC concentration can also be adjusted to improve the resolution and sensitivity.
14. Urea is used as additive to prevent precipitation and aggregation of ADCs during focusing. The concentration of urea in

the final sample or addition of other additives is critical and can be evaluated to improve the resolution and separation for different ADCs.

15. The concentration of ADC in the final composition is typically from 0.1 mg/mL to 0.5 mg/mL. High protein concentration can overload the capillary and cause poor resolution, while low protein concentration can result in low signal. For best results, the recommended protein concentration is 0.2 mg/mL. However, this could be varied and optimized depending on the properties of ADC samples. The application notes for charge heterogeneity analysis of proteins and antibodies using iCE280/iCE3/Maurice can be found on ProteinSimple website.
16. Try to remove bubbles and avoid bubble formation during sample preparation and transfer. The bubbles could interfere with focusing and separation.
17. The focusing time can be evaluated and optimized based on the properties of ADC samples.

References

1. Diamantis N, Banerji U (2016) Antibody-drug conjugates—an emerging class of cancer treatment. Br J Cancer 114:362. https://doi.org/10.1038/bjc.2015.435. https://www.nature.com/articles/bjc2015435#supplementary-information
2. Beck A, Reichert JM (2014) Antibody-drug conjugates. MAbs 6(1):15–17. https://doi.org/10.4161/mabs.27436
3. McCombs JR, Owen SC (2015) Antibody drug conjugates: design and selection of linker, payload and conjugation chemistry. AAPS J 17 (2):339–351. https://doi.org/10.1208/s12248-014-9710-8
4. Beck A, Goetsch L, Dumontet C, Corvaïa N (2017) Strategies and challenges for the next generation of antibody–drug conjugates. Nat Rev Drug Discov 16:315. https://doi.org/10.1038/nrd.2016.268
5. Chudasama V, Maruani A, Caddick S (2016) Recent advances in the construction of antibody–drug conjugates. Nat Chem 8:114. https://doi.org/10.1038/nchem.2415
6. Agarwal P, Bertozzi CR (2015) Site-specific antibody–drug conjugates: the Nexus of bioorthogonal chemistry, protein engineering, and drug development. Bioconjug Chem 26 (2):176–192. https://doi.org/10.1021/bc5004982
7. Panowski S, Bhakta S, Raab H, Polakis P, Junutula JR (2014) Site-specific antibody drug conjugates for cancer therapy. MAbs 6 (1):34–45. https://doi.org/10.4161/mabs.27022
8. Chen T, Chen Y, Stella C, Medley CD, Gruenhagen JA, Zhang K (2016) Antibody-drug conjugate characterization by chromatographic and electrophoretic techniques. J Chromatogr B 1032:39–50. https://doi.org/10.1016/j.jchromb.2016.07.023
9. Gahoual R, Giorgetti J, Beck A, Leize-Wagner E, François Y-N (2018) Chapter 19 - biopharmaceutical applications of capillary Electromigration methods. In: Poole CF (ed) Capillary electromigration separation methods. Elsevier, Amsterdam, pp 453–480. https://doi.org/10.1016/B978-0-12-809375-7.00021-6
10. Dai J, Lamp J, Xia Q, Zhang Y (2018) Capillary isoelectric focusing-mass spectrometry method for the separation and online characterization of intact monoclonal antibody charge variants. Anal Chem 90 (3):2246–2254. https://doi.org/10.1021/acs.analchem.7b04608
11. Gahoual R, Beck A, Leize-Wagner E, François Y-N (2016) Cutting-edge capillary electrophoresis characterization of monoclonal antibodies and related products. J Chromatogr B 1032:61–78. https://doi.org/10.1016/j.jchromb.2016.05.028

12. Redman EA, Mellors JS, Starkey JA, Ramsey JM (2016) Characterization of intact antibody drug conjugate variants using microfluidic capillary electrophoresis–mass spectrometry. Anal Chem 88(4):2220–2226. https://doi.org/10.1021/acs.analchem.5b03866
13. Stolz A, Jooß K, Höcker O, Römer J, Schlecht J, Neusüss C (2018) Recent advances in capillary electrophoresis-mass spectrometry: Instrumentation, methodology and applications. Electrophoresis 40(1):79–112. https://doi.org/10.1002/elps.201800331
14. Wiggins B, Liu-Shin L, Yamaguchi H, Ratnaswamy G (2015) Characterization of cysteine-linked conjugation profiles of immunoglobulin G1 and immunoglobulin G2 antibody–drug conjugates. J Pharm Sci 104(4):1362–1372. https://doi.org/10.1002/jps.24338
15. Valliere-Douglass JF, Lewis P, Salas-Solano O, Jiang S (2015) Solid-state mAbs and ADCs subjected to heat-stress stability conditions can be covalently modified with buffer and excipient molecules. J Pharm Sci 104 (2):652–665. https://doi.org/10.1002/jps.24276

Chapter 18

Characterization of the Primary Structure of Cysteine-Linked Antibody-Drug Conjugates Using Capillary Electrophoresis with Mass Spectrometry

Josiane Saadé, Rabah Gahoual, Alain Beck, Emmanuelle Leize-Wagner, and Yannis-Nicolas François

Abstract

Capillary electrophoresis-mass spectrometry (CE-MS) enables the characterization of the primary structure of ADCs. An analytical method based on a derived bottom up proteomic workflow is designed to provide detailed information about the amino acid sequence, the glycosylation profiling, and the location on the peptide backbone of the conjugated drugs. Here we describe the experimental protocol applied on the characterization of cysteine-linked brentuximab vedotin (Adcetris®).

Key words Antibody-drug conjugate, Brentuximab vedotin, Cytotoxic drug, Capillary electrophoresis–mass spectrometry, Structural characterization, Drug-loaded peptide

1 Introduction

Antibody-drug conjugates (ADCs) represent one of the fastest growing classes of oncology therapeutics. After brentuximab vedotin (Adcetris®) in 2011 and trastuzumab emtansine (Kadcyla, T-DM1) in 2013 [1], recent approval of inotuzumab ozogamicin (Besponsa, IO) [2] and re-approval of gemtuzumab ozogamicin (Mylotarg, GO) in 2017 [3] have opened the way for ongoing clinical trials that include 80 further ADC candidates [4]. In 2019, nine ADCs are in late clinical development [5]. ADCs incorporate highly potent warheads which can be delivered using the specificity provided by mAbs to target tumor cells and limit exposition of healthy cells, therefore optimizing treatment potency and limit the occurrence of side effects [6]. Various conjugation chemistries have been developed mainly based on stochastic conjugation to hinge cysteine residues after mild reduction or on surface-exposed lysine residues.

L. Nathan Tumey (ed.), *Antibody-Drug Conjugates: Methods and Protocols*, Methods in Molecular Biology, vol. 2078,
https://doi.org/10.1007/978-1-4939-9929-3_18,

ADC heterogeneity generated from different number and position of conjugated drugs during production contributes to the intrinsic variability coming from conjugation with mAbs. Compared to unconjugated mAbs, ADCs are much more structurally complex and represent a major challenge for analytical sciences to obtain a deep characterization. Mass spectrometry (MS) has gradually taken a decisive position in structure characterization of biopharmaceutical products [7–9]. MS still often needs to be used in combination with a separation method such as liquid chromatography [10, 11]. Recently, capillary electrophoresis-MS (CE-MS) methods with a sheathless interface have been developed to perform the characterization of mAbs in one injection including amino acid sequence, glycosylation characterization, and other types of post-translational modifications (methionine oxidation, asparagine deamidation...) [12–15]. Indeed, nanoESI, obtained from the ultra-low flow rate generated in CE separation, allows an increase of sensitivity and a decrease of ion suppression phenomenon and makes this interface a tool of choice particularly suitable for biotherapeutic characterization. Based on these works, Said et al. [16] developed a CE-ESI-MS/MS method derived from bottom-up proteomic analysis in order to be fully compatible with the requirement of the analysis of ADCs.

Here, we detail the sheathless CE-ESI-MS/MS method for the characterization of the primary structure of cysteine-linked ADCs with simultaneous determination of the amino acid sequence, the glycosylation profiling, and the identification of drug-loaded peptides. The choice of cysteine-linked ADC was based on the literature describing the robustness and reproducibility of the methodology. However, due to the large structural variability coming from the nature of ADC chemical conjugation, some modifications in the digestion protocol could be performed. Therefore, a bottom-up approach on lysine-linked ADC is under investigation in order to achieve optimal MS characterization.

2 Materials

2.1 Chemicals

Ultrapure water produced from Milli-Q Water System™ (Millipore) (prepared by purifying deionized water, to attain a sensitivity of 18.2 MΩ cm^{-1} at 25 °C). Chemicals used were of analytical grade or high purity grade. Prepare all reagents at room temperature and store the solutions in the fridge (unless indicated otherwise).

1. *Ammonium acetate buffer: 200 mM, pH 4.0.* Add about 10 mL water to a 25 mL volumetric flask. Weigh 0.385 g of ammonium acetate and transfer to the flask. Add 0.996 mL of acetic acid (>99%). Make up to 25 mL with water.

2. *Ammonium acetate buffer: 200 mM, pH 7.0.* Add about 30 mL water to a 100 mL volumetric flask. Weigh 1.54 g of ammonium acetate and transfer to the flask. Add 6.38 μL of acetic acid (1% (v/v)). Make up to 100 mL with water.
3. *Sodium phosphate buffer: 50 mM, pH 7.4, sodium chloride 150 mM.* Add about 30 mL water to a 100 mL volumetric flask. Weigh 0.569 g of disodium hydrogen phosphate and 0.119 g of sodium dihydrogen phosphate, and transfer to the flask. Weigh 0.877 g of sodium chloride and transfer to the flask. Make up to 100 mL with water.
4. *DTT solutions: 1 M.* Weigh 0.154 g of DTT and transfer to a 2.5 mL microtube. Make up to 1 mL of ammonium bicarbonate buffer (50 mM, pH 8.0).

2.2 ADC

Brentuximab vedotin (Adcetris®) was purchased from Takeda Pharma (Danemark). ADC was stored at 4 °C.

2.3 Instrumentation

1. CESI8000 system (Sciex, Brea, CA, USA) was hyphenated using a sheathless nanoelectrospray (nanoESI) interface.
2. Separation was performed using bare fused silica capillaries (total length 100 cm; 30 mm i d.) with characteristic porous tip on its final end on 3 cm.
3. A second capillary (total length 80 cm; 50 mm i.d.) filled during experiments with 10% acetic acid background electrolyte (BGE) allows electric contact.
4. A Triple TOF 5600+ mass spectrometer (Sciex, Darmstadt, Germany) is equipped with a hybrid analyzer composed of a quadrupole followed by a time-of-flight (TOF) analyzer.
5. Calibration solution: Before CE MS analysis, calibrate the Triple TOF 5600+ by the CE-MS separation of digest of *β-galactosidase*. Mix 5 μL of digest of *β-galactosidase* (8 μM) and 15 μL ammonium acetate 200 mM, pH 4.0 to obtain a final concentration of 2.0 μM.

3 Methods

The following protocol details the different steps for the characterization of cysteine-linked brentuximab vedotin using sheathless CE-ESI-MS instrument (*see* **Note 1**).

Carry out all procedures at room temperature unless otherwise specified.

3.1 IdeS Digestion

Store IdeS at −20 °C.

1. Mix 30 μL of ADC at 5 μg/μL and 117.25 μL of 50 mM sodium phosphate, 150 mM sodium chloride, pH 7.4 in a 500 μL microtube.

2. Add 2.25 μL of IdeS (67 U/μL) to the sample (*see* **Note 2**), to obtain a final ADC concentration of 1 μg/μL. Heat at 37 °C for 30 min.
3. After digestion completion, exchange sample buffer with 50 mM ammonium bicarbonate buffer, pH 7.0 using Amicon centrifugal filters 10 kDa (Merck Millipore, Darmstadt, Germany) (*see* **Note 3**) at 10 °C and 14,000 × *g* for 20 min.
4. Evaporate to dryness using speed vacuum instrument and reconstitute in a volume of 10 μL to obtain a final ADC concentration of 12.5 μg/μL (*see* **Note 4**).

3.2 Trypsin Digestion Protocol

Store trypsin and RapiGestSF at −20 °C.

1. Mix 10 μL ADC at 12.5 μg/μL and 10 μL of 0.1% RapidGest surfactant (*see* **Note 5**) in a 500 mL microtube to obtain ADC concentration of 6.25 μg/μL. Heat sample at 40 °C for 10 min (total volume 20 μL).
2. Add 1 μL DTT solution (500 mM) to obtain a concentration of 25 mM (*see* **Note 6**). Heat sample at 80 °C for 10 min (total volume 21 μL).
3. Once cooled down to room temperature, add 2 μL of ACN (10% (v/v)) to conserve hydrophobic drug-loaded peptides in solution (*see* **Note 7**) (total volume 23 μL).
4. Add a first volume of 2 μL of trypsin (0.5 μg/μL). Leave at room temperature for 3 h (total volume 25 μL).
5. Add a second volume of 2 μL of trypsin (0.5 μg/μL). Heat sample overnight at 37 °C (total volume 27 μL).
6. Add 1 μL DTT solution (1 M) to a final concentration of around 35 mM (*see* **Note 6**). Heat sample at 56 °C for 45 min (total volume 28 μL).
7. Once cooled down to room temperature, add 11.5 μL of IPA (40% (v/v)) to conserve hydrophobic drug-loaded peptides in solution (*see* **Note 7**) (total volume 39.5 μL).
8. Add 0.5 μL formic acid solution (1% (v/v)) (*see* **Note 8**). Leave sample at room temperature for 2 h. The final concentration of ADC is 3.1 μg/μL (21 μM) (total volume 40 μL).
9. Before CE-MS analysis, mix 1 μL of ADC sample and 9 μL ammonium acetate 200 mM, pH 4.0 to obtain a final concentration in protein of 2.1 μM (*see* **Note 9**).

3.3 CE-ESI-MS Analysis

1. New capillaries are flushed at 75 psi (5.17 bars) for 10 min with methanol, then 10 min with 0.1 M sodium hydroxide, followed by 10 min with 0.1 M hydrochloric acid and water for 20 min (*see* **Note 10**).

2. Before each analysis, separation capillary is flushed at 50 psi (3.45 bars) for 10 min with the BGE composed of 10% acetic acid. The second capillary for maintaining the electric fields is flushed with the same BGE for 5 min at 50 psi (3.45 bars).
3. After each analysis, separation capillary is flushed at 75 psi (5.17 bars) for 10 min with methanol, then 10 min with 0.1 M sodium hydroxide, followed by 10 min with 0.1 M hydrochloric acid and water for 20 min. The second capillary is flushed with the same BGE for 3 min at 50 psi (3.45 bars).
4. Add 10 μL of ADC sample (2.1 μM) in a microvial (Sciex, Darmstadt, Germany). Place it in the sample platform of the instrument.
5. Perform a hydrodynamic injection of 90 nL by applying 10 psi for 1 min (around 100 nL injected).
6. Perform the separations using a voltage of +20 kV for 50 min (*see* **Note 11**).
7. Set ESI source parameters as follows: ESI voltage—1.45 kV while Gas supplies (GS1 and GS2) were deactivated. Source heating temperature 150 °C and curtain gas value 4 (*see* **Note 12**). Mass/charge (m/z) range was 100–2000 in MS and 50–2000 in MS/MS.
8. Calibrate all spectra by external calibration using a digest of *β-galactosidase*.

3.4 MS and MS/MS Data Analysis

1. Use Analyst software (Sciex, Darmstadt, Germany) to convert your MS-raw data from .wiff format to .mgf format (*see* **Note 13**).
2. Open the .mgf file with a dedicated software (Biotools (Bruker, Germany) in our cases) to perform the identification of the primary structure of the ADC. The mass tolerance for search algorithm identification was set to ±5 ppm for precursor ions and ±0.05 Da for fragmentation ions.
3. For the missing peptides not found by the search algorithm, calculate the theoretical monoisotopic masses using a fragment ion calculator (for instance, Protcomics Toolkit). Extract found masses from the MS-raw data using Peakview software (Sciex, CA) and validate the presence of missing peptide using MS/MS data (Fig. 1).
4. For glycopeptides and drug-loaded peptides characterization, enter the theoretical modification in the search algorithm and perform the identification.
5. For the missing glycopeptides or drug-loaded peptides, follow the same protocol described in **step 3** with the masses of modified peptides (Fig. 2).

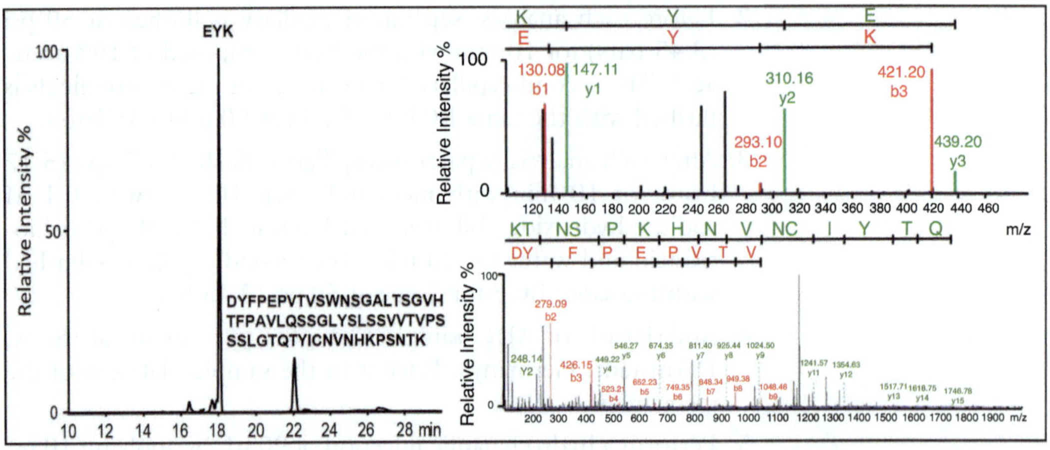

Fig. 1 Ion electropherogram (EIE) corresponding to the mass-to-charge ratios of [EYK] and [DYFPEPVTVSWNSGALTSGVHTFPAVLQSSGLYSLSSVVTVPSSSLGTQTYICNVNHKPSNTK] MS/MS fragmentation spectra for both peaks are shown at right. (Adapted with permission from ref. 16. Copyright (2016) Elsevier)

6. To perform the glycan profiling of each mAb, estimate relative occurrence levels from the sum of isotopic peak intensities, considering all charge states of the ion corresponding to one glycopeptide [17]. Compare the relative abundance of all glycoforms (Fig. 3).

4 Notes

1. The method is dedicated to the primary structure characterization of ADCs conjugated to hinge cysteine residues. Concerning lysine-linked ADC, IdeS digestion could be removed and other enzymes as chymotrypsin could be evaluated.
2. IdeS digestion cleaves the ADC between two consecutive glycine residues present in the hinge region. It results in two types of fragments ($F_{c/2}$ and $F\ (ab')_2$). Particularly in the case of brentuximab vedotin, IdeS digestion prior to trypsin digestion enables the formation of a THTCPPCPAPELLG peptide potentially loaded with 0 to 2 drugs, and then facilitates the characterization of the drug-loaded peptides.
3. Due to the total mass of ADC of around 150 kDa, Amicon centrifugal filter 50 kDa could be used to perform the desalting step. Other manufacturer could be evaluated.
4. Sample volume has to be evaporated to dryness and reconstitute to a volume of 10 μL to get an ADC concentration of 12.5 μg/μL in order to obtain at the end of the digestion protocol a final concentration of 21 μM allowing to inject 200 fmol by CE-ESI-MS analysis.

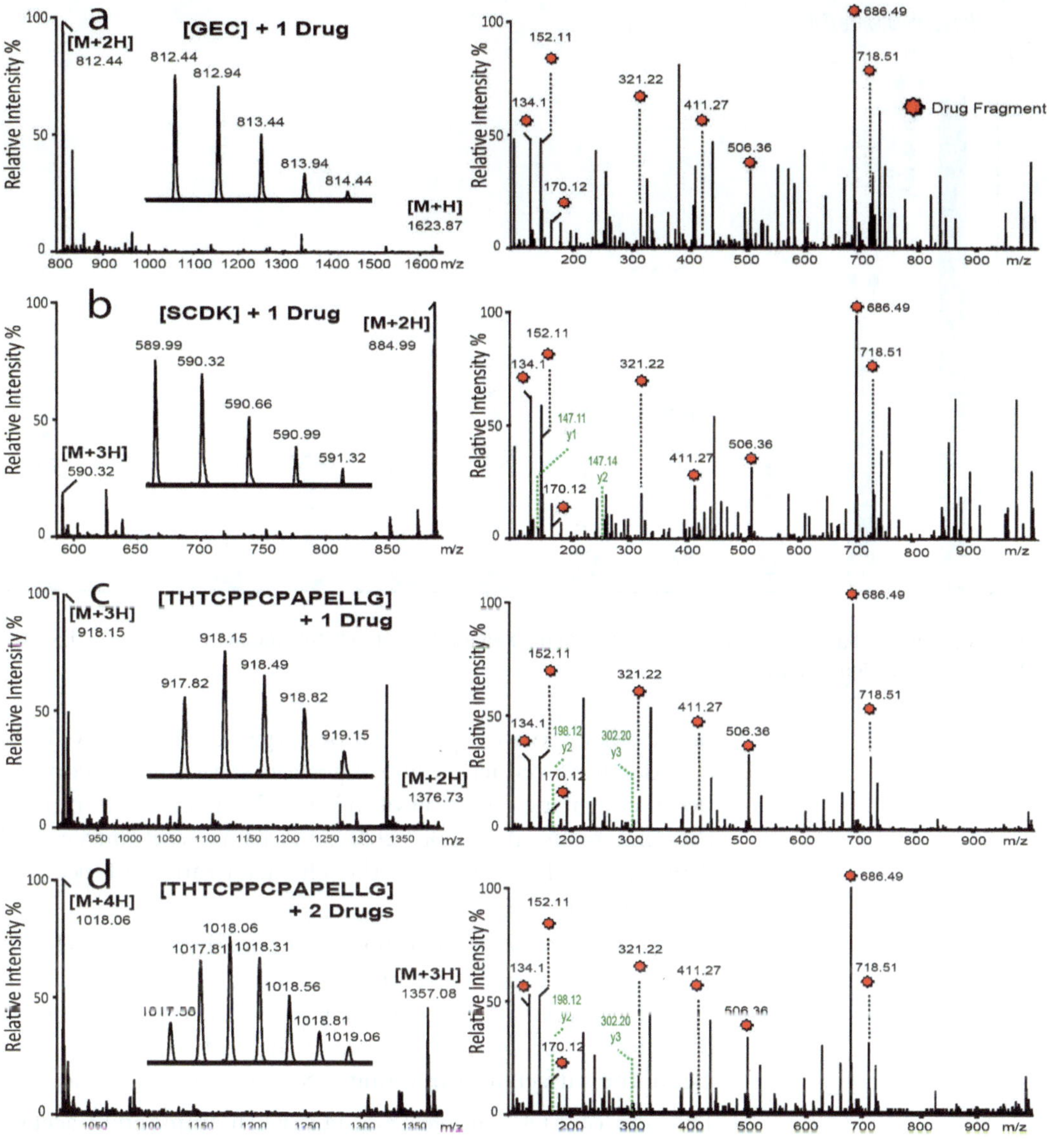

Fig. 2 MS and MS/MS spectra of drug-loaded peptides. (**a**) [GEC] + 1 payload, (**b**) [SCDK] + 1 payload, (**c**) [THTCPPCPAPELLG] + 1 payload, and (**d**) [THTCPPCPAPELLG] + 2 payloads. (Reprinted with permission from ref. [16]. Copyright (2016) Elsevier)

5. Rapigest surfactant is a well-known denaturing agent used in this protocol. Other denaturing agents such as guanidine-HCl or urea could be used [18].
6. DTT is a well-known reducing agent used in this protocol. Other reducing agent as TCEP (tris(2-carboxyethyl) phosphine) could be used.
7. Hydrophobicity of drug molecule induces precipitation of drug-loaded peptides in aqueous buffers such as ammonium

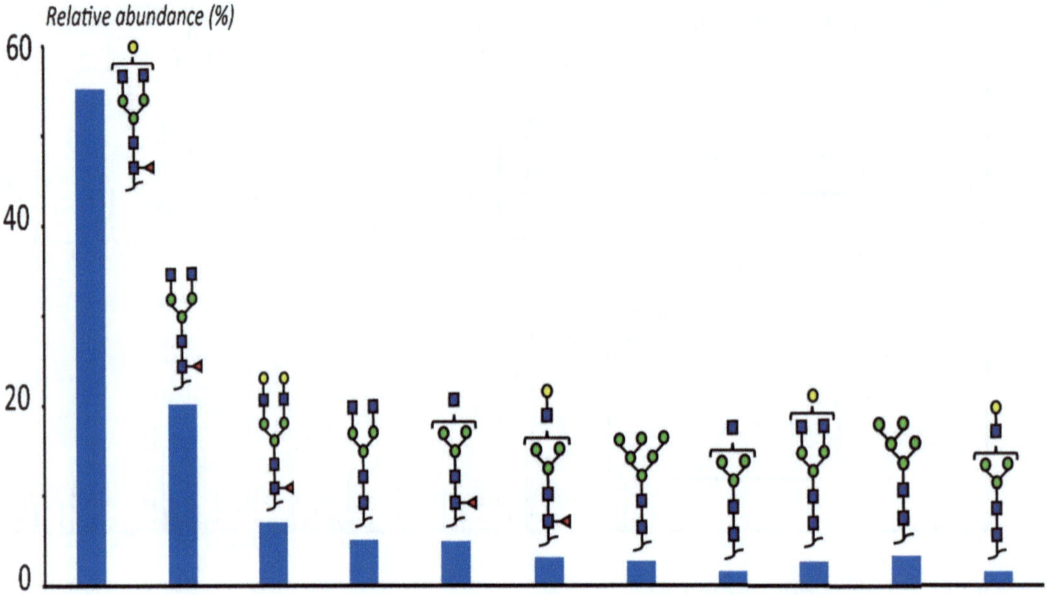

Fig. 3 Glycoform relative abundances determination obtained for brentuximab vedotin using the CE–ESI-MS/MS method in a single analysis

bicarbonate. To avoid precipitation, organic solvents have been added during reduction and digestion steps for the conventional enzymatic digestion of mAbs [12]. The modification of the enzymatic protocol, especially using acetonitrile and 2-propanol, did not affect the characterization of peptides and glycopeptides.

8. Rapigest, also known as sodium 3-[(2-methyl-2-undecyl-1,3-dioxolan-4-yl)methoxy]-1-propanesulfonate, is an acid-cleavable anionic detergent used to enhance the enzymatic digestion of proteins. Addition of an acid is mandatory to cleave the surfactant promoting MS detection of peptides.

9. Dilution of ADC sample (3.1 μg/μL) in ammonium acetate 200 mM, pH 4.0 modifies the sample buffer and allows sample to be in favorable condition to perform online pre-concentration by transient-isotachophoresis during the CE-ESI-MS analysis.

10. A bare fused silica capillary is used in the described protocol. However, in an alternative lysyl endopeptidase C (Lys-C) protocol, Dada et al. propose the use of a neutral linear polyacrylamide capillary [18]. Using this kind of capillary, the washing protocol for the new capillary and the reconditioning step could degrade the quality of coating and thus causes performance degradation.

11. CE instrument allows following the current profile during the separation. If the current drops, this indicates that you have a

loss of separation and therefore a decrease in resolution. Among the most probable causes is the formation of an air bubble at the capillary inlet or the clogging or rupture of the capillary.

12. Due to the ultra-low flow rate obtained with the sheathless CE-ESI-MS interface, curtain gas must be less than 10 to get a stable spray.
13. Each mass spectrometer manufacturer requires obtaining raw data in a proprietary format (e.g., .wiff for Sciex). However, analysis of this data implies the use of dedicated software. The most file formats commonly used in MS proteomics is the Mascot Generic Format (mgf) file. The mgf file was developed by Matrix Science (London, UK), the maker of Mascot, the most widely used commercial search engine, but it is widely supported by many proteomics search engines. Then it allows a better flexibility for data treatment of obtained MS data.

Acknowledgments

The authors would like to thank Sciex separations Inc. for lending a CESI8000 system and a 5600 TripleTOF. They would like to thank Bruker Daltonics for lending a Maxis 4G. They would like also to express their gratitude to Dr. E. Wagner-Rousset, M. C. Janin-Bussat, and O. Colas (Centre d'Immunologie Pierre Fabre, St Julien en Genevois, France) for helpful discussions. This work was supported by the CNRS (UMR 7140) and the University of Strasbourg.

References

1. Beck A, Reichert JM (2014) Antibody-drug conjugates. MAbs 6(1):15–17
2. Tvito A, Rowe JM (2017) Inotuzumab ozogamicin for the treatment of acute lymphoblastic leukemia. Expert Opin Biol Ther 17 (12):1557–1564
3. Jen EY, Ko C-W, Lee JE et al (2018) FDA approval: Gemtuzumab ozogamicin for the treatment of adults with newly-diagnosed CD33-positive acute myeloid leukemia. Clin. Cancer Res 24(14):3242–3246
4. Beck A, Goetsch L, Dumontet C, Corvaïa N (2017) Strategies and challenges for the next generation of antibody–drug conjugates. Nat Rev Drug Discov 16:315
5. Kaplon H, Reichert JM (2018) Antibodies to watch in 2018. MAbs 10(2):183–203
6. Zolot RS, Basu S, Million RP (2013) Antibody-drug conjugates. Nat Rev Drug Discov 12(4):259–260
7. Biacchi M, Gahoual R, Said N, Beck A, Leize-Wagner E, François Y-N (2015) Glycoform separation and characterization of Cetuximab variants by middle-up off-line capillary zone electrophoresis-UV/electrospray ionization-MS. Anal Chem 87(12):6240–6250
8. Stoll DR, Hannes DC, Danforth J et al (2015) Direct identification of rituximab Main isoforms and subunit analysis by online selective comprehensive two-dimensional liquid chromatography-mass spectrometry. Anal Chem 87(16):8307–8315
9. Debaene F, Boeuf A, Wagner-Rousset E et al (2014) Innovative native MS methodologies for antibody drug conjugate characterization: high resolution native MS and IM-MS for

average DAR and DAR distribution assessment. Anal Chem 86(21):10674–10683

10. Janin-Bussat M-C, Dillenbourg M, Corvaia N, Beck A, Klinguer-Hamour C (2015) Characterization of antibody drug conjugate positional isomers at cysteine residues by peptide mapping LC-MS analysis. J Chromatogr B 981:9–13
11. Firth D, Bell L, Squires M, Estdale S, McKee C (2015) A rapid approach for characterization of thiol-conjugated antibody–drug conjugates and calculation of drug–antibody ratio by liquid chromatography mass spectrometry. Anal Biochem 485:34–42
12. Gahoual R, Busnel J-M, Beck A, François Y-N, Leize-Wagner E (2014) Full antibody primary structure and microvariant characterization in a single injection using transient Isotachophoresis and Sheathless capillary electrophoresis-- tandem mass spectrometry. Anal Chem 86 (18):9074–9081
13. Gahoual R, Burr A, Busnel JM et al (2013) Rapid and multi-level characterization of trastuzumab using sheathless capillary electrophoresis-tandem mass spectrometry. MAbs 5(3):479–490
14. Gahoual R, Biacchi M, Chicher J et al (2014) Monoclonal antibodies biosimilarity assessment using transient isotachophoresis capillary zone electrophoresis-tandem mass spectrometry. MAbs 6(6):1464–1473
15. Gahoual R, Beck A, Leize-Wagner E, François Y-N (2016) Cutting-edge capillary electrophoresis characterization of monoclonal antibodies and related products. J Chromatogr B 1032:61–78
16. Said N, Gahoual R, Kuhn L, Beck A, François Y-N, Leize-Wagner E (2016) Structural characterization of antibody drug conjugate by a combination of intact, middle-up and bottom-up techniques using sheathless capillary electrophoresis—tandem mass spectrometry as nanoESI infusion platform and separation method. Anal Chim Acta 918:50–59
17. Giorgetti J, D'Atri V, Canonge J et al (2018) Monoclonal antibody N-glycosylation profiling using capillary electrophoresis—mass spectrometry: assessment and method validation. Talanta 178(Supplement C):530–537
18. Dada OO, Zhao YM, Jaya N, Salas-Solano O (2017) High-resolution capillary zone electrophoresis with mass spectrometry peptide mapping of therapeutic proteins: peptide recovery and post-translational modification analysis in monoclonal antibodies and antibody-drug conjugates. Anal Chem 89 (21):11236–11242

Chapter 19

Purification of ADCs by Hydrophobic Interaction Chromatography

Calvin L. Becker, Robert J. Duffy, Jorge Gandarilla, and Steven M. Richter

Abstract

Antibody-drug conjugate (ADC) in vitro potency has been shown to be dependent on drug load, with higher drug load providing lower IC_{50} values. However, in vivo potency is affected by intrinsic biological effects as well, such as plasma clearance, dose-limiting toxicity, etc. Developing a preparative HIC process for ADC purification to isolate species with a specific drug loading involves several steps including conjugation optimization, resin selection, solubility studies gradient screening, and step gradient development (buffer selection). In this chapter, the rationale and general considerations for developing a preparative hydrophobic interaction chromatography (HIC) method are described for isolation of an example ADC with specific drug load, e.g., two monomethyl auristatin E (MMAE) payloads (E2).

Key words Antibody-drug conjugate (ADC), Hydrophobic interaction chromatography (HIC), Drug-antibody ratio (DAR), Lyotrope, Buffers, Gradient

1 Introduction

HIC chromatography takes advantage of the differences in hydrophobicity of different constituents present in complex protein matrices, such as the drug-loaded species in ADCs, by utilizing a reversible interaction between the proteins and the hydrophobic stationary phase of a HIC resin. The interaction between the ADC and the resin is influenced by the presence of salts in the elution buffer. High salt concentration encourages the interaction while lowering the salt concentration weakens the interaction. The greater the hydrophobicity, the lower the ionic strength of the buffer salt required to maintain the interaction with the resin. Gradients of decreasing ionic strength of the buffer are employed to elute the individual drug-load species in order of increasing hydrophobicity, or in other words those with the lowest drug load to the highest [1].

HIC purification of MMAE ADCs has produced conjugates with a specific drug load. Antibody-drug conjugate potency in vitro

L. Nathan Tumey (ed.), *Antibody-Drug Conjugates: Methods and Protocols*, Methods in Molecular Biology, vol. 2078,
https://doi.org/10.1007/978-1-4939-9929-3_19,

has been shown to be directly dependent on drug load, i.e., IC_{50} values E8 < E4 < E2 where E refers to a MMAE conjugate and the number refers to the number of MMAEs conjugated. However, the in vivo antitumor activity does not follow the same trend. Purified E8 and E4 demonstrated comparable potency at equal mAb doses in vivo. Dosing at equal mAb amounts would provide only half the MMAE for E4 versus E8 yet the antitumor activity is comparable. In addition, MMAE drug load impacts plasma clearance, as E8 cleared three times faster than E4 and five times faster than E2 [2].

In a recent example, LRRC15 (leucine-rich repeat containing 15) was found to be highly expressed on stromal fibroblasts in multiple solid tumor types (e.g., breast, head and neck, lung, pancreatic, sarcoma, melanoma, glioblastoma) with limited expression in normal tissue [3]. This led to evaluation of an ADC containing two MMAE molecules per antibody (E2) targeting LRRC15 optimized for efficacy targeted against stromal fibroblasts with LRRC15 overexpression. The parent LRRC15-targeting antibody is conjugated to the potent cell permeable antimitotic molecule MMAE through a cleavable valine-citrulline dipeptide linker. Following conjugation, a HIC step is used to isolate drug substance containing primarily the E2. The E2 profile was chosen over the broad distribution product with a drug-antibody ratio (DAR) of four, based on the preclinical efficacy data. In this chapter, we describe development of a scalable process for the production of highly enriched individual drug-load species (e.g., E2 or E4 isolates).

1.1 Optimize Conjugation/Reduction for Desired DAR

The first step in the development of a scalable process for isolation of an individual DAR species is to identify the DAR species of interest, for example, a DAR2 species (also referred to as E2). To achieve the maximum yield for an isolation process, an important consideration is optimization of the process to produce the maximum amount of E2 in the crude reaction mixture. Protocols for the development of an ADC synthetic route have been previously described [4]. Crude ADC can be prepared in a two-step, one-pot process via a partial reduction of the mAb (monoclonal antibody) interchain disulfide bridges followed by quantitative alkylation of the resulting thiols by excess drug-linker, such as vc-MMAE. The primary factor controlling DAR in cysteine conjugations is determined by the stoichiometry of the reducing agent, in our case tris (carboxyethyl)phosphine hydrochloride (TCEP•HCl) or dithiothreitol (DTT). The mAb is diluted with a suitable buffer to raise the pH for conjugation such as phosphate buffered saline pH 7.4 (PBS) or sodium borate pH 8 buffer containing a chelator such as ethylenediaminetetraacetic acid (EDTA) to prevent re-oxidation. This is followed by a titration study varying the equivalents of TCEP and temperature to achieve the maximum level of the desired DAR species. After selecting reducing conditions, the partially reduced mAb is then conjugated with a molar excess of drug-linker dissolved in a suitable water miscible co-solvent such as dimethyl sulfoxide or dimethylacetamide [4, 5]. It is important to note that the co-solvent content may impact HIC retention times and should be considered before changing the relative amount of co-solvent in future conjugation optimization. Excess drug-linker is quenched with an aqueous solution of *N*-acetyl-L-cysteine (NAC) [6]. The resulting crude product solution is the source material for HIC method development.

1.2 Gradient Screening

1.2.1 Equipment

One of the first considerations in developing a HIC method is the selection of equipment for the task. There are several column options available, which can be broadly classified into prepacked and self-packed options. Self-packed columns are packed by adding the HIC resin slurry and compressing the bed through a combination of fluid flow and dynamic axial compression. Since most stationary phase options are compressible, this activity must be performed with some care to properly pack the bed according to manufacturer's instructions and avoid overcompression of the HIC resin. As the scale of the column increases, additional precautions are needed to ensure that the bed is packed evenly. Advantages of self-packing columns include increased control over the packing parameters, the potential to reduce lead times for columns by maintaining an inventory of stationary phases, and a reduced cost over the long term by reusing equipment.

A second option is to source prepacked columns from either the manufacturer of the stationary phase or a third party. These are readily available from multiple vendors with a variety of stationary phases, particularly at smaller scales. Advantages of prepacked columns include leveraging the packing expertise and equipment capability of a resin producer or third-party partner and avoiding the processing time to pack and potentially repack a column on site. Prepacked columns also avoid the need to unpack the HIC resin after use, which requires cleaning equipment before reusing and the possibility to expose personnel to resin that has been in contact with ADC and potent drug-linker used in the ADC processes.

1.2.2 Screening and Definition of Operating Parameters

Definition of the operating parameters for a chromatography step is typically done at the small scale and then scaled up based on the small-scale model. Column selection is dependent on the hydrophobicity of the target molecule and the matrix within which it resides, as is the selection of the mobile phases for the separation. A variety of HIC separation media are commercially available in prepacked columns and/or high-throughput screening plate formats.

These stationary phases include a range of hydrophobicity and ligand density and need to be screened to ensure that they can provide the appropriate resolution for the species of interest [7, 8]. Elevated hydrophobicity of the resin can lead to conformational changes in the protein upon adsorption and should be monitored closely [9]. In addition to the chemical composition of the stationary phase, the particle size can play a significant role in resolution of species. Smaller particles can deliver increased resolution but may restrict flow rate due to limitations in the pressure drop across the compressible bed. Larger or less compressible beads allow the use of an increased flow rate and thereby shorter cycle times. This is of particular interest as scale and cost of operation increases.

Because the separation kinetics of a HIC chromatography is somewhat dependent on temperature, the selection and optimization of the stationary and mobile phases of the chromatographic separation should be done at the intended temperature of the final operation. For example, if the separation will be run in a research lab for discovery purposes, development of the step may be done at the ambient temperature of the R&D lab (e.g., 21–22 °C), but temperature control is paramount to ensure process consistency. However, if the final operation space will be a GMP manufacturing space, the space is often kept cooler to accommodate the gowning requirements for the individuals performing the separation (e.g., 19–20 °C). The chromatography temperature can be controlled by careful maintenance of the feed vessels for elution buffers and load, or through the use of an in-line heat exchanger. Automated control of the chromatography step simplifies the operation and can improve reproducibility between experiments using any of the commercially available chromatography workstations, such as an ÄKTA system by GE Healthcare.

As mentioned before, buffer selection for the separation is dependent on the hydrophobicity of the molecule and the stationary phase selected for the separation. The buffers selected for HIC are typically neutral buffering species, such as sodium phosphate. Higher and lower pH conditions can lead to proteins experiencing modifications such as deamidation of susceptible amino acids [10]. Because of this, typical separations are performed between pH 5 and pH 8.

Because HIC is dependent on the polarity of the mobile phase, relative to the stationary phase, there are a variety of lyotropic salts to select from in the binding separation. A lyotropic salt promotes the hydrophobic interaction. One of the most commonly used is ammonium sulfate, which is a stronger lyotrope compared to ammonium chloride according to the Hofmeister series [11, 12]. Either can be utilized for HIC, but it requires a higher concentration of the chloride salt compared to the sulfate salt to enable the binding of the antibody protein to the ligand. For general screening purposes and in the following examples, ammonium sulfate is used in a neutral sodium phosphate buffer solution.

The first step to defining the operating parameters is developing an understanding of load material and at what point it will precipitate out of solution as a function of the salt concentration in the mobile phase, which drives the hydrophobic interaction with the chromatography ligands on the selected column. There are two primary strategies widely used to determine the point at which the protein in solution will precipitate during the HIC load preparation: (1) the direct titration method when the sample availability is very limited, and (2) the screening panel method when there is an ample supply of the starting material. Most large proteins, including antibodies and ADCs, will precipitate once a critical salt concentration is reached. Binding conditions for a HIC column separation are strongest just below the lyotrope concentration at which the protein would precipitate, but remains soluble in solution.

HIC involves binding a protein using an immobilized ligand on the surface of chromatography resin beads. The type and density of the ligand dictate the hydrophobicity of the resin. The binding is enabled through the use of lyotropic salts, such as ammonium sulfate, at high enough concentrations that encourage binding to the ligand on the stationary phase, but the product remains in solution. Column selection should be based on the hydrophobicity of the proteins to be isolated. For strongly hydrophobic molecules, such as MMAE-conjugated antibodies, a hydrophobic ligand stationary phase resin, such as the Butyl Sepharose High Performance resin from GE Healthcare, is a good choice. The column should be equilibrated in a lyotrope concentration equivalent to the concentration in the load. The target molecule is then bound to the column and the column is washed at the same lyotrope concentration to flush out all of the nonbinding components present in the load matrix. Following the wash, a 20 column volume (CV) descending salt concentration gradient elutes the molecule of interest and related other drug-load species from the column. The material that remains on the column can then be removed with a sodium hydroxide clean-in-place (CIP)/sanitization wash. Using the mobile phases described below, the chromatography method would adhere to the description in Table 1, which provides an example of a linear gradient. The residence, or contact time, of the process stream and the resin is controlled by the flow rate, or axial linear velocity, of the pumped solution through the column and is determined by the resin manufacturer's recommendations. For example, the Butyl Sepharose HP resin is recommended to be operated at ≤100 cm/h to avoid overcompression of the resin bed at a back pressure of ≥0.5 MPa, when scaled up to a 20 cm packed bed height [13].

The separation of an MMAE cysteine-conjugated ADC product is shown in Fig. 1. The Butyl Sepharose HP column was loaded

Table 1
Linear gradient example

Step	Volume	% B	Mobile phase
Equilibration	5 CV	33.3% B	25 mM Na_2PO_4, 1.0 M $(NH_4)_2SO_4$
Load	–	0% B	25 mM Na_2PO_4, 1.0 M $(NH_4)_2SO_4$
Wash	5 CV	33.3% B	25 mM Na_2PO_4, 1.0 M $(NH_4)_2SO_4$
Elution	30 CV	33.3% to 100% B	25 mM Na_2PO_4, 1.0 M $(NH_4)_2SO_4$ 25 mM Na_2PO_4, 0.0 M $(NH_4)_2SO_4$
Post-elution wash	3 CV	100% B	25 mM Na_2PO_4, 0.0 M $(NH_4)_2SO_4$
CIP/sanitization	3 CV	0% B	0.5 N NaOH
Storage	4 CV	0% B	20% EtOH

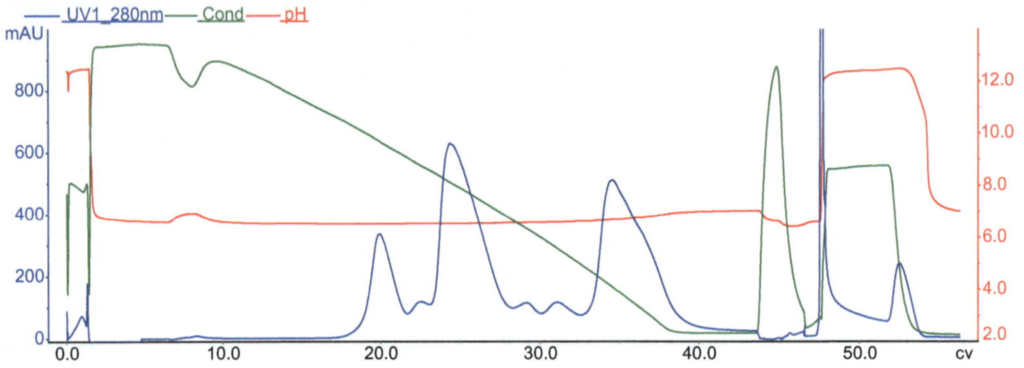

Fig. 1 Chromatogram of a Butyl Sepharose HP separation of a conjugated antibody including UV (blue), pH (red), and conductivity (green)

to a protein binding capacity of 20 mg/mL of resin. All species were bound to the column, including the unconjugated mAb. As the gradient proceeded, the lyotropic salt concentration decreased and the different drug-load species were eluted in order of the fewest drug per antibody to the most. The first major absorbance (blue) peak to elute was the unconjugated antibody, followed by E2 and then E4. The peaks of E6 and E8 were more hydrophobic and eluted in the CIP/sanitization wash and the storage wash. Minor peaks eluting between the major peaks are likely odd species of conjugates including E1 and E3.

1.3 Microbial and Endotoxin Controls

If the product being generated by the HIC step is intended to be used for testing in live organisms, microorganisms, such as bacteria and viruses, as well as pyrogens (endotoxin), must be controlled. All surfaces that will contact the product stream need to be sanitized (*See* Note Section 4.1). While some contact surfaces may be autoclaved (e.g., glass and stainless steel) to control adventitious biological organisms [14], the products from those organisms such as lipopolysaccharides (endotoxins) remain on their surface. These can be removed by either high temperature exposure or chemical exposure over time [15, 16]. The latter is preferred for controlling both organisms and endotoxins on the surfaces of non-metal (e.g., plastic, etc.) or glass. For example, the contact surfaces in a flow path of a chromatography workstation and column, including the resin if it is caustic stable, can be treated with 0.5 M NaOH for 30 min at ambient temperature to both control microbes and destroy endotoxin [17]. *Note: Some bacteria spores* (e.g., *Bacillus subtilis) may survive the treatment with 0.5 M NaOH, so it is recommended that the system and column be sanitized prior to use, as well as after. If this is a routine problem, 30 mM peracetic acid exposure for 1 h would be sufficient to eliminate the spores* [18].

Process solutions are potentially an additional source of bioburden and endotoxin and are thus prepared with WFI (water for injection), or equivalent quality water. The preparation of the solutions to be used in chromatography should be filtered through a 0.2 μm filter to establish sterility by removing bacteria. When the solutions are prepared and filtered, they should be tested for endo toxin prior to use. There are multiple commercially available options for endotoxin testing including, but not limited to, the Endosafe® Nexgen-PTS system from Charles River (cat# PTS150K). If endotoxin is found to be present in a solution after 0.2 μm filtration, it can be filtered through a depyrogenated, 10 kDa molecular weight cut-off membrane in either direct or tangential flow according to the manufacturer's instructions. *Be sure to collect the filtrate in a sterile depyrogenated/non-pyrogenic container.*

1.4 Temperature Dependence and Impact on Loading

A warning frequently offered by chromatography experts with hydrophobic interaction chromatography is the sensitivity observed to temperature [19]. Hydrophobic interaction is often described as an entropy-driven effect and changes in the order of the system. Hydrophobic components tend to associate among themselves and exclude more hydrophilic components, which in turn associate themselves. The addition of ions further promotes the association between the hydrophobic ligand of the resin and hydrophobic regions of the protein. The opposite is true, as decreasing ion concentration weakens the interactions. As temperature increases, collisions also increase and further enhance the hydrophobic interaction. This has a counterintuitive effect. as temperature increases the hydrophobic interaction between ligand and hydrophobic protein increases, which is manifested as an increase in binding and/or loading capacity. Since various DAR components are closely related, the impact of temperature on binding strength can cause significant changes in the separation. As temperature increases, increased hydrophobic interactions lead to broader

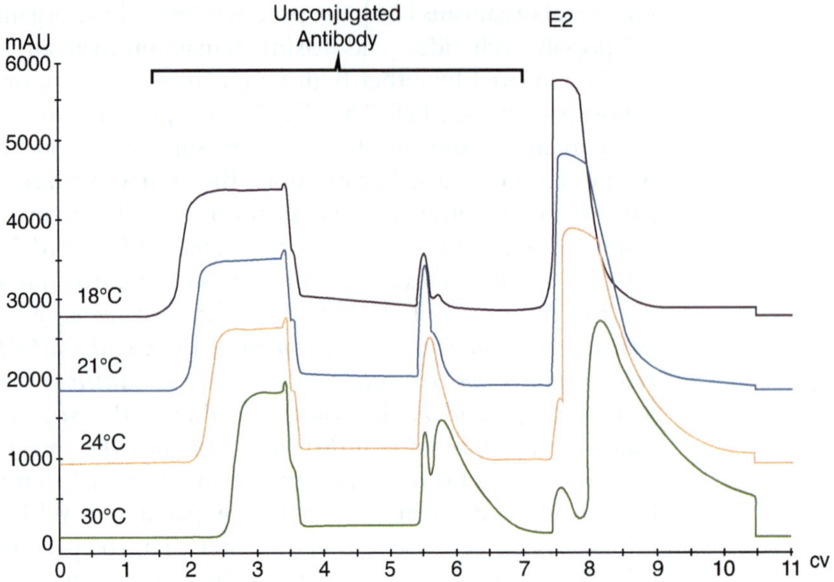

Fig. 2 Elution chromatogram of a preparative separation of a vcMMAE conjugate and the effect of temperature

peaks and increasing tailing under the same load (*see* Fig. 2). In the example shown, the goal was to isolate enriched 2-drug species (E2) and the small peak around 7.5 CVs is residual unconjugated mAb and E1 species. Table 2 shows the observed decrease in E2 peak area (pa%) as temperature increases.

1.5 Preparative Hydrophobic Interaction Chromatography

1.5.1 Column Qualification

Column packing is the introduction of the separation resin into a column housing in a way that particles are evenly distributed in a packed resin bed in the column and minimizes physical separation of resin based on gravity. It is often described as an art, as the level of experience of the person, or team, packing the column can influence the quality of the packed bed. Available equipment may dictate the method used to pack a column. For example, to pack small columns in the lab, constant flow, or constant pressure, may be the most accessible options to cover a wide range of column diameters. Larger columns may use the same techniques and more sophisticated equipment may be available to ensure reproducible packing and minimizing buffer usage. The column packing process may be automated depending on equipment availability. Each HIC resin has different manufacturer's packing recommendations and requirements based on their specific physicochemical properties that give their particle rigidness. It is a best practice to follow the manufacturer's recommendations when handling the resin. Once a column has been packed, it is recommended to evaluate the packing efficiency through the use of a small nonbinding molecule, such as sodium chloride, using an injection volume of 0.0025–0.3 CV, passed through the packed resin bed. The resulting peak shape

Table 2
Effect of temperature

	Eluate attributes			
Temperature (°C)	HIC (E2 pa %)	Eluate (mg/mL)	Eluate (CVs)	Recovery (%)
18	99.6	9.0	1.6	40.2
21	97.5	7.2	1.9	39.5
24	96.5	5.3	2.6	39.6
30	93.3	3.8	3.0	32.1

and retention are evaluated for asymmetry and HETP (Height Equivalent Theoretical Plates) to identify gross packing errors and other potential flaws before introducing valuable material.

1.5.2 Selection of Gradient or Step Elution

A linear gradient elution was described in Table 1. It is a good choice for initial purification screening efforts and it also allows identification of the ionic strength to develop a step elution gradient. The particular ionic strength or mobile phase concentration at which a component begins to elute provides the desired buffer concentration to elute a particular component. A step elution is determined based on this phenomenon. For example, a 2 × 1 mL Butyl Sepharose HP HiTrap column with 30 g/L load was equilibrated and loaded at 0.8 M $(NH_4)_2SO_4$, 25 mM Na_2PO_4, pH 7.1 and eluted over a 24 CV gradient to 25 mM Na_2PO_4, pH 7.1. Figure 3 presents the results from that separation. Based on the leading edges of the key peaks in the gradient separation, it was determined that E0 could be eluted without impacting the E2 peak at approximately 115 mS/cm and that E2 could be eluted at approximately 90 mS/cm. From these conductivities, the salt concentration in the mobile phase can be optimized for step elution balancing multiple considerations including the purity of the desired component, the number of column volumes required to elute a desired component, and the sensitivity to breakthrough of the more strongly retained components under a given set of elution conditions. There may be advantages in selecting one mode of operation over the other. For instance, a linear gradient may be less susceptible to temperature effects but produce larger amounts of waste. Additionally, there are cases when a step elution can offer greater resolution of peaks poorly separated by a linear gradient. Because of this, a step gradient is favored for scale-up since buffers can be specifically prepared within narrow specifications, decreasing burden on equipment performance.

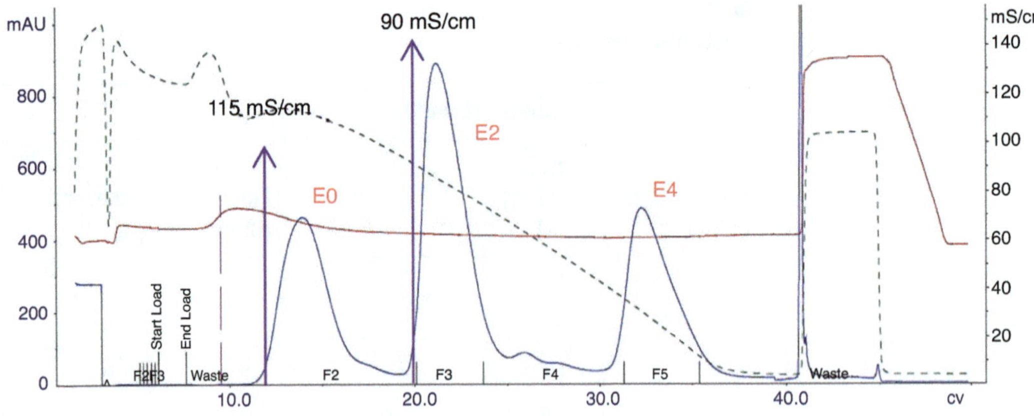

Fig. 3 Gradient elution showing conductivities of leading peak edges

1.6 Step Gradient Example

If necessary, the room temperature is adjusted to the desired elution temperature allowing time for buffer temperatures to equilibrate, or an in-line heat exchanger can be employed. Figure 4 illustrates a step gradient elution of a MMAE conjugate on a Butyl Sepharose HP column with a 20 cm bed height and 30 g/L loading, where the column is equilibrated and loaded at 0.8 M ammonium sulfate. Unconjugated antibody is eluted with 0.65 M ammonium sulfate, and the desired E2 conjugate elutes with 0.425 M ammonium sulfate. Table 3 shows the steps and column volumes employed for elution. At the start of the purification cycle the column is sanitized with 4 CVs (column volumes) of 0.5 N sodium hydroxide, and then equilibrated with 3–4 CVs of 0.8 M ammonium sulfate using a linear flow rate of 75 cm/h. The product is then loaded onto the column at about 38 cm/h, or about half the linear flow rate. The load wash, 2 CVs of 0.8 M ammonium sulfate, follows at the linear flow rate of 75 cm/h; this serves to displace co-solvent and other unbound species before the start of the step gradient. Unconjugated monoclonal antibody (E0) is eluted with 3 CVs of 0.65 M ammonium sulfate. The conductivity is further dropped using 0.425 M ammonium sulfate to elute the desired product. Collection is based on UV signal at 280 nm and collection starts using a 150 mAU trigger at the start and end of the peak based on UV. The product fraction is collected in a suitable sterile container and stored cold awaiting completion of any remaining cycles. The resin undergoes regeneration with 4 CVs of 0.5 N sodium hydroxide and 4 CVs of 25% isopropanol in phosphate buffer which serves as the short-term column storage solution if multiple cycles are performed. Additional cycles, starting with sanitization, are repeated until all the load solution has been processed. Each product fraction is analyzed for product concentration and density to calculate yield and analytical HIC for purity. Product fractions from multiple cycles are then pooled and carried through

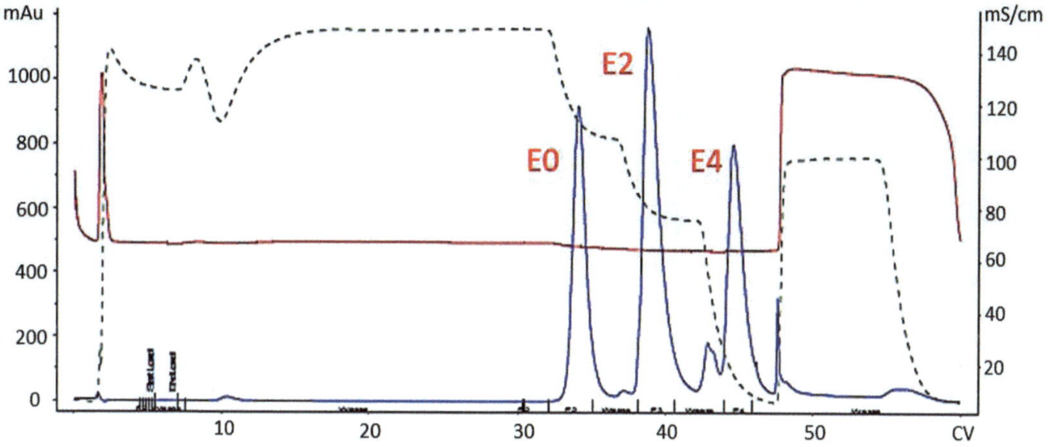

Fig. 4 Step gradient elution of a vcMMAE conjugate

Table 3
Step gradient elution

Step	Volume	Mobile phase
Equilibration	4 CV	0.8 M $(NH_4)_2SO_4$, 25 mM Na_2HPO_4, pH 7.1
Load	–	ADC reaction 0.8 M $(NH_4)_2SO_4$, pH 7.2
Wash	2 CV	0.8 M $(NH_4)_2SO_4$, 25 mM Na_2HPO_4, pH 7.1
E0 elution	2 CV	0.65 M $(NH_4)_2SO_4$, 25 mM Na_2HPO_4, pH 7.1
E2 elution	4 CV	0.425 M $(NH_4)_2SO_4$, 25 mM Na_2HPO_4, pH 7.1
>E2 flush	4 CV	0.5 N NaOH
>E2 flush	4 CV	25% IPA, 25 mM Na_2HPO_4, pH 7.1

the remaining process. Figure 5 shows an example of the analytical HIC of the crude load solution and purified E2 product solution after following a procedure similar to that described above. Consistent product quality is achieved across scales when the bed height is kept constant but column diameter is varied by maintaining the same linear velocity across the bed. If bed height is changed, linear velocity is modified to maintain a constant residence time.

Ultimately, the goal of HIC scale-up purification of an ADC is to produce material of equivalent quality to that achieved in the lab and/or sufficient quality for its intended use. For an effective scale-up, it is necessary to maintain the operating parameters identified at the lab scale (e.g., buffer composition, linear flow velocity (residence time), bed height, loading, sample preparation, and gradient while column diameter increases proportionally with scale). Following the general considerations outlined in this chapter, separation of individual DAR species of an ADC, with a suitably hydrophobic payload, is feasible at a production scale.

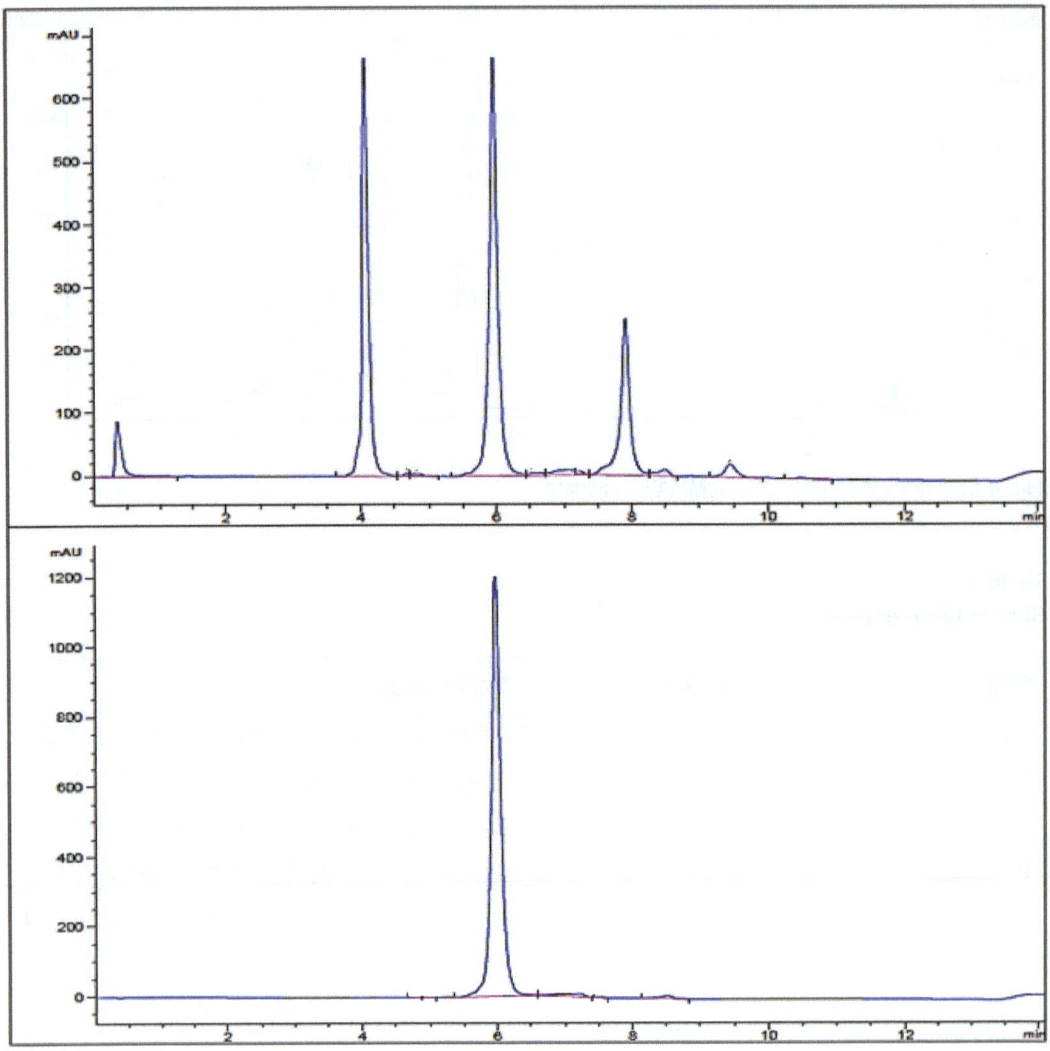

Fig. 5 Before and after preparative HIC (top chromatogram—load solution, bottom chromatogram—product pool)

2 Materials

The buffer recipes presented here are for one liter of solution. Multiple liters, or fractions thereof, can be prepared as multipliers of these recipes. Depending on the purpose of the isolated product, care should be taken to use the proper quality of water to prevent introduction of undesired contaminants like endotoxin, bacteria, or other pathogens. For in vivo testing, WFI (water for injection) or equivalent water quality is preferred.

HIC Load Diluent: 25 mM Sodium Phosphate, 3.0 M Ammonium Sulfate, pH 7.0

1. Add 800 mL water to a suitable mixing vessel (e.g., glass beaker).
2. Add 396.4 g of ammonium sulfate (FW 132.14 g/mol).
3. Add 6.7 g of Sodium Phosphate, Dibasic, 7-hydrate, crystals (FW 268.07 g/mol).
4. Mix until salts are fully dissolved.
5. Titrate buffer to pH 7.0 using 1.0 M HCl.
6. Adjust to the final volume of 1.0 L, or 1.20 kg with water (*density = 1.20 g/mL*).
7. Mix until homogeneous.

Mobile Phase A: 25 mM Sodium Phosphate, 1.0 M Ammonium Sulfate, pH 7.0

1. Add 800 mL water to a suitable mixing vessel (e.g., glass beaker).
2. Add 132.1 g of ammonium sulfate (FW 132.14 g/mol).
3. Add 6.7 g of Sodium Phosphate, Dibasic, 7-hydrate, crystals (FW 268.07 g/mol).
4. Mix until salts are fully dissolved.
5. Titrate buffer to pH 7.0 using 1.0 M HCl.
6. Adjust to the final volume of 1.0 L, or 1.10 kg with water (*density = 1.10 g/mL*).
7. Mix until homogeneous.

Mobile Phase B: 25 mM Sodium Phosphate, pH 7.0

1. Add 800 mL water to a suitable mixing vessel (e.g., glass beaker).
2. Add 6.7 g of Sodium Phosphate, Dibasic, 7-hydrate, crystals (FW 268.07 g/mol).
3. Mix until salts are fully dissolved.
4. Titrate buffer to pH 7.0 using 1.0 M HCl.
5. Adjust to the final volume of 1.0 L, or 1.0 kg with water (*density = 1.00 g/mL*).
6. Mix until homogeneous.

Sanitization Buffer: 0.5 N Sodium Hydroxide

1. Add 800 mL water to a suitable mixing vessel (e.g., glass beaker).
2. Add 20 g of Sodium Hydroxide pellets (FW 40.0 g/mol).
3. Mix until pellets are fully dissolved. *This is an exothermic reaction.*
4. Adjust to the final volume of 1.0 L, or 1.02 kg with water (*density = 1.02 g/mL*).
5. Mix until homogeneous.

Storage Buffer: 20% Ethanol

1. Add 200 mL 200 Absolute Ethanol to a suitable mixing vessel (e.g., glass beaker).
2. Adjust to a final volume of 1.0 L or 0.98 kg with water (*density = 0.98 g/mL*).
3. Mix until homogeneous.

3 Methods

3.1 Load Solubility Screening and Preparation Methods

Techniques described here are presented assuming that 500 μL crude ADC solution is available at pH 7. Volumes can be adjusted according to available sample volumes.

3.1.1 Direct Titration Method

1. Transfer 500 μL of sample to a clear 1.5 mL Eppendorf tube.
2. Add 100 μL of HIC Load Diluent to the tube to adjust to 0.5 M $(NH_4)_2SO_4$.
3. Thoroughly mix by tube inversion or vortexing.
4. Centrifuge at ≥3000 × *g* for ≥2 min.
5. Inspect the base of the tube for pellet.
6. If there is a pellet, dilute the solution by 10% using Mobile Phase B and vortex thoroughly until the pellet is fully suspended, or dissolved. Centrifuge again. If after centrifugation the pellet reappears, repeat this step until the pellet is dissolved.
7. If there is no pellet, repeat **steps 2–6** adding HIC Load Diluent in sequence 25 μL (0.60 M), 27 μL (0.70 M), 30 μL (0.80 M), 33 μL (0.90 M), 35 μL (1.00 M), 40 μL (1.10 M), 43 μL (1.20 M), 50 μL (1.30 M), 55 μL (1.40 M), 62 μL (1.50 M).

3.1.2 Screening Panel Method

1. Label 11 clear 1.5 mL Eppendorf tubes from 0.5 to 1.5 in increments of 0.1.
2. Transfer 500 μL of sample to each tube.

   Add HIC Load Diluent buffer to each tube according to the following table.

Tube (M)	μL Diluent
0.5	0.100
0.6	0.125
0.7	0.152
0.8	0.182
0.9	0.215
1.0	0.250

(continued)

Tube (M)	μL Diluent
1.1	0.290
1.2	0.333
1.3	0.383
1.4	0.438
1.5	0.500

Thoroughly mix by tube inversion, or vortexing.

3. Centrifuge tubes at ≥3000 × *g* for ≥2 min.
4. Inspect the base of the tube for pellet. Alternatively, the supernatant may be measured for absorbance at 280 nm and compared to the expected concentration to determine when the precipitation has occurred.
5. The highest molar (M) concentration of ammonium sulfate without a pellet should be used to prepare the load.

3.2 Gradient Development

1. Temper Mobile Phase A and B to room temperature.
2. Adjust the ADC load solution to an ammonium sulfate concentration defined in Subheading 3.1.
3. Perform the linear gradient in Table 1 using a HiScreen Butyl HP column (additionally, other resins may be screened).
4. Following the linear gradient elution, determine mixture points from the gradient where individual drug-load species begin to elute as illustrated in Fig. 3.
5. Define a step gradient method comparable to Table 3 designed to isolate each species targeting mixtures of Mobile Phase A and Mobile Phase B at the proper conductivity points defined in **step 4** for the E0, E2, and E4. E6 through E8 species are washed off the column using 100% Mobile Phase B, followed by the CIP described in Table 1.
6. Use the gradient mixing capabilities on a chromatography workstation or prepare buffers at these conductivity points by adding Mobile Phase A to Mobile Phase B with mixing until the proper conductivity is reached.
7. Execute the step gradient at 20 g/L loading using a HiScreen Butyl HP column and verify the performance of the designed elution steps. *In this example we describe a 20 g/L load on a HiScreen Butyl HP column. Any appropriate HIC resin would follow a similar strategy,* (e.g., *Phenyl, Octyl,* etc.)
8. Analyze product pool for purity and recovery. Adjust the ionic strength for each of the gradient steps based on the results from the fraction pool analysis.

Optimize parameters including, but not limited to, loading, buffer ionic strength, temperature, pH, lyotrope selection, and resin functionality until the method is optimal with respect to purity, recovery, and throughput.

4 Notes

4.1 Microbial and Pyrogen Control Methods

4.1.1 Autoclave

Autoclaves are commercially available and use of such equipment should be done according to the manufacturer's instructions. Before committing articles to the autoclave, ensure that they are autoclavable. Some plastics, for example, will melt in the autoclave.

1. Thoroughly clean and rinse all articles to be placed in the autoclave.
2. Cover openings to glassware and autoclavable plasticware with autoclave paper. *Caution: never create an airtight seal over a container opening; this can result in destruction of equipment and/or serious injury.*
3. Wrap utensils with autoclave paper or autoclave pouches.
4. Use autoclave tape to secure autoclave paper and wrappings.
5. Place items in the autoclave and start the cycle according to the manufacturer's instructions.
6. Autoclave should reach not less than 121 °C at 15 psi above atmospheric pressure for at least 15–20 min.
7. Use caution and heat-resistant gloves when removing items from the autoclave; they will be hot and may cause burns.

4.1.2 Dry Heat by Depyrogenation Oven

Dry heat depyrogenation ovens are commercially available and use of such equipment should be done according to the manufacturer's instructions. Before committing articles to the autoclave, ensure that they can withstand the temperatures anticipated in the oven. Plastics, for example, will melt in the oven and paper may combust at high temperatures. Depyrogenation ovens are effective according to the European Pharmacopeia at 250 °C for 30 min or 200 °C for 60 min [20].

1. Thoroughly clean, rinse, and dry all articles to be placed in the oven.
2. Cover openings to metal and glassware with aluminum foil. *Caution: never create an airtight seal over a container opening; this can result in destruction of equipment and/or serious injury.*
3. Wrap utensils with aluminum foil.
4. Depyrogenation oven should be preheated to 250 or 200 °C and items should be left in the oven for not less than 30 or 60 min, respectively.

5. Use caution and heat-resistant gloves when depositing and removing items from the oven; they will be hot and may cause burns.

4.1.3 Chemical Exposure

All caustic stable surfaces, such as chromatography columns, resins, and workstations, may be depyrogenated by the following method [17]. Other equipment can be soaked and then rinsed with sterile pyrogen-free purified water.

1. 1. For chromatography systems, place the system's inlet line (s) into a vessel filled with 0.5 N NaOH. Ensure that the outer surface of the inlet tubing is also submerged in the 0.5 M NaOH. *This can be done with the chromatography column inline, as well.*
2. Flow the 0.5 NaOH through the system ensuring that all flow path surfaces are in contact with the 0.5 N NaOH. Include all valve positions and pump interfaces, as well.
3. 3. Allow the surfaces to be in contact with the 0.5 N NaOH for not less than 30 min at ambient temperature.
4. Flush the hydroxide from the system using sterile pyrogen-free purified water or buffer.

References

1. McCue JT (2009) Theory and use of hydrophobic interaction chromatography in protein purification applications. Methods Enzymol 463:405–414
2. Hamblett KJ, Senter PJ et al (2004) Effects of drug loading on the antitumor activity of a monoclonal antibody drug conjugate. Clin Cancer Res 10:7063–7070
3. Purcell JW, Tanlimco SG et al (2018) LRRC15 is a novel Mesenchymal protein and stromal target for antibody–drug conjugates. Cancer Res 78:4059–4072
4. Stump B, Steinmann J (2013) Conjugation process development and scale-up. Methods Mol Biol 1045:235–247
5. Hutchison MH, Hendricks RS et al (2018) Chapter 40: process development and manufacturing of antibody-drug conjugates. In: Biopharmaceutical processing, pp 813–836
6. Torgov FG, Handley PD et al (2005) Reduction alkylation strategies for the modification of specific monoclonal antibody disulfides. Bioconjug Chem 16(5):1282–1290
7. Application note 28-9964-49 AA, High-throughput screening of HIC media in PreDictor™ plates for capturing recombinant Green Fluorescent Protein from *E. coli* (2011). GE Healthcare Bio-Sciences AB. http://www.processdevelopmentforum.com/files/articles/28996449AA.PDF
8. Machold C, Deinhofer R et al (2002) Hydrophobic interaction chromatography of proteins: I. comparison of selectivity. J Chromatogr A 972(1):3–19
9. Jungbauer A, Machold C et al (2005) Hydrophobic interaction chromatography of proteins: III. Unfolding of proteins upon adsorption. J Chromatogr A 1079 (1–2):221–228
10. Aditya AW, Ronald TB (2006) Formulation considerations for proteins susceptible to asparagine Deamidation and aspartate isomerization. J Pharm Sci 95(11):2321–2336
11. Hofmeister F (1888) Zur Lehre von der Wirkung der Salze. Archiv für experimentelle Pathologie und Pharmakologie 24 (4–5):247–260
12. Kunz W, Henle J et al (2004) Zur Lehre von der Wirkung der Salze' (about the science of the effect of salts): Franz Hofmeister's historical papers. Curr Opin Colloid Interface Sci 9 (1–2):19–37
13. Phenyl Sepharose™ High Performance Butyl Sepharose High Performance (2018). https://cdn.gelifesciences.com/dmm3bwsv3/AssetStream.aspx?mediaformatid=10061&destinationid=10016&assetid=13968

14. <1211>Sterilization and Sterility Assurance of Compendial Articles (2011) United States Pharmacopeia (USP35-NF30) 863–867
15. Salama SEM, Mobarez EA (2015) Depyrogenation methods. Egypt J Chem Environ Health 1(1):540–551
16. Salama SEM, Mobarez EA (2015) Depyrogenation methods. Egypt J Chem Environ Health 1(1):540–551
17. Application note 18-1124-57 AI, Use of sodium hydroxide for cleaning and sanitization of chromatography media and systems (2014.) GE Healthcare Bio-Sciences AB: https://www.gelifesciences.co.jp/catalog/pdf/18112457AI_AppNote_NaOHforCIP_SIP_final_1.pdf
18. Impact of sporicidal agent on MabSelect SuRe™ protein A resin lifetime, 29262168 AA (2014.) GE Healthcare Bio-Sciences AB: https://cdn.gelifesciences.com/dmm3bwsv3/AssetStream.aspx?mediaformatid=10061&destinationid=10016&assetid=18576
19. Carta G, Jungbauer A (2010) Protein chromatography: process development and scale-up. Wiley-VCH, Weinheim
20. Hecker W, Witthauer D et al (1994) Validation of dry heat inactivation of bacterial endotoxins. PDA J Pharm Sci Technol 48(4):197–204

Chapter 20

Detection and Removal of Small Molecule and Endotoxin Contaminants in ADC Preparations

Jeffrey Casavant, Anokha S. Ratnayake, Sujiet Puthenveetil, and L. Nathan Tumey

Abstract

Incomplete removal of free (unconjugated) drug or drug-linker species used to prepare ADCs results in contaminated ADC samples which may pose a risk for toxicity. Due to the extreme potency of typical small molecule toxins employed in ADCs, even relatively low levels of free drug contaminants in ADC samples have been hypothesized to result in nonspecific (i.e., off target) activity in biological systems. It is possible for trace levels of certain free drug species to persist in final ADC samples despite the inclusion of common purification steps during the preparation processes. Therefore, methods for the detection, quantification, and removal of residual free drug present in ADC samples are ultimately required for the preparation of safe and efficacious final ADC drug products. Herein we report general methods for the detection and removal of such contaminants.

Key words ADC, Free drug, Endotoxin, Biobeads, HPLC, Detoxi-Gel

1 Introduction

ADCs typically consist of an antibody that is covalently bound to a linker-drug species. During the manufacturing process, it is typical to use a large excess of the linker-drug in order to drive the conjugation reaction to completion. This excess free drug is typically removed from the ADC by buffer exchange methods such as gel filtration, tangential flow filtration, ultracentrifugation, or dialysis. However, it is common for trace levels of certain free drug species to persist in final ADC samples despite the inclusion of such purification steps. Due to the extreme potency of typical small molecule toxins employed in ADCs, even relatively low levels of free drug contaminants in ADC samples have been hypothesized to result in nonspecific (i.e., off-target) activity in biological systems. Therefore, methods for the detection, quantification, and removal of residual free drug present in ADC samples are often required for the preparation of safe and efficacious final ADC drug products.

L. Nathan Tumey (ed.), *Antibody-Drug Conjugates: Methods and Protocols*, Methods in Molecular Biology, vol. 2078, https://doi.org/10.1007/978-1-4939-9929-3_20,

Herein we report general methods for the detection and removal of such contaminants.

In addition to free drug contamination, the preparation of ADCs for in vivo analysis requires a method that avoids endotoxin contamination. Endotoxin, also known as lipopolysaccharide (LPS), is a membrane component of gram negative bacteria that acts as a strong immunostimulant. Endotoxin can be inadvertently introduced into protein samples due to bacterial contamination or due to contact with surfaces that have previously been in contact with bacteria. Avoiding endotoxin contamination typically requires the diligent use of rigorous decontamination and cleaning procedures for all equipment and vessels that come in contact with the antibody during the conjugation and purification procedures. Due to the high intrinsic value of the antibody and linker-payload, we found it necessary at times to employ a method to remove endotoxin that was unintentionally introduced during the ADC preparation and isolation process. This method has been successfully used to "rescue" endotoxin-contaminated batches of ADCs in advance of in vivo studies.

1.1 Free Drug Detection

An ideal method for the detection of free drug will:

1. Be useful for a wide variety of drug-linkers and not require re-optimization for each different linker-drug being conjugated.
2. Require little or no sample preparation in order to avoid any potential release of free drug from the ADC during the sample preparation process.
3. Rely on UV absorbance thereby allowing unknown or unexpected impurities to also be detected alongside the free drug or drug-linker.

Previous technology to detect free drug typically relies on MS-based detection which is targeted to known contaminants and requires the generation of an authentic standard for quantitation [1]. We describe a general liquid chromatography (LC) method that has proven very useful in the detection and quantitation of both known and unknown free drug impurities in ADC samples. This analytical method provides adequate sensitivity to accurately detect free drug-linker related contaminants down to levels that are deemed to be inconsequential for in vitro cytotoxicity measurements. Using this method, we have determined that trace amounts of drug-linker can occasionally contaminate final ADC samples despite the use of purification processes such as size-exclusion chromatography (SEC), hydrophobic interaction chromatography (HIC), or tangential flow filtration (TFF).

The HPLC method utilizes reverse phase column chromatography, which reliably separates antibodies from small molecule

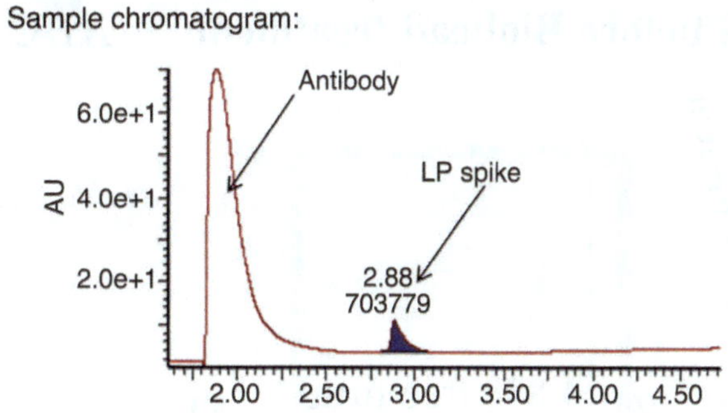

Fig. 1 Representative example of typical free link-drug detection (at 220 nM)

contaminants (Fig. 1). The AUC of the small molecule peak is used to quantitate the amount of small molecule impurity present in the ADC by comparison to positive controls. In order to establish the level of sensitivity necessary for small molecule detection, we performed a "back of the envelope" estimation assuming that bound drug should generally be >100-fold higher concentration than free drug (*see* **Note 1**). Given that most ADCs are stored as stock concentrations at ~5 mg/mL with a DAR of 2–4 (~70–140 μM bound drug), we generally aim to have a free drug concentration of <1 μM. With this in mind, the typical procedure calls for preparation of stock solutions in which 1 μM or 5 μM LP is spiked into a naked antibody matrix. This gives a suitable positive control that was directly compared to the small molecule AUC obtained through the ADC injection (*see* **Note 2**).

1.2 Free Drug Removal

Using the method described in Subheading 1.1, we find that particular linker-payloads (especially those that are very hydrophobic) are often not removed during typical buffer exchange purification methods. Initial attempts to remove these hydrophobic molecules through dialysis, ultrafiltration, or desalting cartridges ultimately proved unsuccessful. This suggests that the contamination is the result of low-affinity, nonspecific interactions between the drug-linker and the antibody conjugate. Thus, a suitable method requires the small molecule drug to be actively sequestered in order to remove the contaminant. Both hydrophobic resins and activated charcoal are reported for such purposes. For example, Smith describes a hydrophobic polymeric resin for the removal of detergents from protein preparations and Meyer reports the use of activated charcoal for capturing excess benzodiazepine during process-scale ADC preparations [2, 3]. However, to our knowledge there are no reports of these methods being employed for routine ADC purification. Thus, we describe a convenient and high-throughput method that employs a macroporous polystyrene resin ("Bio-Beads") for the removal of free drug-linker contaminants that otherwise tend to noncovalently "stick" to the desired

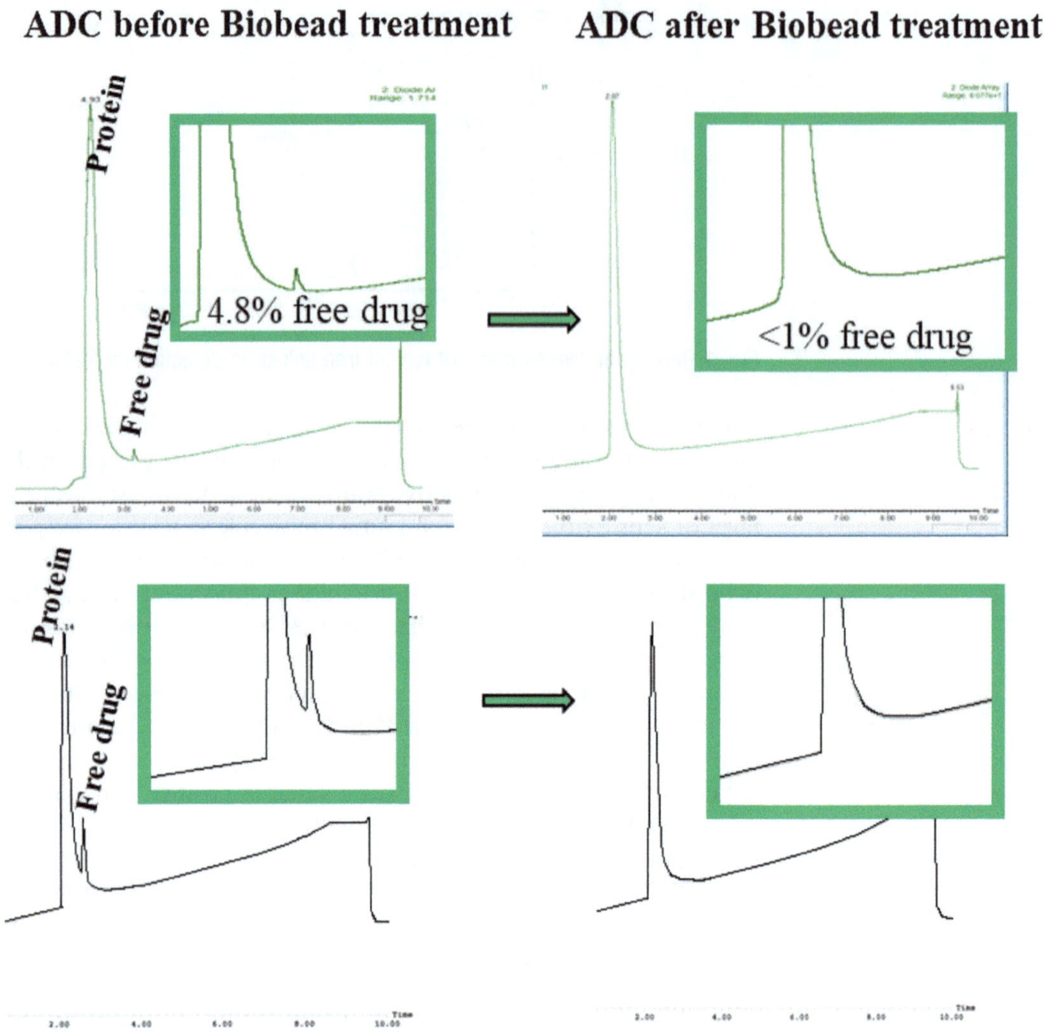

Fig. 2 ADCs contaminated with free drug (left panels) were treated with biobeads. Free drug was undetectable following treatment (right panels)

ADC product. This method has proven invaluable in the delivery of high-quality ADC samples for in vitro and in vivo testing (Fig. 2).

Biobeads are a hydrophobic macroporous polystyrene resin designed to adsorb hydrophobic molecules while having minimal adsorbance of proteins. The Biobeads must be washed with methanol prior to use in order to prevent endotoxin contamination of the ADC sample. Washed biobeads can be stored frozen until needed. The beads are typically gently shaken in the presence of the ADC for 2–24 h in order to remove free drug from the sample. The method outlined in Subheading 3.2 has been used to remove trace amounts of linkers-payloads of a variety of structural classes. Not surprisingly, the method appears to be most successful with hydrophobic drug-linkers. On occasion it is necessary to gently heat the sample overnight in the presence of biobeads in order to facilitate complete drug removal. In these cases, small increases in the amount of ADC aggregation are sometimes observed, thus necessitating further purification by SEC to remove the newly formed aggregate from desired monomeric ADC product. In most cases ADC recovery is ≥75%.

1.3 Endotoxin Removal

The preparation of ADCs for in vivo analysis requires a preparation that is free from endotoxin contamination. This necessitates the diligent use of rigorous decontamination and cleaning procedures for all equipment and vessels that come in contact with the antibody during the conjugation and purification procedures. Typically, consumable items used during ADC preparation should be freshly opened and labeled as "non-pyrogenic." Equipment and nonconsumable items should be thoroughly decontaminated using dilute sodium hydroxide (0.1 M) and ethanol. However, endotoxin contamination can continue to be a problem even when such precautions are taken. Due to the high intrinsic value of the antibody and linker-payload, we developed a method to remove endotoxin from ADC preparations that were inadvertently contaminated with endotoxin during the preparation and isolation process. This method has been successfully used to "rescue" endotoxin-contaminated batches of ADCs in advance of in vivo studies.

2 Materials

2.1 Free Drug Detection

1. Reagent grade formic acid and DMSO.
2. Dulbecco's Phosphate Buffered Saline (DPBS, 1×, 9.5 mM PO_4 without Calcium or Magnesium).
3. HPLC grade acetonitrile and water.
4. UPLC system: Waters Acquity UPLC with a PDA detector and a high sensitivity flow cell.
5. Column: Agilent Zorbax 300SB-CN, 4.6 × 150 mm, 3.5 μm (P/N: 863973–905).
6. Linker-payload (LP) stock solutions are typically stored at 10 mM in DMSO or DMA at −80 °C.
7. Unconjugated antibody stock solution is formulated at 2 mg/mL in PBS stored at 4 °C.
8. ADC samples are stored at 2–5 mg/mL in PBS at 4 °C.

2.2 Free Drug Removal

1. Bio-Beads™ SM-2 non-polar polystyrene adsorbent, 20–50 mesh (Bio-Rad).
2. Reagent grade methanol.

3. Cellulose-acetate centrifugal filter (such as Spin-X® Centrifuge Tube Filters, part# 8160).

2.3 Endotoxin Removal

1. Detoxi-Gel Endotoxin Removing Columns (Thermo Scientific, PN 20344, 1 mL, Polymixin B ligand immobilized on beaded affinity resin).
2. Dulbecco's Phosphate Buffered Saline (DPBS, 1×, 9.5 mM PO_4 without calcium or magnesium).
3. 1% solution of sodium deoxycholate in water (Thermo Scientific).
4. Endosafe PTS instrument (Charles River).
5. Endosafe LAL disposable test cartridges (Charles River).

3 Methods

3.1 Free Drug Detection

Set up UPLC method as shown below:

- Column temperature: 80 °C.
- Buffer A: 97.9% water +2% acetonitrile +0.1% formic acid.
- Buffer B: 99.9% acetonitrile +0.1% formic acid.
- Gradient: 5% B to 95% B over 8 min, hold at 95% B for 1 min, then 2 min re-equilibration at 5% B. Total run time 11 min.
- Flow rate: 1 mL/min.
- Injection: 25 μL.
- PDA parameters: 3D data collection enabled (210–350 nm), 80 pts/s sample rate, 4.8 nm resolution, fast filter time constant.

Using the HPLC method outlined, the antibody (or ADC) typically elutes at ~2 min while the small molecule contaminants elute between 2.5 and 3.5 min. Quantitation of the free drug is performed using the following method:

1. Dilute the initial LP stock solutions (10 mM) to 100 μM in DMSO:water 1:1 (v/v) by mixing 1 μL of the initial LP stock with 49.5 μL each of DMSO and PBS.
2. Prepare a 1 μM LP standard by spiking 1 μL of the LP stock (100 μM, DMSO:PBS 1:1 v/v) into 99 μL of an antibody solution (2 mg/mL in PBS).
3. Prepare a 5 μM LP standard by spiking 5 μL of the LP stock (100 μM, DMSO:PBS 1:1 v/v) into 95 μL of an antibody solution (2 mg/mL in PBS).
4. Inject samples in the following order, 25 μL per injection:

   (a) Blank PBS—single injection.

   (b) ADC injection 1—record AUC (*see* **Note 3**).

(c) ADC injection 2—record AUC.
(d) Blank PBS—single injection (*see* **Note 4**).
(e) mAb (2 mg/mL) + 1 μM LP spike (prepared in **step 2**)—record AUC.
(f) mAb (2 mg/mL) + 1 μM LP spike (prepared in **step 2**)—record AUC.
(g) mAb (2 mg/mL) + 5 μM LP spike (prepared in **step 3**)—record AUC.
(h) mAb (2 mg/mL) + 5 μM LP spike (prepared in **step 3**)—record AUC.

5. Estimate the free drug concentration by comparing the average AUC for the test sample (injection b and c) to the AUC for the 1 μM and 5 μM spikes (injection e–h).

3.2 Free Drug Removal [4]

1. Methanol (2 mL) is added to Bio-Beads (~250–300 mg) and gently shaken (600–800 rpm) at room temperature for a few minutes. Solvent is removed by pipette.
2. The beads are resuspended in 2 mL of fresh methanol and gently shaken (600–800 rpm) at 37 °C overnight. The MeOH is removed and the beads are rinsed (RT, 600–800 rpm, ~30 min) successively in distilled water (1 × 2 mL) and PBS (2 × 2 mL).
3. The final PBS suspension is filtered to afford dry beads. Beads are used immediately or are frozen for long-term storage.
4. The ADC sample (~5–10 mg/mL) is treated with ~50 mg of pre-washed Bio-Beads™ per mL of sample. The sample is gently agitated (600 rpm) at 37 °C for ~3 h. An aliquot is taken, filtered through a 0.2 μm cellulose acetate filter, and analyzed by LCMS (Subheading 3.1) to confirm removal of free drug (*see* **Note 5**).
5. Once removal of the free drug is confirmed, the beads are removed using a centrifugal sterile filter unit with a 0.2 μm membrane (such as Spin-X® centrifuge tube filters) by spinning for ~30 s at 300 rpm to remove Bio-Beads. The beads are washed once with a minimal amount of PBS and filtering process repeated. The filtrate is concentrated by ultrafiltration as necessary.

3.3 Endotoxin Removal

1. 4.2 mL of an ADC in DPBS buffer (1.73 mg/mL concentration, 7.26 mg) was tested via Endosafe PTS instrument to contain endotoxin at >25 EU/mL (endotoxin units/mL) (*see* **Note 6**).
2. Two separate 1 mL Detoxi-Gel prepacked columns were washed with 5 resin bed volumes each of 1% sodium

deoxycholate solution to regenerate the active resin. The eluent was discarded.

3. The columns of activated Detoxi-Gel were equilibrated with 6 resin bed volumes each of DPBS. The eluent was discarded.
4. The ADC solution (2.1 mL per column) was loaded onto each column and gravity eluted.
5. Column flow-through was recycled through each column 3× to increase exposure time of conjugate to resin (*see* **Note 7**).
6. Finally, columns were washed with additional 2 mL of DPBS each. This afforded diluted ADC sample in approximately 8 mL total volume.
7. Diluted ADC sample was re-concentrated via 50KD ultrafiltration device to afford 2.5 mL final ADC (2.42 mg/mL, 6.05 mg, 83% recovery).
8. The purified ADC sample was tested to contain endotoxin at 2.13 EU/mL. The entire process could be repeated as necessary to further decrease the endotoxin load (*see* **Note 8**).

4 Notes

1. A variety of experiments were performed in which 1–5 mol% free payload or free payload-linker was spiked into various ADCs. The cytotoxicity of these ADCs was evaluated in antigen-expressing and antigen-null cell lines and found to have negligible differences from uncontaminated ADCs [data not shown]. Thus, the prevailing consensus is to ensure that free drug concentration is >100-fold lower concentration than bound drug.
2. The limit of detection (LOD) and limit of quantitation (LOQ) were established using two prototypical linker-payloads. The LOQ using the described method was determined to be ~0.3–0.8 μM while the LOD was determined to be 0.1–0.3 μM. Thus, the method was deemed "fit for purpose" for routine ADC analysis. Improved sensitivity could easily be obtained by injecting a more concentrated sample of the ADC.
3. The ADC typically elutes at ~2 min while the small molecule contaminants elute between 2.5 and 3.5 min, depending on their polarity. On rare occasions the small molecule peak overlaps the ADC/antibody peak thus preventing quantitation. The AUC is typically measured using a wavelength known to be absorbed by the payload class in question (often 220 or 254 nM). The antibody peak for hinge-conjugated ADCs is sometimes "lumpy" due to partial separation of HC and LC

species. This typically does not interfere with the free drug analysis.

4. A PBS-blank is injected in between ADC sample injections in order to prevent cross-contamination due to potential ADC carryover.
5. Aliquots are typically removed and monitored by HPLC in "real time" to determine when complete removal of drug-linker contaminant has been achieved. Typical removal requires 2–24 h of agitation.
6. According to manufacturer's specifications, 1 mL of Detoxi-Gel resin removes >9995 EU (endotoxin units) from a 5 mL sample challenge containing 10,000 EU. In the example procedure outlined, the resin was conservatively loaded with contaminated sample as the exact total amount of endotoxin present in the sample was not known.
7. As an alternative to recycling eluent through the resin bed multiple times to increase exposure of sample to resin, it is also possible to stop elution once sample has been applied to the column and incubate the sample on the resin for up to 1 h before ultimately collecting the sample.
8. Per manufacturer's specifications, the resin may be used at least ten times without loss of activity given proper regeneration, washing, and storage.

References

1. Birdsall RE, McCarthy SM, Janin-Bussat MC et al (2016) A sensitive multidimensional method for the detection, characterization, and quantification of trace free drug species in antibody-drug conjugate samples using mass spectral detection. MAbs 8:306–317. https://doi.org/10.1080/19420862.2015.1116659
2. Smith SA, Morrissey JH (2004) Rapid and efficient incorporation of tissue factor into liposomes. J Thromb Haemost 2:1155–1162. https://doi.org/10.1111/j.1538-7836.2004.00772.x
3. Meyer D, Sun M (2016) Activated carbon filtration for purification of benzodiazepine ADCs. United States Patent US 9,453,046 B2
4. Tumey LN, Leverett CA, Vetelino B et al (2016) Optimization of Tubulysin antibody-drug conjugates: a case study in addressing ADC metabolism. ACS Med Chem Lett 7:977–982. https://doi.org/10.1021/acsmedchemlett.6b00195

Chapter 21

Physical Stability Studies of Antibody-Drug Conjugates (ADCs) Under Stressed Conditions

Yilma T. Adem

Abstract

The conjugation of cytotoxic drugs to monoclonal antibodies (mAbs) generates heterogeneous drug load distribution. Antibody-drug conjugates (ADC) are physically less stable as compared to their parent molecule due to modifications made in order to link drugs to the interchain sulfhydryl groups of monoclonal antibodies. The conjugation of small molecule drugs to mAbs alters the physicochemical properties of mAbs and also impacts their degradation profile. The use of appropriate analytical tools to monitor physical stability changes is necessary to identify key product quality attributes such as aggregation. This chapter discusses suitable stress conditions and the use of stability indicating analytical methods to detect degradation products.

Key words Monoclonal antibody, Antibody-drug conjugate, ADC, Cytotoxic drug, Physical stability, Thermal stress, Analytical methods

1 Introduction

Conjugation of cytotoxic drugs to antibodies generates heterogeneous ADC species with different physical stabilities. Instability of proteins refers to degradation due to denaturation, aggregation, fragmentation, and adsorption to surfaces. Factors that impact physical instability of proteins that leads to physical stress include temperature, agitation, and formulation conditions such as pH and ionic strength [1, 2]. Physical instability such as aggregation affects in vitro stability of a drug product as well as in vivo pharmacokinetics [3]. Solvent exposure of hydrophobic surfaces of proteins due to stress can cause protein-protein interactions leading to aggregate formation. The conjugation of the cytotoxic small molecule drugs to antibodies results in a species that has an overall higher hydrophobic character as compared to the unconjugated parent antibodies. In general, ADCs are less stable than their parent antibodies because their molecular surface properties are altered due to the conjugation of cytotoxic agents. This is primarily due to the linking

L. Nathan Tumey (ed.), *Antibody-Drug Conjugates: Methods and Protocols*, Methods in Molecular Biology, vol. 2078, https://doi.org/10.1007/978-1-4939-9929-3_21, © Springer Science+Business Media, LLC, part of Springer Nature 2020

of cytotoxic drugs via the interchain sulfhydryl groups of monoclonal antibodies. This approach has a tendency to affect the overall structure of ADCs leading to physical stability challenges [4].

Commonly used stress conditions include exposure to high temperature, agitation, freeze-thaw, high and low pH, and oxidation, to mention a few [5].The use of these stress conditions form the basis for forced degradation studies that are integral to the development of therapeutic antibodies. These studies are used to understand manufacturability, to support formulation development, to evaluate batch to batch comparability, to develop analytical methods, and to understand degradation pathways [5].

To monitor physical stability changes after stress and long-term storage, the application of appropriate analytical methods is crucial. For instance, assessing the thermodynamic and colloidal stability of ADCs before setting up thermal stress studies using differential scanning calorimetry (DSC) provides information on the thermal unfolding behavior of ADCs [6]. This technique has utility to screen for excipients during formulation studies of ADCs. DSC also can be used in selecting suitable thermal stress temperature. For example, the thermal melting (T_m) onset temperature that is close to the stress temperature means that the stress condition is not representative of the expected real-time storage conditions [4]. In other words, if the T_m onset of an ADC is low (e.g., 45–50 °C), a stress temperature of 25 and 30 °C should be used to gain representative degradation profile whereas 40 °C can be too close to the T_m onset temperature. However, if the intention of the stress study is to compare degradation pathways of drug product batches but not to use the degradation data to predict long-term stability, aggressive storage conditions such as 40 °C can still be used. Overall, care must be taken when selecting a thermal stress temperature and the use of DSC provides useful insights.

Analytical method such as size exclusion high performance liquid chromatography (SE-HPLC) is a well-established technique that helps to monitor size variant distribution of ADCs, especially aggregates (high molecular species) [7]. Another critical attribute for ADCs is the drug-to-antibody ratio (DAR). The unwanted de-conjugation of the cytotoxic drugs from the antibody can lead to changes in the DAR distribution. Stress conditions of ADCs can lead to the breaking of covalent bonds between the cytotoxic drugs and the antibody resulting in changes in the DAR. For ADCs with high DAR (i.e., DAR4 and above), the mAb in the hinge region and the light and heavy chains are primarily held together via electrostatic and hydrophobic interactions due to the fact that the cytotoxic drugs are linked to the native cysteine residues that would otherwise form the disulfide bonds. The de-conjugation or breaking off of drugs from the mAbs' conjugation sites brings product quality changes that impact the efficacy and safety of ADCs to patients [8]. Hydrophobic interaction chromatography (HIC) is the most commonly used analytical technique that separates each DAR species based on their drug load to monitor changes during stress or during the shelf life of a molecule [9].

In addition, other stability indicating assays that are not discussed in the methods section of this chapter can be used to understand other product quality properties of ADCs such as a potency assay to measure biological activity and a free drug assay to monitor the presence of free cytotoxic drug in the drug product solution. Capillary electrophoresis sodium dodecyl sulfate (CE-SDS), though an analytical assay that is used to detect and quantify fragmented low molecular species, is not useful in assessing fragmentation in ADCs that have intentionally disrupted interchain disulfide bonds as the presence of disodium sulfate (SDS) dissociates the electrostatic and hydrophobic interaction between the light and heavy chain of ADCs [4]. However, this assay can be used to assess fragmentation in Thiomabs wherein the payload is bound to an engineered cysteine residue in the Fab region of the antibody [10]. Other high order structure analysis such as circular dichroism (CD) and Fourier-transform infrared spectroscopy (FTIR), though less sensitive, can also be utilized to monitor structural or conformational changes in ADCs due to physical stress.

The understanding of the physical stability of ADCs and the assessment of product quality attributes using appropriate analytical techniques provide knowledge necessary in order to manufacture well-controlled products that are safe and efficacious to the end users. This chapter focuses on stability indicating analytical methods and also other tools, such as DSC, to determine thermodynamic stability of ADCs.

2 Materials

All mobile phases and buffers should be prepared using analytical grade reagent and purified water, and filtered using a 0.22 μm filter membrane before storage. It is a good practice to store the antibody or ADC samples at 2–8 °C prior to analysis. ADC solutions should be handled with care, and personal protection equipment (glove, goggles, and lab coats) should be worn due to the presence of cytotoxic agents.

1. Protein samples (e.g., antibody, ADC).
2. Agilent 8453 spectrophotometer or equivalent to measure protein concentration.
3. 1 cm quartz cuvette for protein concentration measurement.
4. Agilent 1200 HPLC system or equivalent.
5. SE-HPLC stationary phase (column): A Tosoh TSK G3000 SW_{XL}, 7.8 mm × 30 cm, 5 μm particle size column or equivalent.

6. Purified water to prepare mobile phases.
7. Organic solvent: Isopropyl alcohol and Methanol.
8. SE-HPLC mobile phase: 0.2 M potassium phosphate and 0.25 M potassium chloride, pH 6.95.
9. HIC mobile phase A: 1.5 M ammonium sulfate, 25 mM sodium phosphate, pH 6.95.
10. HIC mobile phase B: 25 mM sodium phosphate, pH 6.95 with 25% (v/v) IPA (*see* **Note 1**).
11. HIC stationary phase (column): butyl-NPR 4.6 mm ID × 3.5 cm, 2.5 μm or equivalent.
12. HPLC vials and aluminum flip off caps.
13. VP Capillary DSC (MicroCal, Northampton, MA) or equivalent.
14. Malvern Panalytical Inc. 96-well plate and cover for VP-capillary.
15. ChemStation software (Agilent Technologies) or Chromeleon software (Dionex Corporation).

3 Methods

3.1 Preparation of Thermally Stressed Samples

Stability of biotherapeutic antibodies is a critical product quality attribute that is required to determine shelf life. Thermal stress is one of the relevant conditions for providing information about potential long-term stability at the intended storage condition [5]. A stress or forced degradation at elevated temperature (e.g., at greater than the intended storage temperature) is considered a way to generate degradation within a short time, such as weeks. The purpose of thermal stress is to generate degradation (such as aggregation), to develop formulation, and to develop assays that support the characterization of degradation products. Formulating mAbs conjugated with toxins in the hinge region (e.g., vcMMAE) has been shown to aggregate more quickly than the parent antibody when formulated in high ionic strength buffer and when thermally stressed. Therefore, formulating ADCs in a high ionic strength buffer and then thermally stressing them is useful for evaluating ADC stability (Fig. 3) [11]. Elevated temperature stress study can be achieved as follows:

1. Aliquot formulated antibody sample into glass vials, stopper and crimp (*see* **Note 2**).
2. Prepare several aliquots filled in same glass vial size and same fill volume (*see* **Note 3**).
3. Store glass vials at an upright position boxed in appropriate thermal stress temperature, e.g., 30 or 40 °C for up to 8 weeks,

with appropriate light protection. Store unstressed control ($T = 0$) sample at −70 °C for future analysis.

4. Pull out samples from stress temperature storage based on the desired time points (e.g., 1, 2, 4, 6, 8 weeks or as necessary) and test immediately or freeze at −70 °C until analysis (*see* **Note 4**).

3.2 Protein Concentration Measurement (UV-Vis Spectrophotometer)

Measuring protein concentration using appropriate methods is important in order to know the starting protein concentration and also to monitor the stability of the molecule during thermal stress or storage at various temperatures. This method also helps to monitor protein loss due to binding to surfaces, precipitation, or insoluble aggregate formation.

UV-Vis Method Steps

1. Dilute protein sample with formulation buffer or water so that the absorbance maximum around 280 nm is between 0.5 and 1.0 absorbance unit. Mix protein sample gently by inverting tubes several times. Volumetric or gravimetric sample dilution can be applied as needed (*see* **Note 5**).
2. If the protein sample's UV absorbance is between 0.5 and 1 absorbance unit, dilution is not necessary.
3. Use a cuvette (e.g., 1-cm quartz cuvette) to load samples with appropriate sample volume. Make sure to fill the cuvette above the light path window with sample (*see* **Note 6**).
4. Wash cuvettes with water and dry before use and in between samples. Use 100% organic solvent (e.g., methanol) to dry the cuvettes fast.
5. Get rid of bubbles that may be introduced in the cuvette during sample loading by gently tapping the sides of the cuvette.
6. Use formulation buffer or water to blank the system or the instrument.
7. Use spectrophotometer with diode array (e.g., Agilent 8453 or equivalent) instrument to measure protein concentration.
8. Use appropriate extinction or absorptivity coefficient of the protein sample in order to calculate protein concentration in milligram per milliliter (mg/mL).
9. Multiply with the dilution factor to get the final protein concentration value.
10. Calculate protein concentration using the Beer-Lambert law (Eq. 1) [12].

$$\text{Protein conc.}\left(\frac{\text{mg}}{\text{mL}}\right) = \frac{\text{Maximum absorbance}}{\text{Extinction coefficient} \times \text{cell pathlength (cm)}} \times \text{Dilution factor} \qquad (1)$$

3.3 Differential Scanning Calorimetry (DSC)

Differential scanning calorimetry is a biophysical characterization tool that is used for direct assessment of the heat energy uptake by a molecule in order to determine thermal-induced transitions. Thermal-induced transition temperatures can be measured in liquid, solid, or suspensions. The formulation and composition of an antibody determines its thermal-induced unfolding. Changes in the heat capacity can originate from the disruption of the forces that stabilize native protein structure. These forces can include van der Waals, hydrophobic, and electrostatic interactions, hydrogen bonds, hydration of the exposed residues, conformational entropy, and the physical environment (i.e., pH, buffer, ionic strength, and excipient). As such, DSC studies can allow comparison of stabilities across formulations and molecule variants [13] and are also a useful tool for selecting appropriate thermal stress temperature by identifying the unfolding temperature (T_m) of mAbs (Fig. 1) [4, 14].

DSC Method Steps

1. Prepare a minimum of 500 μL of protein sample at 1 mg/mL protein concentration diluted in formulation buffer.
2. Prepare a reference solution (e.g., formulation buffer of the test sample) and make sure it exactly matches the protein sample dilution buffer.
3. Load samples on a 96-well plate that is provided by the vendor (MicroCal, Northampton, MA).
4. Each sample requires four wells in the 96-well plate. One protein sample, one reference solution, and two sets of reference solution to subtract background noise from the instrument.

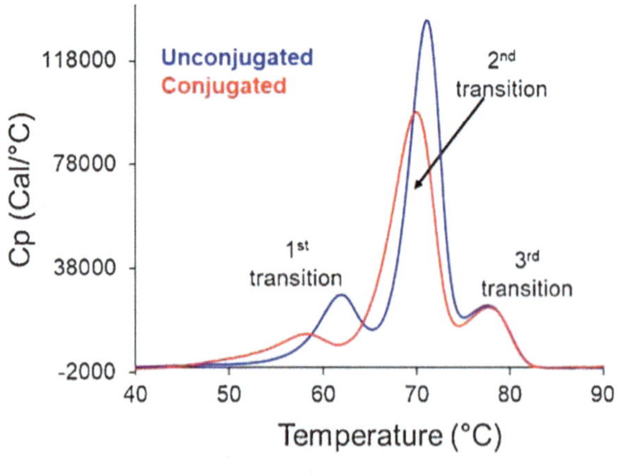

Fig. 1 DSC thermograms of unconjugated (blue line) and conjugated (red line) antibodies formulated in high ionic strength buffer. Overall, the conjugated antibody unfolds at lower T_m when compared with the unconjugated antibody

5. Protein samples that have the same dilution buffer/formulation buffer can share the same reference solution.
6. Run 2 reference solution sets for each buffer system to ensure a good blank.
7. Scan each sample-buffer pair over the temperature range 15–95 °C at a rate of 1 °C per minute.
8. Analyze data and determine T_m onset and other thermal transition temperatures using appropriate computer software (e.g., *Origin* software (OriginLab; Northampton, MA)).

3.4 Size Exclusion Chromatography High Performance Liquid Chromatography (SE-HPLC)

SE-HPLC is a conventional technique that helps to monitor the size distribution of antibodies. SE-HPLC is effective to monitor changes in high molecular weight species (aggregate) formation and it can also be used to monitor low molecular weight formation (fragments) [7]. ADCs are more hydrophobic compared to their parent molecule due to the presence of hydrophobic small molecules linked to the native cysteine residues in the hinge region (e.g., vcMMAE); the addition of organic solvent (e.g., isopropyl alcohol) in the mobile phase solution is common to prevent nonspecific hydrophobic interaction between the ADC and the stationary phase [15] (Figs. 2 and 3).

SE-HPLC Method Steps

1. Prepare mobile phase (e.g., 0.2 M potassium phosphate and 0.25 M potassium chloride, pH 6.95, then add 5% (v/v) Isopropyl Alcohol) (*see* **Note 1**).

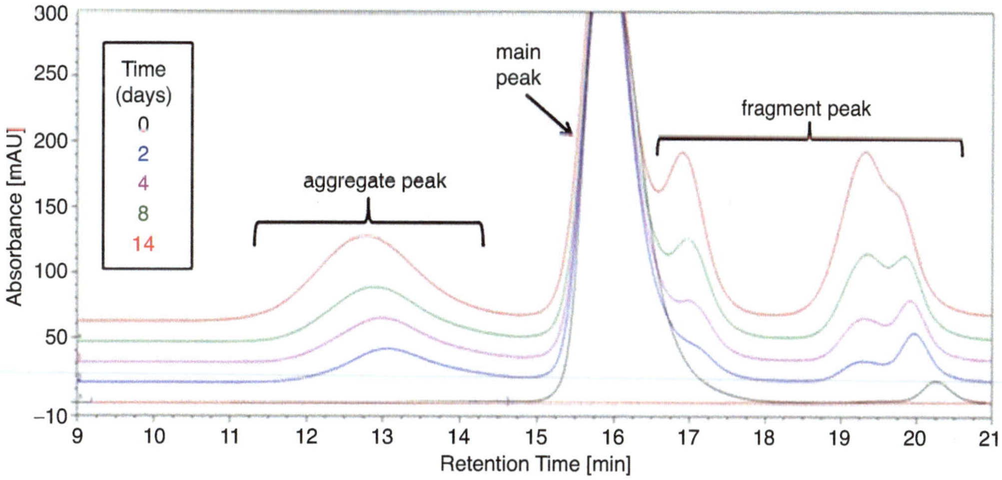

Fig. 2 Thermal stability chromatography of an antibody conjugated with vcMMAE. Isolated DAR 6 species formulated in high ionic strength buffer and stored at 40 °C for up to 14 days. The HMWS and LMWS increase in a time-dependent manner as shown by SE-HPLC

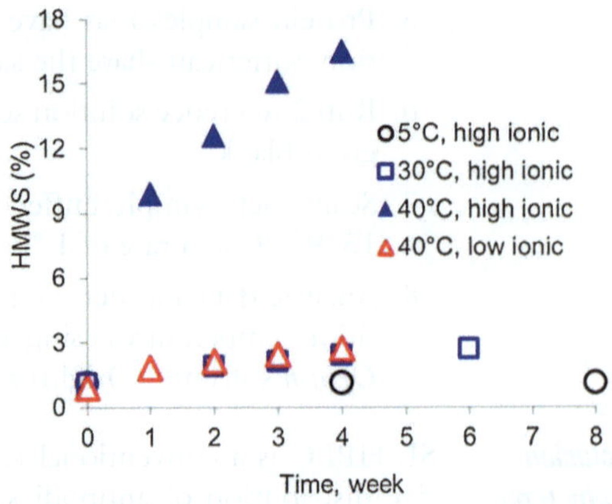

Fig. 3 Thermal stability of an ADC formulated in low and high ionic strength buffers and then stored at 5, 30, or 40 °C for up to 8 weeks (SE-HPLC)

2. Use a liquid chromatographic system (HPLC) (e.g., Agilent 1200, Waters, or equivalent) with multiple wavelength detector that has in-line UV detection capability to monitor 280 nm.
3. Use TSKgel G3000 or G2000 SEC columns (e.g., TSKgel G3000SWXL, 7.8 mm × 30 cm, 5 μm particle size) [7], maintain ambient column temperature and 2–8 °C autosampler temperature.
4. Equilibrate stationary phase (column) with mobile phase until stable baseline is reached using a flow rate of 0.5 mL per minute (*see* **Note** 7).
5. Dilute protein test sample to 1–2 mg/mL with mobile phase if desired and inject between 20 and 50 μg (*see* **Note** 7).
6. Prepare assay controls and blanks in a similar fashion as the test sample.
7. Load samples into appropriate SE-HPLC vials and inject samples using the autosampler. Employ isocratic elution at a flow rate of 0.5 mL/min for a minimum run time of 30 min (*see* **Note** 7).
8. Analyze data using a suitable electronic integrator or computer system.
9. Exclude from integration any peaks that are present in the blank.
10. Integrate protein-related peaks and classify them as HMWS, monomer, and LMWS.
11. Report the percentage of peak areas for the HMWS, main peak, and LMWS.

12. Use the following equation to calculate percent peak area (Eq. 2):

$$\text{Percent peak area of peak of interest} = \frac{(\text{Area of peak of interest})}{(\text{Total area of protein peak})} \times 100 \quad (2)$$

3.5 Hydrophobic Interaction Chromatography (HIC)

HIC is one of the commonly used methods to determine the drug-to-antibody ratio (DAR) and drug load distribution during the manufacturing release of drug product and during stability [4]. The ADC conjugation to the native cysteine residues of mAbs using the maleimide chemistry generates heterogeneous mixture of DAR species, i.e., DAR 0, 2, 4, 6, or 8 (e.g., conjugation of vcMMAE to mAbs). Hydrophobicity of ADCs increases with increasing the DAR species and ADC peaks elute from the HIC column based on the number of drug attached to the mAb, such that the no drug species (DAR0) elute first and the highest drug load species elute last (DAR8) (Fig. 4). Reversed-phase high-performance liquid chromatography (RP-HPLC) offers an orthogonal method to obtain DAR for ADCs but it will not be discussed in this section [9]. When there are changes due to physical stress, the peak profile and the relative percent area of each DAR species will also change. The experimental conditions are listed below.

HIC Method Steps [10, 11, 16]

1. Prepare mobile phases: buffer A (1.5 M ammonium sulfate, 25 mM sodium phosphate, pH 6.95) and buffer B (25 mM sodium phosphate, pH 6.95 with 25% (v/v) IPA) (*see* **Note 1**).
2. Use an HPLC system (e.g., Agilent, Waters, or equivalent) with diode array detector that has in-line UV detection capability to monitor 280 nm.
3. Keep the column temperature at 25 °C during equilibration and throughout chromatography run.
4. Equilibrate stationary phase (e.g., TSKgel, butyl-NPR 4.6 mm ID × 3.5 cm, 2.5 μm, or equivalent) with buffer A until steady baseline is obtained (*see* **Note 7**).
5. Inject a maximum of 5–10 μL (50–100 μg) neat protein sample on the column using the autosampler.
6. Run a linear gradient from 100% mobile phase A to 100% mobile phase B over 18 min with a flow rate of 0.8 mL/min (*see* **Note 8**).
7. Analyze data by integrating each DAR species peak to determine percent peak area of peaks of interest.
8. A typical HIC chromatogram is shown in Fig. 4.

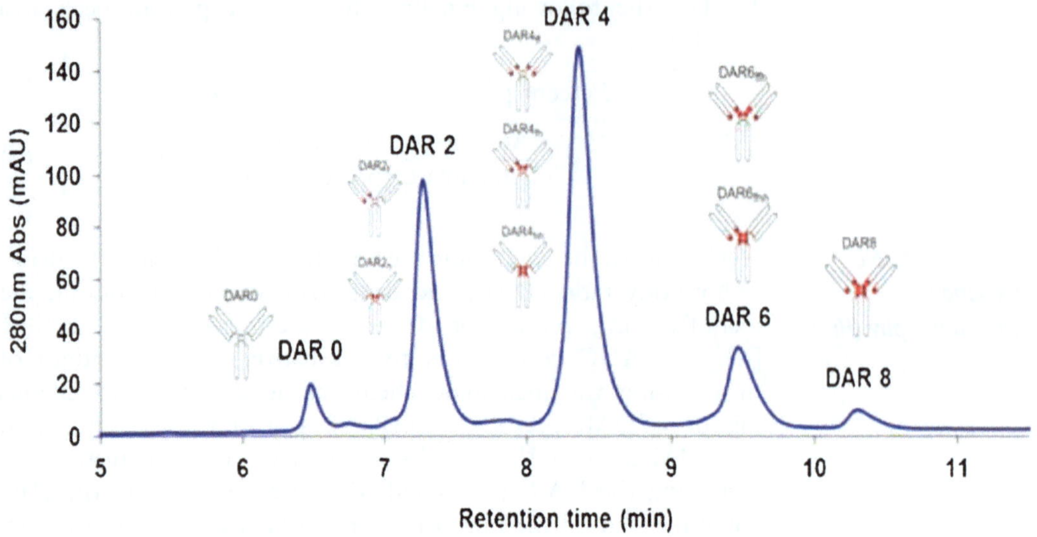

Fig. 4 Hydrophobic interaction chromatography (HIC) of an ADC molecule showing drug (cytotoxic agent, vcMMAE) load distribution (red dots indicate cytotoxic drugs)

9. Calculate the percent peak area of each DAR species using the equation below (Eq. 3) [9]:

$$\text{Percent peak area of DAR}'' \times '' = \frac{(\text{Peak area of DAR}'' \times '')}{(\text{Total peak area of all DAR})} \times 100 \qquad (3)$$

4 Notes

1. ADCs are more hydrophobic than the parent antibody and the addition of IPA in the SE-HPLC mobile phase prevents non-specific hydrophobic interaction between the column and the ADC. The percentage of IPA in the mobile phase needs to be determined in a case by case basis.
2. Autoclave glass vials and rubber stoppers before filling protein samples to keep protein samples sterile.
3. Label each vial with relevant information, e.g., name of product, formulation, time point, etc.
4. Aliquot starting material ($T = 0$) and thermal stressed samples in smaller volumes prior to freezing and then thaw required amount for testing. Samples can be batch tested to avoid run to run variability.

5. Gentle mixing of protein samples is recommended. Vigorous agitation of samples during mixing can induce aggregate formation.
6. Put enough sample in the cuvette to cover the light pathway; otherwise erroneous reading can occur.
7. Follow column vendor's manual for recommended flow rate, equlibration time and protein load amount as a starting point.
8. The gradient conditions may need to be optimized depending on the nature of the ADC molecule.

References

1. Mahler HC, Friess W, Grauschopf U, Kiese S (2009) Protein aggregation: pathways, induction factors and analysis. J Pharm Sci 98 (9):2909–2934. https://doi.org/10.1002/jps.21566
2. Cromwell ME, Hilario E, Jacobson F (2006) Protein aggregation and bioprocessing. AAPS J 8(3):E572–E579. https://doi.org/10.1208/aapsj080366
3. Hollander I, Kunz A, Hamann PR (2008) Selection of reaction additives used in the preparation of monomeric antibody-calicheamicin conjugates. Bioconjug Chem 19(1):358–361. https://doi.org/10.1021/bc700321z
4. Galush WJ, Wakankar AA (2013) Formulation development of antibody-drug conjugates. Methods Mol Biol 1045:217–233. https://doi.org/10.1007/978-1-62703-541-5_13
5. Nowak C, J KC SMD, Katiyar A, Bhat R, Sun J, Ponniah G, Neill A, Mason B, Beck A, Liu H (2017) Forced degradation of recombinant monoclonal antibodies: a practical guide. MAbs 9(8):1217–1230. https://doi.org/10.1080/19420862.2017.1368602
6. Vermeer AW, Norde W (2000) The thermal stability of immunoglobulin: unfolding and aggregation of a multi-domain protein. Biophys J 78(1):394–404. https://doi.org/10.1016/S0006-3495(00)76602-1
7. Hong P, Koza S, Bouvier ES (2012) Size-exclusion chromatography for the analysis of protein biotherapeutics and their aggregates. J Liq Chromatogr Relat Technol 35 (20):2923–2950. https://doi.org/10.1080/10826076.2012.743724
8. Hinrichs MJ, Dixit R (2015) Antibody drug conjugates: nonclinical safety considerations. AAPS J 17(5):1055–1064. https://doi.org/10.1208/s12248-015-9790-0
9. Ouyang J (2013) Drug-to-antibody ratio (DAR) and drug load distribution by hydrophobic interaction chromatography and reversed phase high-performance liquid chromatography. Methods Mol Biol 1045:275–283. https://doi.org/10.1007/978-1-62703-541-5_17
10. Beckley NS, Lazzareschi KP, Chih HW, Sharma VK, Flores HL (2013) Investigation into temperature-induced aggregation of an antibody drug conjugate. Bioconjug Chem 24 (10):1674–1683. https://doi.org/10.1021/bc400182x
11. Adem YT, Schwarz KA, Duenas E, Patapoff TW, Galush WJ, Esue O (2014) Auristatin antibody drug conjugate physical instability and the role of drug payload. Bioconjug Chem 25(4):656–664. https://doi.org/10.1021/bc400439x
12. Grimsley GR, Pace CN (2004) Spectrophotometric determination of protein concentration. Curr Protoc Protein Sci. Chapter 3:Unit 3.1. https://doi.org/10.1002/0471140864.ps0301s33
13. Ionescu RM, Vlasak J, Price C, Kirchmeier M (2008) Contribution of variable domains to the stability of humanized IgG1 monoclonal antibodies. J Pharm Sci 97(4):1414–1426. https://doi.org/10.1002/jps.21104
14. Gill P, Moghadam TT, Ranjbar B (2010) Differential scanning calorimetry techniques: applications in biology and nanoscience. J Biomol Tech 21(4):167–193
15. Wakankar A, Chen Y, Gokarn Y, Jacobson FS (2011) Analytical methods for physicochemical characterization of antibody drug conjugates. MAbs 3(2):161–172
16. Chen T, Chen Y, Stella C, Medley CD, Gruenhagen JA, Zhang K (2016) Antibody-drug conjugate characterization by chromatographic and electrophoretic techniques. J Chromatogr B Analyt Technol Biomed Life Sci 1032:39–50. https://doi.org/10.1016/j.jchromb.2016.07.023

Chapter 22

Biophysical Methods for Characterization of Antibody-Drug Conjugates

Vamsi Krishna Mudhivarthi and Jianxin Guo

Abstract

Antibody-drug conjugates (ADC) are made up of three components: (1) a mAb specific to cells of choice, (2) a small molecule with desired end goal, and (3) a linker to covalently link drug molecule to the antibody. Bringing together the mAb, drug molecule, and the linker results in the formation of an immunoconjugate designed to selectively deliver the drug molecule to a cell of interest. Synergic effects of the mAb and drug molecule lead to destroying the target tumor cells while leaving the normal cells unharmed. However, the development of ADCs is associated with challenges due to the heterogeneity of the ADC molecules created from the conjugation process. Addition of the linker and drug moieties during processing as well as the hydrophobicity of the drug itself can lead to structural changes that may affect the stability and functional profile of the conjugated molecule. Furthermore, linkers site of attachment plays a major role in determining the conformational and colloidal properties of the ADCs. In this chapter, several characterization methods are introduced to determine the biophysical characteristics of the ADC. Protocols, data analysis as well as notes for circular dichroism, intrinsic fluorescence, ANS fluorescence, differential scanning calorimetry, and dynamic scanning fluorimetry are outlined in detail.

Key words ADC, Hydrophobicity, ANS, Intrinsic fluorescence, Extrinsic fluorescence, Dynamic scanning fluorimetry, Differential scanning colorimetry

1 Introduction

Antibody-drug conjugates (ADC) are made up of three components: (1) a mAb specific to cells of choice, (2) a small molecule with desired end goal, and (3) a linker to covalently link drug molecule to the antibody [1, 2]. Bringing together the mAb, drug molecule, and the linker results in the formation of an immunoconjugate designed to selectively deliver the drug molecule to a cell of interest. Synergic effects of the mAb and drug molecule lead to destroying the target tumor cells while leaving the normal cells unharmed [3]. However, the development of ADCs is associated with challenges due to the heterogeneity of the ADC molecules

L. Nathan Tumey (ed.), *Antibody-Drug Conjugates: Methods and Protocols*, Methods in Molecular Biology, vol. 2078,
https://doi.org/10.1007/978-1-4939-9929-3_22, © Springer Science+Business Media, LLC, part of Springer Nature 2020

created from the conjugation process [3–5]. The addition of the linker and drug moieties during processing as well as the hydrophobicity of the drug itself can lead to structural changes that may affect the stability and functional profile of the conjugated molecule. Furthermore, linkers site of attachment plays a major role in determining the conformational and colloidal properties of the ADCs. In this chapter, several characterization methods are introduced to determine the biophysical characteristics of the ADC. Protocols, data analysis as well as notes for circular dichroism, intrinsic fluorescence, ANS fluorescence, differential scanning calorimetry, and dynamic scanning fluorimetry are outlined in detail.

2 Materials

2.1 Circular Dichroism

1. Pure N2 gas to purge the optics while running the instrument.
2. Cuvettes ranging from 0.01 cm to 1 cm path length, to be used according to the requirement.

2.2 Intrinsic Fluorescence

1. 1 cm cuvette made out of Quartz to minimize the absorbance around 280 nm.

2.3 ANS Fluorescence

1. 80 μM of 1-anilino-8-naphthalene dye solution was prepared prior to the analysis of ANS spectroscopy.

2.4 Differential Scanning Calorimetry

1. 5% contrad detergent to wash cells free of protein adsorption and copious amounts of water to rinse the cells, in case of hard to remove impurities.

2.5 Differential Scanning Fluorimetry

1. Sypro Orange stock solution: The Sypro Orange dye is typically supplied as a 5000× concentrated solution in dimethyl sulfoxide (DMSO).
2. DCVJ stock solution: 4-(dicyanovinyl)Julolidine (DCVJ) concentrate solution (4 mM) is prepared by dissolving the DCVJ powder in DMSO.
3. Thioflavin T stock Solution: Thioflavin T concentrate solution (4 mM) is prepared by dissolving the Thioflavin powder in DMSO.

3 Methods

3.1 Circular Dichroism

3.1.1 Introduction

Targeted delivery of anticancer drugs and radioactive isotopes is being studied extensively. In doing so, hydrophobic payloads are conjugated to antibodies to make ADCs. Conjugation of the hydrophobic drug to the antibody may alter the chemical and physical properties of the antibody. Changes in physical properties of the antibody can be determined by measuring the near UV, far UV CD spectra. In certain circumstances, induced CD spectra can also be used to determine the change in structure over a period of time [6].

3.1.2 Sample Preparation

Absorbance, path length, concentration of the protein, and the choice of buffer or excipient have a significant effect on the quality of the collected data.

1. Circular dichroism (CD) analysis of the antibody and ADC was performed using Chirascan (Applied Photophysics Ltd., UK) (*see* **Note 1**).
2. A subtle balance between light striking the detector vs. concentration of the sample should be maintained to obtain good signal to noise ratio. For the same reason it is preferred that total absorbance of the cuvette+ buffer+ sample does not exceed 0.8.
3. In cases where the concentration of the protein is high or the buffer absorbs significantly in the given region of interest, it is recommended to use cuvettes of small path length (e.g., 0.01 cm).
4. It is preferred to use buffers with least absorbance when analyzing in the far UV region. Phosphate and Tris buffers are known to have low absorbance in the far UV region at the pH range of 6–10. Halogens are known to absorb significantly in this region; therefore phosphate buffer or Tris buffer with chloride ions will also lead to higher absorbance in the far UV region and should be avoided where possible. Zwitterionic buffers such as IPES, MOPS, MES, and HEPES exhibit high absorbance in the far UV region.

3.1.3 Experiment Setup

Scan rate, number of scans, time constant, and bandwidth play a significant role in the quality of the results [7].

1. In general a bandwidth of less than or equal to 1 nm is sufficient with routine CD spectra. For resolution of CD spectra related to phenylalanine, a lower bandwidth of 0.1 nm is recommended.
2. Time constant is a measure of time over which the data are averaged and scan rate is the number of nanometer's per given

time. Both parameters are important to obtain results with high fidelity. In general a scan rate of 0.2–0.5°/min is used for good signal to noise ratio.

3. Signal to noise is proportional to square root of the number of scans; therefore more scans will result in an improved signal.

3.1.4 Data Analysis

Signature CD bands related to different secondary and tertiary structures of the proteins are mentioned below [8–11].

1. α-Helixes exhibit three major absorbance bands with two negative minima at approximately 208 and 222 nm and a positive maxima between 190 and 195 nm.
2. β-Sheets are recognized by two signature peaks with negative minima between 217 and 218 nm and positive maxima between 195 and 197 nm (Fig. 1).
3. Random coil is typically represented by negative minima around 200 nm.

Apart from the above-mentioned commonly observed peaks, few other peaks representative of type I and type II beta sheets are mentioned below.

1. Peaks in the region of 250–270 nm are attributable to phenylalanine residues.
2. Peaks from 270 to 290 nm are attributable to tyrosine residues.
3. Peaks from 280 to 300 nm are attributable to tryptophan residues.
4. Disulfide bonds have weak broad peaks throughout the near UV region (260–300 nm).
5. Apart from the above-mentioned signal, linking small molecules to protein or mAb can also induce CD peaks specific to the conjugate.

3.2 Intrinsic Fluorescence

3.2.1 Overview

Tyrosine (Tyr), Tryptophan (Trp), and Phenylalanine (Phe) are three amino acids in protein with intrinsic fluorescence properties, but in practice studies are typically restricted to Tyr and Trp residues because of their high quantum yields in hydrophobic conditions compared to hydrophilic conditions. Thus, only proteins with either Tyr and/or Trp residues can be studied using intrinsic fluorescence. Trp emission is widely used because of its higher stoke shift leading red shift or blue shift of the peak maxima. Conjugation of drugs with antibodies might result in micro- or macro-structural changes that can lead to change in the micro-environment of the Trp residues that could lead to increase or decrease in intensity or shift in the peak maxima. Therefore, steady-state Trp fluorescence can be utilized for rapid and robust screening of protein conformations in ADC formulations [12–14].

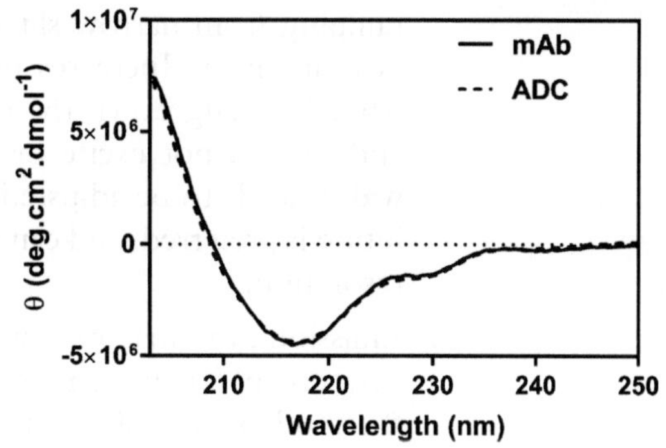

Fig. 1 Circular dichroism spectra of mAb and ADC are presented. mAb represented by solid line shows peak maxima at 217 nm; similarly ADC also has its peak maxima at 217 nm. Both the mAb and ADC spectra overlap with each showing no major conformational changes due to the conjugation of small molecule to the antibody

3.2.2 Sample Preparation

1. Cuvettes made out of quartz do not absorb and/or exhibit minimum absorbance at or around 280 nm, which is essential for excitation of the protein samples in the range of 280–295 nm. Typically 10 × 10 mm cuvettes are used for this purpose. In the case of high absorbance samples, cuvettes of lower path length are suggested (*see* **Note 2**).
2. Typically optical density of less than 0.05 is preferred to avoid inner filtration effect [15]. Care should be taken in placing the cuvette, so that right angle surface of the cuvette is facing the detector.
3. Cuvettes should be cleaned thoroughly to get rid of any protein residues by thoroughly rinsing with water and soaking in a detergent, strong acid, base, or protease-based solution. Thoroughly rinse after taking the cuvette out of the solution.

3.2.3 Experiment Setup

1. Fluorescence spectra were obtained using Varian Cary Eclipse Fluorescence Spectrophotometer (Palo Alto, CA).
2. Switch on the Xenon lamp and wait for 15 min before turning on the photomultiplier tube (PMT) module and electronics. A water bath with preferred temperature setup should also be turned on.
3. Excitation parameters can be set to either 280 nm or 295 nm depending on the emission spectra that needs to be obtained. Excitation at 295 nm (>95% Trp emission) can be set up for Trp emission, with emission recorded from 300 to 400 nm. Optimal excitation for Tyr is at 280 nm, with emission recorded from 290 to 390 nm.
4. Excitation and emission slit widths typically are set to ±5 nm. Slit width can also be set based on the detector saturation, by

ramping from narrow slit to slit width with desired emission peak intensity. Increases in slit width improve the sensitivity while bringing down the resolution and vice versa. Phe, Trp, and Tyr do not excite or emit with same efficiency, and slit width needs to be adjusted accordingly. In general 1 nm resolution is preferred, and can increase or decrease to fine-tune the resolution.

5. Emission peak maxima can be measured as a function of temperature, pH, concentration, or ionic strength to determine the thermodynamics of denaturation.

3.2.4 Data Analysis

Raw data can be analyzed using any commercially available graphing software and comparing the fluorescence spectra pre- and post-conjugation to determine the change in micro-environment of the Trp residues in mAb (Fig. 2).

3.3 ANS Fluorescence

3.3.1 Overview

Several dyes can noncovalently bind to proteins, including compounds from the naphthylamine sulfonic acids family. The most commonly used fluorophores in this class are 1-anilinonaphthalene-6-sulfonic acid (ANS) and 2(p-toluidinyl)naphthalene-6-sulfonic acid (TNS). In general these probes fluoresce weakly in aqueous environment, while fluorescing strongly when bound to hydrophobic regions of the protein. ANS when bound to protein can also quench the intrinsic fluorescence of the Trp [13, 14, 16].

3.3.2 Sample Preparation

1. 80 μM of ANS and 0.4 mg/mL mAb are mixed thoroughly and equilibrated for half hour before use. ANS can be added in excess to bind all the protein present in the solution.
2. A Quartz cuvette does not absorb and/or exhibit minimum absorbance at or around 280 nm which is essential for excitation of the protein samples in the range of 280–295 nm. Typically 10 × 10 mm cuvettes are used for this purpose. In the case of high absorbance samples cuvettes of lower path length are suggested.
3. Typically optical density of less than 0.05 is preferred to avoid inner filtration effect [15]. The cuvette should be placed in a position that is correctly aligned with the detector (that is, the right angle surface faces the detector).
4. Cuvettes should be cleaned thoroughly to get rid of any protein residues by thoroughly rinsing with water and soaking in a detergent, strong acid, base, or protease-based solution. Thoroughly rinse after taking the cuvette out of the solution.

3.3.3 Experiment Setup

1. ANS Fluorescence spectra were obtained using Varian Cary Eclipse Fluorescence Spectrophotometer (Palo Alto, CA).

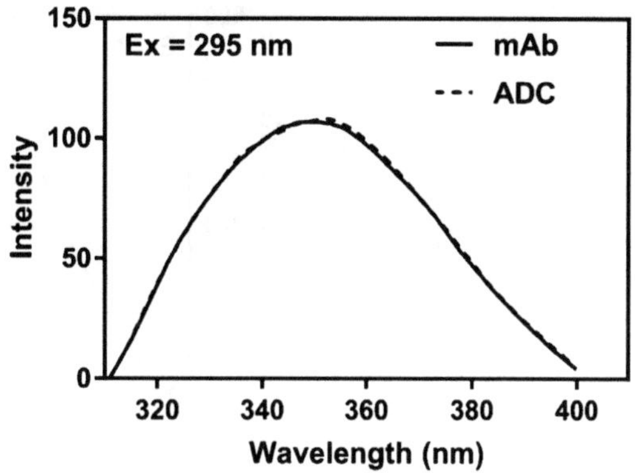

Fig. 2 Intrinsic fluorescence spectra of mAb and ADC are presented. Excitation wavelength of 295 nm was utilized and the emission spectrum was recorded from 305 to 400 nm. Emission spectra of mAb and ADC overlap with each other and no major changes in conformation are observed

2. Switch on the Xenon lamp and wait for 15 min before turning on the PMT module and electronics. Water bath with preferred temperature setup should also be turned on.
3. Excitation wavelengths of 280 or 372 nm are utilized for ANS-bound ADC samples. Excitation of Trp at 280 nm leads to emission in the range of 290–300 nm. Binding of ANS to ADC quenches the emission from Trp. Note that ANS alone exhibits emissions in the region of 400–600 nm. In the absence of aromatic amino acid residues, ANS can be directly excited at 372 nm to result in emission in the region of 390–600 nm. Excitation parameters can be set to either 280 or 372 nm depending on the preference. Excitation at 280 or 372 nm can be set up for Trp emission, which is recorded from 290 to 600 nm or 390 to 600, respectively.
4. Excitation and emission slit widths typically are set to ±5 nm. Slit width can also be set based on the detector saturation, by ramping from narrow slit to slit width with desired emission peak intensity.
5. To determine the thermodynamics of denaturation, emission peak maxima can be measured as a function of temperature, pH, concentration, and ionic strength.

3.3.4 Data Analysis

Raw data can be analyzed using any of the graphing software and comparing the fluorescence spectra pre- and post-conjugation to determine the change in micro-environment of the ANS bound to protein (Fig. 3).

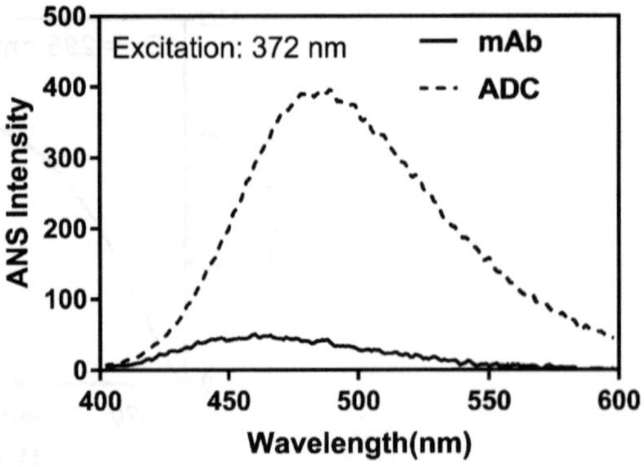

Fig. 3 ANS fluorescence spectra of mAb and ADC are presented. ANS in the presence of mAb and ADC was excited at 372 nm and the resulting emission was recorded from 400 to 600 nm. No significant peak is observed for ANS emission in the presence of mAb itself, while an emission peak is observed when mAb is conjugated with small molecules

3.4 Differential Scanning Calorimetry

3.4.1 Overview

Antibodies show strong structure to function relationship. Depending on the conjugation chemistry or the type of linker-payload, the stability of antibodies may increase or decrease or the antibody may undergo a change in conformation. Differential scanning calorimetry is a powerful tool to evaluate thermal stability. In general, unmodified antibodies undergo a cooperative denaturation process. Thermogram of antibodies typically shows three distinct peaks after deconvolution. The initial peak or bump observed in the range of 60–70 °C is representative of the CH_2 domain, followed by sharp increase in the heat capacity, Cp, or a major peak around 80 °C representative of the Fab, which can bind specifically to the antigen. The final peak in the range of 80–100 °C is representative of CH_3 domain. DSC helps in determination of stability or instability of each of these domains after conjugation of the drug substance [17–19].

3.4.2 Sample Preparation

1. DSC was performed using a high-throughput MicroCal VPDSC with autosampler (MicroCal, LLC, Northampton, MA).
2. Buffer should exhibit low pH dependence on temperature. Glycine, phosphate, acetate, sodium citrate, and sodium cacodylate buffers are appropriate because of their low dependence on temperature [20].
3. The protein sample should be dialyzed with the corresponding buffer to prevent incorrect slope or heat capacity profile.
4. After dialysis, the sample should be filtered through a 0.22–0.45 μm filter or centrifuged for ~15 min at ~8000 × *g* at the temperature where protein is most stable (typically at 2–8 °C).

5. Measure the exact concentration of protein after filtering or centrifugation of the sample.
6. While the sample preparation is going on, the DSC sample cell and reference cell should be rinsed with one syringe volume of concentrated detergent, 1 M HCl, or 1 M NaOH and then the cell should be rinsed with ~ 1 L of water.

3.4.3 Experiment Setup

1. Enter the exact concentration of the protein sample into the analysis software. Exact concentration of the sample is important in determining the thermodynamic parameters of the protein unfolding.
2. A cell cleaning detergent should be used and ensure there is no residual protein left in the cells. Alternatively when using manual mode 1 M HCl, 1 M NaOH, 10% formic acid, or 95% ethanol could be used. In the case of difficult to clean proteins, cells can be heated to 60–70 °C and then cooled to 20 °C. Once cleaned, the cells should be thoroughly rinsed with copious amounts of water to ensure removal of the cleaning agent. In general, a 20 °C starting temperature could be used, but this may vary depending on the onset of the melting temperature of the sample.
3. If an autosampler is available, a final set point temperature of 90 to 100 °C should be utilized. The final set point can be further increased to 120 °C by using a flange (manual mode) to increase the pressure to 3 atm (*see* **Note 3**). Higher final temperature set point helps in obtaining stable baseline specifically for proteins with high melting temperature.
4. In general scan rate is set to 1 °C/min. In the cases where denaturation kinetics is to be determined, thermal denaturation at different scan rates can be measured.
5. In cases where reversibility of the denaturation is expected, the sample is cooled from the final set temperature of 100 to 20 °C (*see* **Note 4**).
6. For proteins which can undergo reversible denaturation, reversible denaturation is determined by setting the final temperature of the second heating cycle to 90 °C or higher depending on the induced pressure (*see* **Note 4**).
7. After determining the concentration of the protein, the sample is placed under vacuum while stirring (stir bar) slowly to eliminate or purge any dissolved gas.
8. The sample cell can be filled using disposable plastic syringes or Pasteur pipette (manual loading). DSC cells have an inlet and outlet or have inlet and outlet ports. The reservoir is connected to the outlet before injecting the sample. Sample is slowly injected into the cell until the solution appears in the reservoir.

Once the solution is seen in reservoir, briskly pump in and out the solution several times to eliminate air bubbles in the sample cell. Repeat the above procedure with reference cell using the same buffer that is used to dialyze protein. At the end of loading cell, carefully place the cap provided by the vendor on the outlet without introducing bubbles in the sample or buffer solution.

9. Apply pressure using flange to at least 1.5 atm to a max of 3 atm. Increasing the pressure increased the boiling point of water and the maximum temperature can be set to as high as 120 °C, providing a broader range of operating temperatures in the determination of the enthalpy or entropy of denaturation.

3.4.4 Data Analysis

1. Extract the raw data either single or multiple samples and subtract the reference thermogram from sample thermogram (Fig. 4, [17]).
2. In general, the heat capacity of the unfolded protein should be higher than that of the folded protein. Linear or cubic curve fitting can be used depending on the thermogram of protein unfolding curve. Enter protein concentration in case it is not included during setting up of the experiment. The same type of peak fitting should be used for all the samples to obtain reproducible thermodynamic parameters.
3. Peak integration is performed using nonlinear square fit applying either two-state or non-two-state model. A two-state model should be used for thermograms with cooperative transition observed represented by a single peak, and non-two-state model should be used for thermograms with multiple peaks or for unknown samples.
4. Denaturation onset (T_{onset}), melting temperature T_{m}, and enthalpy of denaturation (ΔH) are the end results derived from these thermograms.

3.5 Differential Scanning Fluorimetry

3.5.1 Overview

The screening method differential scanning fluorimetry (DSF) represents a powerful technique in understanding ADC stability. DSF is an excellent method to identify solution conditions and excipients that stabilize ADCs. In DSF, the protein solution is heated by a multiwall RT PCR instrument in the presence of a fluorescence dye to monitor thermally induced conformational changes or the formation of aggregates. Fluorescence dyes such as Sypro Orange, 4-(dicyanovinyl)Julolidine (DCVJ), and Thioflavin T are commonly used in DSF experiments to monitor thermal unfolding and formation of aggregates. Sypro Orange shows high specificity and sensitivity to surface-exposed hydrophobic residues or patches. In aqueous solutions, the fluorescence emission from free probes is negligible, but in the presence of unfolded proteins,

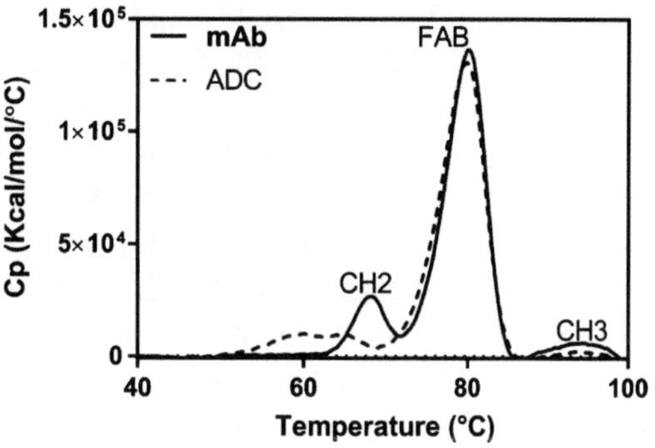

Fig. 4 Thermogram of mAb and ADC measured using differential scanning calorimetry. Thermogram of mAb shows three distinct peaks representing CH_2, FAB, and CH_3 domains. While mAb conjugated with drug molecule shows decrease in peak intensity of CH_2 domain and shifting it to lower temperature, peak representative of FAB domain largely remains unperturbed

the fluorescence intensity increases significantly due to the increased exposure of the hydrophobic protein interior, which provides hydrophobic regions to which the probe can bind [21]. The use of Sypro Orange is however limited to formulations without surfactants, since interactions with the highly hydrophobic tails of surfactants interfere with the use of Sypro Orange-based DSF.

On the other hand, another class of fluorophores known as fluorescent molecular rotors was shown to be able to detect protein aggregation in the presence of surfactants without high background fluorescence [22]. In contrast to Sypro Orange, fluorescence molecular rotors are primarily sensitive to the viscosity of the environment and to a lesser extent to changes in solvent polarity. Examples of molecular rotors include 9 (2 carboxy 2 cyanovinyl) julolidine (CCVJ), DCVJ, and Thioflavin T. When CCVJ or DCVJ binds to aggregates, the dye becomes partially immobilized, accompanied by an increase in quantum yield [23, 24]. Studies have shown that DCVJ responds to the early stages of aggregation and, thus, has a strong preference for oligomeric aggregates [24]. The formation of cross-β steric zipper motif [25, 26] mediated aggregates that can potentially form amyloid-like fibrils is monitored by means of Thioflavin T fluorescence [27, 28]. Thioflavin T recognizes certain features of the amyloid-type protein aggregates, e.g., ß-sheets and the surfaces formed by tyrosine residues and between the protofilaments, with nonspecific interactions [27].

3.5.2 Experiment Setup

1. Prior to use, Sypro Orange concentrate solution is diluted 2000-fold into the assay samples (*see* **Notes 6** and 7). With excitation set at 560–590 nm, the fluorescence emission is collected using a ROX filter (600–630 nm).

2. Both DCVJ and Thioflavin T concentrated solutions are diluted 200-fold to 20 μM working concentration in the assay samples (*see* **Notes 5**, **6**, and **8**). With excitation at 450–490 nm, the fluorescence emissions are collected using a FAM filter (515–530 nm).
3. Various ADC solutions are prepared in a PCR plate. Each cell is filled with 25 μL of sample solution in triplicate. The typical sample concentration can range from 0.5 mg/mL to 50 mg/mL. The plate is sealed with optically clear adhesive film.
4. The fluorescence can be monitored by a PCR Thermal Cycler.
5. The sample plates are subject to a temperature ramp from 5 to 95 °C at an increment of 1 °C. At each temperature, the plate is equilibrated for 1 min prior to measurement. Ramping protocol including temperature range, increment, and equilibrium time can be adjusted based on study need.
6. The fluorescence data and the second derivatives obtained from the built-in software are exported as a CSV file into Microsoft Excel (Microsoft Corporation, Redmond, WA) or another graphing software for further data analysis.

3.5.3 Data Analysis

1. The midpoint of the fluorescence curve of Sypro Orange is defined as temperature of hydrophobic exposure (T_h); the midpoint of the DCVJ fluorescence curve is defined as temperature of aggregation (T_{agg}); and the midpoint of Thioflavin T fluorescence curve is defined as temperature of formation of amyloid-like fibrils. These midpoints can be obtained by software that uses a mathematical derivative method to determine the inflection point of the curve.
2. Figure 5 depicts the fluorescence intensity profile as well as mathematical derivative of intensity profile as a function of temperature.
3. In Fig. 5, panels a and b use Sypro Orange dye, panels c and d use DCVJ while panels e and f use Thioflavin T. Panels a, c, and e show fluorescence intensity profiles while panels b, d, and f show the mathematical derivative of corresponding intensity profiles.
4. The midpoints of transition can be obtained from the peaks in the derivative curves.
5. After derivative treatment, the temperature of hydrophobic exposure is determined to be 60 °C as detected by Sypro Orange. The temperatures of aggregation are determined to be 65 °C and 76 °C by DCVJ. The temperature of formation of amyloid-like fibrils is determined to be 73 °C as detected by Thioflavin T.

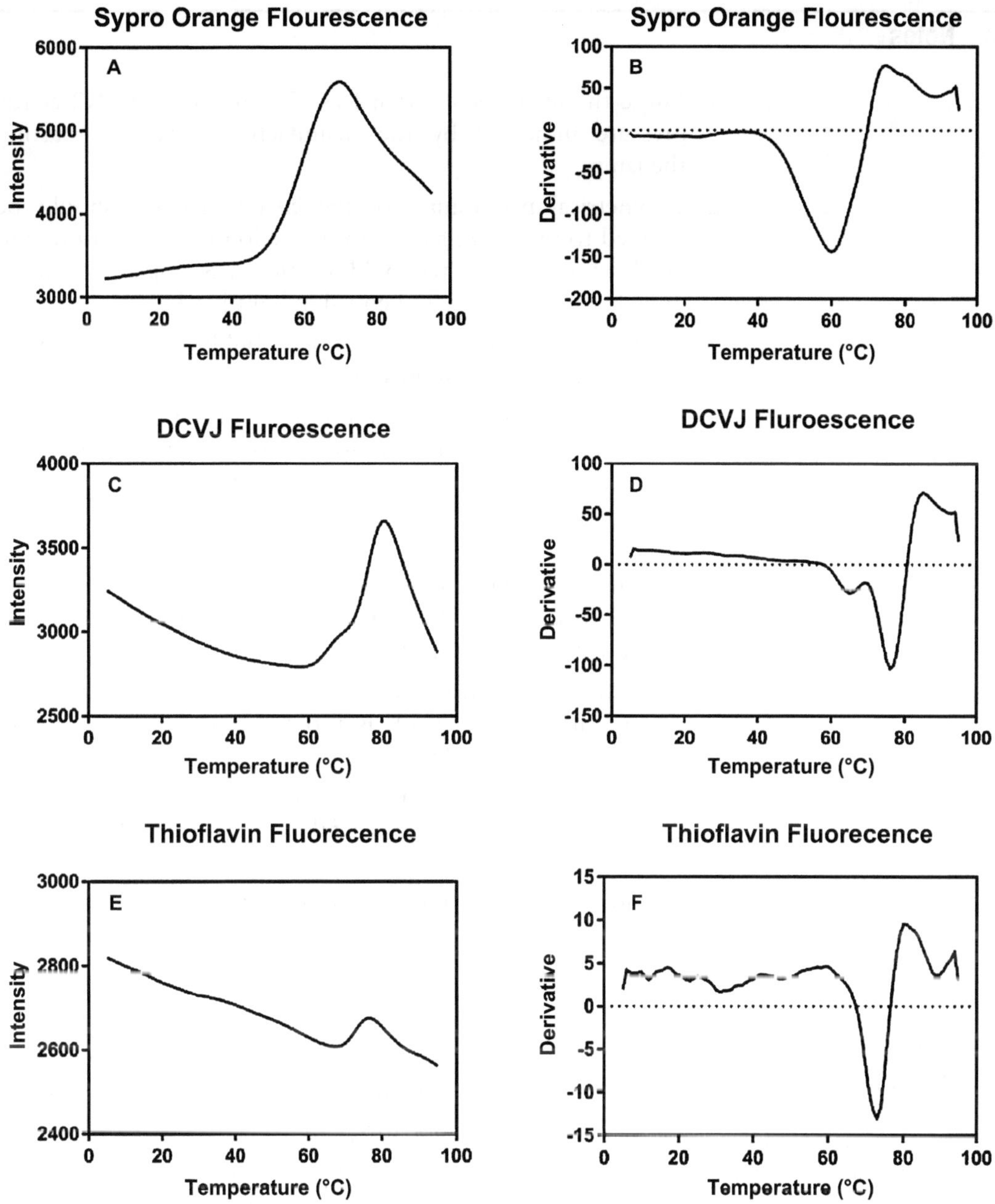

Fig. 5 Fluorescence intensity profile as well as mathematical derivative of intensity profile as a function of temperature. (**a**) Sypro Orange fluorescence intensity; (**b**) Derivative of Sypro Orange fluorescence intensity; (**c**) DCVJ fluorescence intensity: (**d**) Derivative of DCVJ fluorescence intensity; (**e**) Thioflavin T fluorescence intensity; (**f**) Derivative of Thioflavin T fluorescence intensity

4 Notes

1. Purge the instrument for at least 5 min with pure N2 at the pressure indicated by the manufacturer prior to starting the lamp.
2. Geometrical positioning of the cuvette to 45° should be avoided to minimize stray light reflection to monochromator. Smaller volume cuvettes could be utilized as long as it does not impede the excitation and emission light [16].
3. Care should be taken to get rid of air bubbles if the analysis is performed under high pressure.
4. Using a protein concentration of 1 mg/mL will prevent protein-protein interaction, with fewer artifacts in the end result. In general at the end of melting temperature heat capacity (Cp) of the denatured protein is higher than that of the native protein.
5. Dye should be diluted in the assay samples immediately before the thermal cycle study starts to avoid quench of fluorescence due to environmental factors.
6. Other fluorescent molecular rotor such as 9-(2-carboxy-2-cyanovinyl) julolidine (CCVJ) is also reported to be used under similar conditions as DCVJ [29].
7. For Sypro Orange to generate a strong fluorescent signal, the dilution factor is the range of 1:5000 to 1:1000 fold dilution of the original reagent.
8. The lowest concentration for fluorescent molecular rotors to generate a strong fluorescent signal is reported to be 10 μM [29].

References

1. Chari RVJ (2008) Targeted Cancer therapy: conferring specificity to cytotoxic drugs. Acc Chem Res 41:98–107
2. Wu AM, Senter PD (2005) Arming antibodies: prospects and challenges for immunoconjugates. Nat Biotechnol 23:1137
3. Sun MMC, Beam KS, Cerveny CG et al (2005) Reduction–alkylation strategies for the modification of specific monoclonal antibody disulfides. Bioconjug Chem 16:1282–1290
4. Baldwin AD, Kiick KL (2011) Tunable degradation of Maleimide–Thiol adducts in reducing environments. Bioconjug Chem 22:1946–1953
5. Chih H-W, Gikanga B, Yang Y et al (2011) Identification of amino acid residues responsible for the release of free drug from an antibody–drug conjugate utilizing lysine–Succinimidyl Ester chemistry. J Pharm Sci 100:2518–2525
6. Johnson WC Jr (1988) Secondary structure of proteins through circular dichroism spectroscopy. Annu Rev Biophys Biophys Chem 17:145–166
7. Venyaminov SY, Vassilenko KS (1994) Determination of protein tertiary structure class from circular dichroism spectra. Anal Biochem 222:176–184
8. Johnson WC (1999) Analyzing protein circular dichroism spectra for accurate secondary structures. Proteins Struct Funct Genet 35:307–312
9. Levitt M, Chothia C (1976) Structural patterns in globular proteins. Nature 261:552–558

10. Rodger A, Marrington R, Roper D et al (2005) Circular Dichroism spectroscopy for the study of protein-ligand interactions. In: Ulrich Nienhaus G (ed) Protein-ligand interactions: methods and applications. Humana Press, Totowa, NJ, pp 343–363
11. Sreerama N, Venyaminov S, Woody RW (2001) Analysis of protein circular Dichroism spectra based on the tertiary structure classification. Anal Biochem 299:271–274
12. Garidel P, Hegyi M, Bassarab S et al (2008) A rapid, sensitive and economical assessment of monoclonal antibody conformational stability by intrinsic tryptophan fluorescence spectroscopy. Biotechnol J 3:1201–1211
13. Guo J, Kumar S, Chipley M et al (2016) Characterization and higher-order structure assessment of an Interchain cysteine-based ADC: impact of drug loading and distribution on the mechanism of aggregation. Bioconjug Chem 27:604–615
14. Guo J, Kumar S, Prashad A et al (2014) Assessment of physical stability of an antibody drug conjugate by higher order structure analysis: impact of Thiol- Maleimide chemistry. Pharm Res 31(7):1710–1723
15. Kubista M, Sjöback R, Eriksson S et al (1994) Experimental correction for the inner-filter effect in fluorescence spectra. Analyst 119:417–419
16. Anonymous (2006) Protein Fluorescence. In: Lakowicz JR (ed) Principles of fluorescence spectroscopy. Springer US, Boston, MA, pp 529–575
17. Wakankar AA, Feeney MB, Rivera J et al (2010) Physicochemical stability of the antibody–drug conjugate Trastuzumab-DM1: changes due to modification and conjugation processes. Bioconjug Chem 21:1588–1595
18. Wen J, Arthur K, Chemmalil L et al (2012) Applications of differential scanning calorime try for thermal stability analysis of proteins: qualification of DSC. J Pharm Sci 101:955–964
19. Freire E (1995) Differential scanning Calorimetry. In: Shirley BA (ed) Protein stability and folding: theory and practice. Humana Press, Totowa, NJ, pp 191–218
20. Bastiansen O (1977) J. J. Christensen, L. D. Hansen, and R. M. Izatt: Handbook of proton ionization heats and related thermodynamic quantities. J. Wiley and Sons, New York 1976. 269 Seiten, Preis: $28.50. Berichte der Bunsengesellschaft für physikalische Chemie 81:540–540
21. He F, Hogan S, Latypov RF et al (2010) High throughput thermostability screening of monoclonal antibody formulations. J Pharm Sci 99:1707–1720
22. Samra HS, He F (2012) Advancements in high throughput biophysical technologies: applications for characterization and screening during early formulation development of monoclonal antibodies. Mol Pharm 9:696–707
23. Kung CE, Reed JK (1989) Fluorescent molecular rotors: a new class of probes for tubulin structure and assembly. Biochemistry 28:6678–6686
24. Lindgren M, Sorgjerd K, Hammarstrom P (2005) Detection and characterization of aggregates, prefibrillar amyloidogenic oligomers, and protofibrils using fluorescence spectroscopy. Biophys J 88:4200–4212
25. Nelson R, Sawaya MR, Balbirnie M et al (2005) Structure of the cross-beta spine of amyloid-like fibrils. Nature 435:773–778
26. Sawaya MR, Sambashivan S, Nelson R et al (2007) Atomic structures of amyloid cross-beta spines reveal varied steric zippers. Nature 447:453–457
27. Kayser V, Chennamsetty N, Voynov V et al (2011) Conformational stability and aggregation of therapeutic monoclonal antibodies studied with ANS and Thioflavin T binding. MAbs 3:408–411
28. Brummitt RK, Nesta DP, Chang L et al (2011) Nonnative aggregation of an IgG1 antibody in acidic conditions, part 2: nucleation and growth kinetics with competing growth mechanisms. J Pharm Sci 100:2104–2119
29. Ablinger E, Leitgeb S, Zimmer A (2012) Differential scanning fluorescence approach using a fluorescent molecular rotor to detect thermostability of proteins in surfactant-containing formulations. Int J Pharm 441(1-2):255–260

Chapter 23

Determination of ADC Cytotoxicity in Immortalized Human Cell Lines

Shengjia Wu and Dhaval K. Shah

Abstract

Cytotoxicity assays are a necessary first step to triage ADC molecules before moving them forward to relatively time-consuming and expensive in vivo studies. When cells are exposed to ADC molecules, antigen expressing cells can effectively take up those molecules and eventually die as a result of the released payload. This cytotoxic property of ADCs can be evaluated by measuring the percentage of living cells at the end of the incubation period. Tetrazolium colorimetric assay (MTT) is a widely used method that can be used to measure cell viability. Here we describe how to use an MTT assay to measure the cytotoxic effect of ADCs and calculate the corresponding IC_{50}. Besides the cytotoxic behavior on antigen expressing cells, ADCs can also demonstrate bystander killing of antigen negative cells in the vicinity of antigen expressing cells. Here, we report how to use a co-culture experiment to evaluate the bystander effect of ADC with the help of fluorescent protein transfected antigen negative cells.

Key words Antibody-drug conjugate (ADC), Cytotoxicity assay, MTT assay, Bystander effect, Co-culture system, Cell viability assay

1 Introduction

Cytotoxicity assays are an essential experiment during the development of drug molecules like antibody-drug conjugate (ADC), which influence cell proliferation or demonstrate direct killing effects. It is an essential tool to triage promising ADC candidates, predict in vivo efficacy of ADCs, and evaluate the cell specificity of ADCs. The most important outcome of cytotoxicity assay is the information about remaining number of viable or dead cells at the end of the experiment. Several types of methods can be used to measure this outcome, including tetrazolium reduction, resazurin reduction, protease markers, and ATP detection [1]. In this chapter, we describe the use of an MTT [(3-(4,5-dimethylthiazol-2-yl)-2,5-diphenyltetrazolium bromide) tetrazolium] assay, which is one of the most commonly used cytotoxicity assays. This assay, first developed by Mosmann [2], is typically performed in a 96-well

L. Nathan Tumey (ed.), *Antibody-Drug Conjugates: Methods and Protocols*, Methods in Molecular Biology, vol. 2078, https://doi.org/10.1007/978-1-4939-9929-3_23, © Springer Science+Business Media, LLC, part of Springer Nature 2020

plate. It relies on the ability of mitochondrial NADH to transfer electrons to MTT, thus actively converting the MTT into purple needle-like formazan crystals [3, 4]. The purple color generated by these crystals is then used to assess the quantity of living cells in a well using two assumptions: (1) the reduction reaction happens only in viable cells, and (2) the formazan production is directly proportional to the number of living cells [5].

In order to conduct a thorough cytotoxicity assessment of ADCs, it is ideal to use both antigen positive (Ag+) and antigen negative (Ag−) cell lines. Since ADC molecules are large and relatively polar, they are not readily permeable through the cell membrane, and rely instead on binding to cell surface antigens to gain entry into the cell. Consequently, one would expect much more toxicity (i.e., lower IC_{50}) of ADCs in Ag+ cells compared to Ag− cells. As such, ADCs are designed to provide advantage by targeting Ag+ tumor cells and sparing the damage to Ag− healthy cells. However, some ADCs can also kill Ag− cells that are in the vicinity of Ag+ cells by an effect known as the bystander effect [6]. This phenomenon stems from the diffusion of cytotoxic payload, which is generated by degradation of ADC in Ag+ cells, into the media and ultimately into the cytoplasm of Ag− cells. ADCs with cleavable linkers and hydrophobic payloads, such as brentuximab vedotin (SGN-35) which contains a val-cit linker and MMAE as the payload, are known to demonstrate the bystander effect [7, 8]. In order to evaluate the potential safety concerns of ADCs it is also important to assess their bystander effect in vitro.

There are two different types of assays that can be used to evaluate the bystander effect of ADCs in vitro: (1) co-culture assay [8, 9], and (2) medium transfer assay [10]. The medium transfer method is performed by treating Ag+ cells with a certain amount of ADC first, and then transferring the conditioned medium to wells with Ag− cells after a certain period of time. If the medium taken from Ag+ cells shows more killing than treating Ag− cells directly with the same concentration of ADC, then there is a confirmation of the bystander effect. The co-culture method starts with culturing of Ag+ and Ag− cells together, and comparing the viability of Ag− cells in the co-culture system with the viability in Ag− monoculture system at the same ADC concentrations. If Ag− cells are killed to a greater extent in the co-culture system compared to the monoculture system at the same ADC concentrations, then there is a conformation of the bystander effect. The viability of Ag− cells in the co-culture system can be measured by either flow cytometer, where the Ag− cells are detected using fluorescently labeled antibody targeting an antigen specifically expressed on these cells, or fluorescent plate reader that can selectively quantify Ag− cells that are transfected with a fluorescent protein.

In order to provide methodological details of routinely preformed cytotoxicity experiments with ADCs, here we have demonstrated how to evaluate cytotoxicity of ADC in a monoculture system using MTT assay, and how to evaluate in vitro bystander effect of ADCs in a co-culture system using green fluorescence protein transfected Ag– cells.

2 Materials

1. Cell lines (MCF7 and N87 cells).
2. Cell culture medium (Roswell Park Memorial Institute (RPMI) 1640 Medium, supplemented with 100 U/mL penicillin, 100 μg/mL streptomycin, and 10% fetal bovine serum (FBS)).
3. Dulbecco's phosphate-buffered saline (DPBS), pH 7.4.
4. 0.25% Trypsin-EDTA (1×).
5. Pipette or multichannel pipette.
6. Reagent reservoirs for multichannel pipette.
7. Hemocytometer or cell counting machine.
8. Tissue culture treated 96-well plate with clear wall and clear bottom (flat bottom).
9. Tissue culture treated 96-well plate with black wall and clear bottom (flat bottom).
10. Plate reader equipped with the filters for required wavelength.
11. 5 mg/mL MTT solution: Dissolve MTT (thiazolyl blue tetrazolium bromide) in sterile DPBS to 5 mg/mL; filter the prepared MTT solution through a 0.2 μM filter into a sterile, light protected container (*see* **Note 1**).
12. Solubilization solution: 10% (w/v) SDS solution with 0.01 M HCL: Dissolve sodium dodecyl sulfate (SDS) in sterile DI water and make the final concentration as 10% (w/v) (*see* **Notes 2** and **3**).

3 Methods

All agents used in the assay should be sterile, and all the steps before reading the plate should be conducted in a biosafety cabinet.

3.1 Determining Optimal Cell Counts and Incubation Time

1. Prepare cells for the assay. Harvest suspension cells by centrifugation. If cells are adherent, detach them by trypsinization (*see* **Note 4**).
2. Resuspend cells at a density of 1×10^6 per mL.

3. Prepare serial dilution of cells from 1×10^6 per mL to 1×10^3 per mL.
4. Add 100 μL of the dilutions into wells in triplicate. Leave three wells of medium only as blank control (background control) (*see* **Note 5**).
5. Incubate the plate at 37 °C for 6–24 h for cell adaptation (*see* **Note 6**).
6. Add 20 μL of 5 mg/mL MTT solution into each well.
7. Incubate at 37 °C for 1–4 h (*see* **Note 7**).
8. Add 100 μL 10% SDS-HCL solution and incubate the plate in the dark at 37 °C overnight (*see* **Note 8**).
9. Read the absorbance at 570 nm using a plate reader (*see* **Note 9**).
10. Get the average absorbance values from each cell number group and subtract the average value of the blank. Plot the absorbance vs. cell numbers, a suitable working range should lie within the linear portion of the curve. Determine the initial seeding number for the cytotoxicity assay based on doubling time and the desired duration of the assay.

3.2 Monoculture Cytotoxicity Study Using MTT Assay

1. Seed the cells in a 96-well plate at a density of 1000–10,000 cells/well (actual seeding number depends on the optimal assay result) in 50 μL media volume. Arrange the plate as shown in Fig. 1 with six main groups: Blank medium for Ag+ and Ag− cells, Ag+ control, Ag− control, and ADC-treated antigen positive and negative groups. Treat the "Blank" wells with 50 μL fresh medium instead (*see* **Note 10**).
2. Incubate the plate at 37 °C with 5% CO_2 overnight to let cell attach.
3. Prepare the ADC with different concentrations, while keeping each dilution one time more concentrated than the desired concentration in the well. Add 50 μL of prepared ADC solution into each drug treatment well. Add 50 μL of fresh medium into blank and control wells (*see* **Notes 11** and **12**).
4. Incubate the plate at 37 °C for 48–144 h (*see* **Note 13**).
5. Add 20 μL of 5 mg/mL MTT solution into each well.
6. Incubate at 37 °C for 1–4 h depending on the optimal assay result (as determined in Subheading 3.1).
7. Add 100 μL 10% SDS-HCL solution and incubate at 37 °C overnight.
8. Read the absorbance at 570 nm.
9. Calculate the cell viability at different ADC concentrations. Plot the data as % viability vs. ADC concentration, and fit the data to sigmoidal curve to get IC_{50} value (Figs. 2 and 3) (*see* **Note 14**).

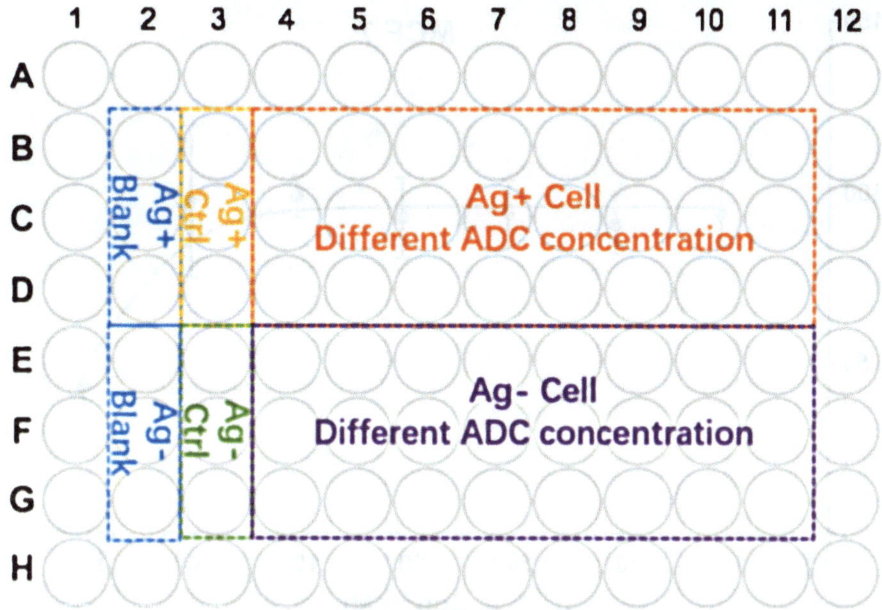

Fig. 1 Typical plate format for monoculture MTT assay. The groups are set in triplicate. For each cell line, there are three main groups: Blank (medium only); untreated cell control, and cells treated with ADC

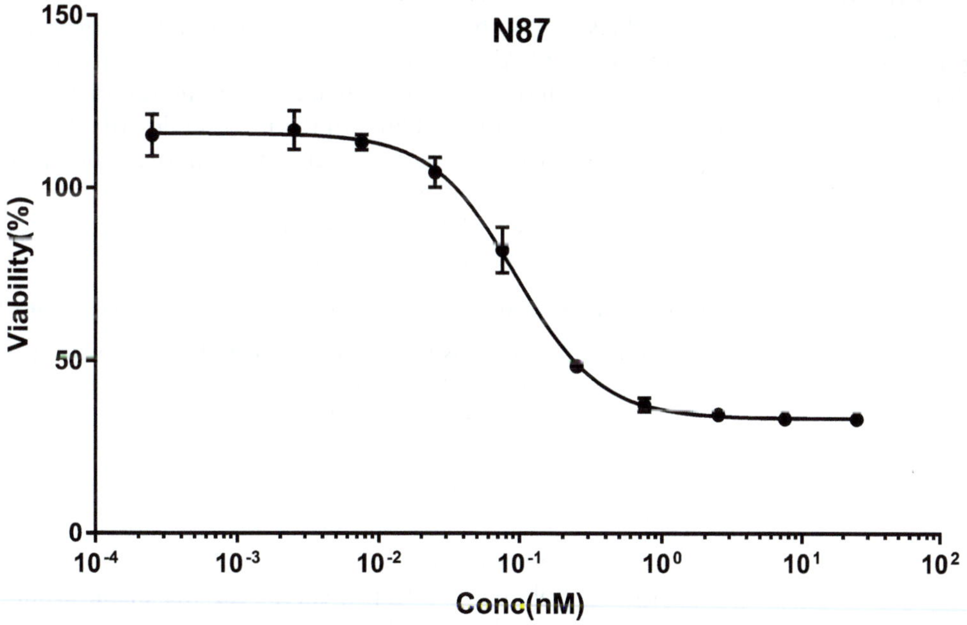

Fig. 2 N87(Ag+) viability curve following treatment with Trastuzumab-vc-MMAE

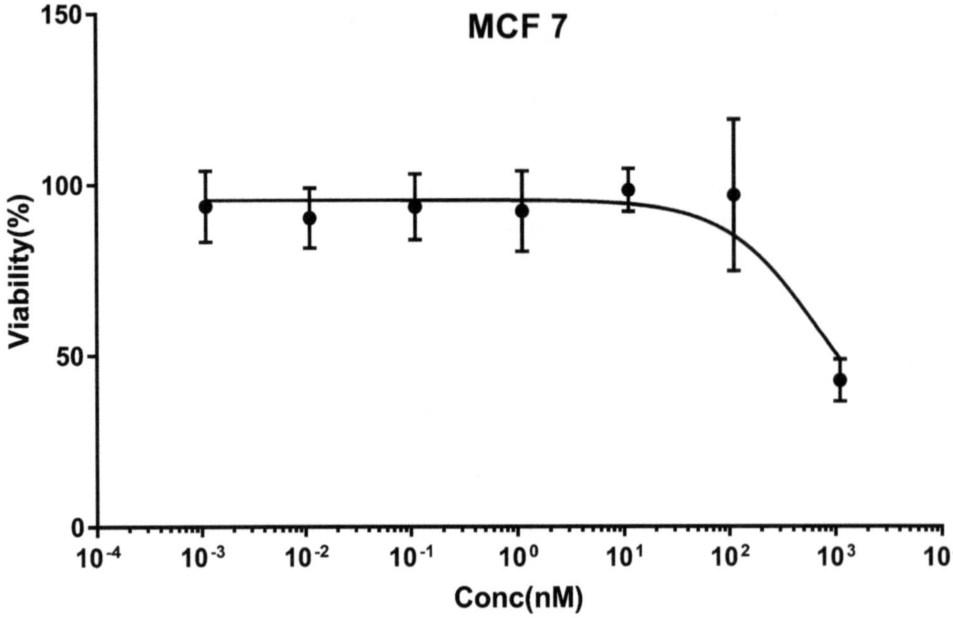

Fig. 3 MCF7(Ag−) viability curve following treatment with Trastuzumab-vc-MMAE. Data digitized from Singh et al. [9]

3.3 Co-culture Study to Determine Bystander Effect of ADC

From the results of cytotoxicity assay on monoculture cell lines, the IC_{50} values for both Ag+ and Ag− cells can be achieved. The concentration of ADC used for bystander effect should be larger than the IC_{90} in the antigen positive cell line, and less than the IC_{50} in the antigen negative cell line. In the method described here, the Ag− cell line needs to be transfected with fluorescence protein. Below, we have demonstrated a co-culture method using green fluorescence protein (GFP) transfected cell line, which was developed by Singh et al. [9] (*see* **Note 15**).

1. Prepare both Ag+ and GFP-transfected Ag− cells (*see* **Note 16**).
2. Arrange the plate as shown in Fig. 4 with seven main groups: Blank (background control), Ag− cell only group, and 5 co-culture groups with different antigen negative cell percentage: 90%, 75%, 50%, 25%, 10% (*see* **Note 17**). Divide the Ag− only and co-culture groups further into two arms: ADC-non-treated (control) and ADC-treated.
3. Seed cells at a density of total 10,000 cells/well at a final medium volume of 100 μL, except for the blank group (*see* **Note 18**). Add only 100 μL of fresh medium into the blank group.
4. Incubate the plate at 37 °C with 5% CO_2 overnight.
5. Remove the old medium in each well. Add 100 μL of ADC containing medium to each ADC treatment well, and 100 μL fresh medium to control wells (*see* **Note 19**).

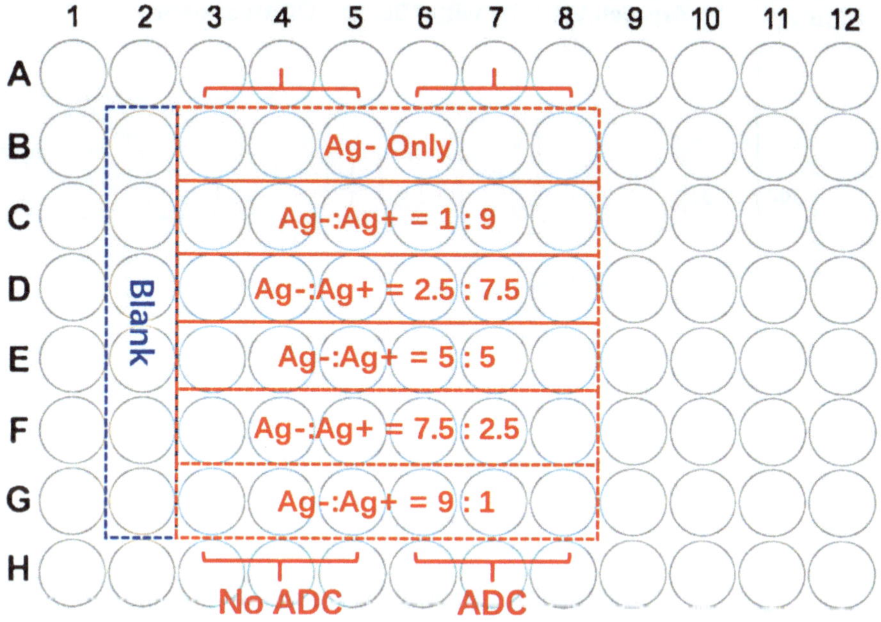

Fig. 4 Typical plate format for co-culture bystander effect assay. It contains: Blank (medium only), untreated co-culture control, and ADC-treated co-culture with different ratios of Ag+ and Ag− cells

6. Incubate the plate at 37 °C with 5% CO_2 for 48 h.
7. Read the plate at 485/535 nm (excitation/emission) (*see* **Note 20**).
8. Repeat **steps 6** and 7 at 96 h and 144 h after ADC treatment (*see* **Note 21**).
9. Normalize the fluorescence intensity value in each well by subtracting the reading from blank group. Divide fluorescence values of ADC-treated wells with the value from non-treated wells to get % viability (*see* **Note 22**) (Fig. 5).

4 Notes

1. MTT dissolves in DPBS slowly and it takes about 5–10 min by vortex or stirring. The sterilized MTT solution can be stored away from light, at 4 °C for short-term usage or at −20 °C for long-term storage up to one month. The easiest way to make a light protected container is wrapping an aluminum foil outside a conical tube.
2. Various agents can be used to solubilize the formazan product, including organic solvent like dimethyl sulfoxide (DMSO), dimethylformamide (DMF), and isopropanol; and detergent like sodium dodecyl sulfate (SDS) and combinations of organic solvent and detergent [1, 11, 12]. Many media used for cell

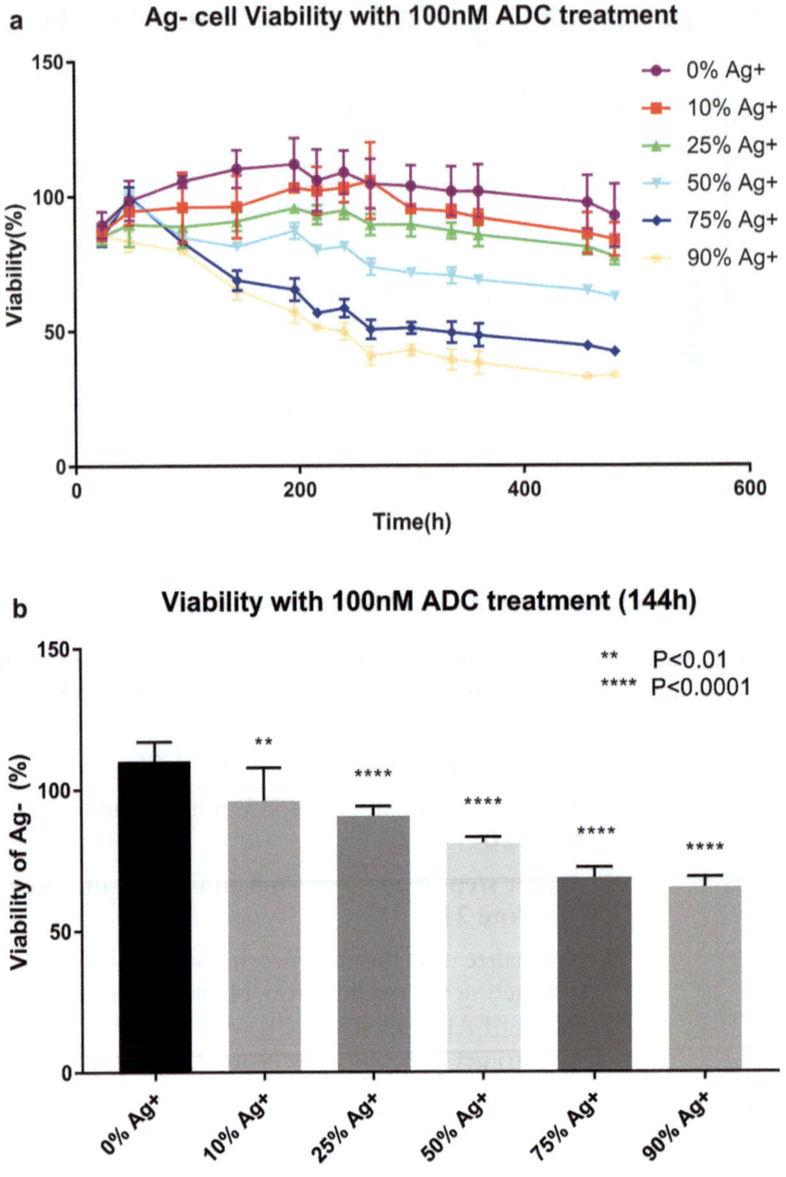

Fig. 5 (**a**) Ag− cell viability over time in N87(Ag+) and MCF7(Ag−) co-culture system with different ratios of the cells. Data digitized from Singh et al. [9]. With higher percentage of Ag+ cells, the bystander effect is more obvious. (**b**) Viability of Ag− cell at a single time point (144 h). Each co-culture group shows statistically significant higher cytotoxicity than Ag− monoculture cells. A one-way ANOVA with multi-comparison was used in this case to determine the significance

culture have phenol red (a pH indicator) in their ingredients, which can affect the absorbance [11]. HCl can help to get rid of its influence [12], and we have found that 0.01 M is the optimal concentration of HCl that can effectively reduce the influence of phenol red and provide maximum absorbance for MTT assay [13]. While dissolving formazan with DMSO provides a purple color, using 10% SDS (w/v) with 0.01 M HCL gives a dark yellow color.

3. Since SDS is a detergent, dissolving this chemical generates bubbles. To avoid these bubbles, avoid heavy vortexing or stirring. Heating can also help dissolve SDS. In general, HCl is added to 0.01 M concentration after the 10% SDS is prepared. This solution can be stored at room temperature.
4. Cells should be maintained at good condition (more than 95% live) before they are used for cytotoxicity assays. Do not use the cell immediately after thawing. Cells should be sub-cultured for at least one passage before using for the MTT assay.
5. Make sure the cells evenly seed inside the well and form a single layer if using adherent cells. To have even seeding, put pipette tip at the wall of the well and form an angle around 30° before pipetting the cells slowly. If multichannel pipette is used to seed the cells, about 1–2 mL more cell suspension is needed in the reagent reservoir. Pay attention to the difference between cells/well and cells/mL notations.
6. The recovery time can vary between cell types. For most of the cells 12–16 h is sufficient.
7. Evaluation of different MTT incubation times (e.g., 1, 2, and 4 h) during assay optimization can be helpful. Within a certain range, the longer the incubation time with MTT the higher the absorbance and resolution that can be obtained. However, when the cell density is too high, the MTT substrate can run out and the linear relationship between formazan production and cell viability can deviate. When conducting an MTT assay, an absorbance of 0.75–1.25 for the control group at the end-point is optimal.
8. Using 10% SDS-HCL solution as solubilization solution takes more time than DMSO to totally dissolve formazan crystal. A relatively longer incubation time provides higher and more stable absorbance. 12–18 h will be enough for most cases.
9. The greatest absorbance for formazan is at 570 nm. However, some plate readers with filter channels do not have the exact wavelength. In this case, choose a reading wavelength within 550–600 nm.
10. When doing cytotoxicity assay using a 96-well plate, the plates are incubated at 37 °C for several days. This leads to an evaporation problem, where the medium around the perimeter evaporates faster than the inner wells, which can cause unwanted noise and is known as edge effect. To minimize this, one solution can be leaving the outermost wells unused and filling them with 200 μL DPBS. If doing this, take into consideration

that only 60 wells are available from a single 96-well plate when designing the experiment.

11. The concentration range of ADC is designed based on ADC efficacy. The range should cover the concentrations with no killing effect on Ag+ and Ag− cells and have concentrations which saturate killing capacity on at least Ag+ cell. When screening the ADC efficacy, a dilution factor of ten is a good start. After understanding the ADC working range, a smaller dilution factor can be applied to get a more precise estimation of IC50, since this will offer more points at log-linear phase of Hill equation.
12. Drug-to-antibody ratio (DAR) is also important to consider while deciding the concentration range of ADC in the experiment. An ADC with a DAR value of four shows more cytotoxicity in vitro than the one with a DAR of 2. Therefore, payload concentration (ADC concentration * DAR value) rather than ADC concentration is more relevant when using payload IC_{50} as a reference to set up the concentration range.
13. The incubation time depends on the type of toxic payload the ADC has and the cytotoxic mechanism-of-action for the payload. If the payload is a tubulin inhibitor (e.g., MMAE or MMAF), 72 or 96 h is better to evaluate cytotoxicity for these agents, since these payloads require cell cycle arrest and cause delayed cell killing. DNA damaging payloads (e.g., PBD or calicheamicin) can induce cell death more quickly.
14. To process the data, the absorbance obtained from all the seeded wells should be subtracted by the average value of blank group. The percentage of live cells is then calculated by dividing the normalized absorbance of ADC-treated groups with the normalized absorbance from control group. The equation is:

$$\text{Viability}(\%) = \frac{\text{OD}_{\text{Treated}}}{\text{OD}_{\text{control}}} \times 100\% \tag{1}$$

Plot data with % viability on y-axis and concentration of ADC on x-axis in log scale. Fit the data using a dose-response equation with four parameters:

$$\text{Viability} = \text{Boundary}_{\text{low}} + \left(\text{Boundary}_{\text{high}} - \text{Boundary}_{\text{low}}\right) \Big/ \left(1 + \frac{\text{Concentration}_{\text{ADC}}{}^{\gamma}}{\text{IC50}^{\gamma}}\right) \tag{2}$$

$\text{Boundary}_{\text{low}}$ is the lowest viability when treated with drug, while the $\text{Boundary}_{\text{high}}$ represents the highest viability that one can get. γ is the hill slope. IC_{50} stands for the ADC concentration that can have 50% of maximum killing. Software such as GraphPad Prism can be used for the curve fitting by choosing the nonlinear regression option. While typically the IC_{50} value is used to evaluated ADC toxicity, sometimes an IC_{90} value is also used instead. IC_{90} is the concentration that induced 90% of maximum killing. From Eq. 2, we can get IC_{90} by making the viability value equal to $Boundary_{low} + 0.1 \times (Boundary_{high} - Boundary_{low})$. Therefore, the IC_{90} equals to $(9 \times IC50^{\gamma})^{1/\gamma}$. IC_{10} can also be calculated by the same way, which equals to $(1/9 \times IC50^{\gamma})^{1/\gamma}$. Figures 2 and 3 show a viability curve for N87 and MCF7 cells after the treatment with Trastuzumab-vc-MMAE ADC. Of note, the %viability can sometimes be higher than 100% at low drug concentration. This may be due to increased metabolism of cells at low concentrations, as this treatment could create stress instead of killing the cells.

15. Other fluorescence protein can also be used for this co-culture method. The cell line needs to be stably transfected, which means the fluorescence protein expression per cell needs to remain unchanged, as the fluorescence intensity must be correlated with cell number.
16. Different cell lines sometimes have different recommended medium. Normally, when doing this co-culture method, mixing two different mediums does not significantly affect the cell growth. If the transfection of Ag− cells is performed in-house, the medium may contain selection antibiotic. Before conducting the co-culture assay, these cells need to be acclimated in normal medium without antibiotic.
17. A tissue culture treated black plate with clear bottom is the most suitable plate type for this kind of assay. The black wall absorbs light, which helps reduce background noise and interference from nearby wells. With a clear bottom, the fluorescence signal can be read from the bottom, which provides better resolution when reading fluorescence from adherent cells. The material of the bottom is not much crucial in this kind of assay; Either plastic or glass bottom works.
18. It requires time to observe the bystander effect compared to the direct cytotoxicity assay, and sometimes it can take up to 3 weeks [9]. The initial seeding density can be adjusted considering the incubation and doubling time. Bystander effect requires the payload to be cleaved from the ADC and penetrate into the nearby Ag− cells. Therefore, adding media during the assay will influence the bystander effect by diluting the free payload concentration, and thus it is not advised.
19. The volume of medium added per well can go up to 200 μL if the assay needs an extended period of incubation.
20. GFP has a maximum excitation wavelength at 488 nm and a maximum emission wavelength at 510 nm. As mentioned in

Note 15, reading from bottom may provide better signal-to-noise ratio.

21. The reading time points and the duration of the assay are adjustable. As long as the initial seeding number is proper, the assay can go up to 20 days according to Singh et al. [9].

22. To evaluate the bystander effect, compare the viability of co-culture system with Ag− cell only. If the difference is statistically significant and less viability is observed in co-culture system, the ADC molecule has bystander activity. For some ADCs, the bystander effect can only be observed when the ratio of Ag+ cell is larger than 50%.

References

1. Riss TL, Moravec RA, Niles AL, Duellman S, Benink HA, Worzlla TJ, Minor L (2013) Cell viability assays. In: Sittampalam GS, Coussens NP, Nelson H et al (eds) Assay guidance manual. Eli Lilly & Company and the National Center for Advancing Translational Sciences, Bethesda, MD
2. Mosmann T (1983) Rapid colorimetric assay for cellular growth and survival: application to proliferation and cytotoxicity assays. J Immunol Methods 65:55–63
3. Liu Y, Peterson DA, Kimura H, Schubert D (1997) Mechanism of cellular 3-(4,5-dimethylthiazol-2-yl)-2,5-diphenyltetrazolium bromide (MTT) reduction. J Neurochem 69:581–593
4. Marshall NJ, Goodwin CJ, Holt SJ (1995) A critical assessment of the use of microculture tetrazolium assays to measure cell growth and function. Growth Regul 5:69–84
5. Sylvester PW (2011) Optimization of the tetrazolium dye (MTT) colorimetric assay for cellular growth and viability. Methods Mol Biol 716:157–168
6. Kovtun YV, Audette CA, Ye Y, Xie H, Ruberti MF, Phinney SJ, Leece BA, Chittenden T, Blattler WA, Goldmacher VS (2006) Antibody-drug conjugates designed to eradicate tumors with homogeneous and heterogeneous expression of the target antigen. Cancer Res 66:3214–3221
7. Younes A, Bartlett NL, Leonard JP, Kennedy DA, Lynch CM, Sievers EL, Forero-Torres A (2010) Brentuximab vedotin (SGN-35) for relapsed CD30-positive lymphomas. N Engl J Med 363:1812–1821
8. Okeley NM, Miyamoto JB, Zhang X, Sanderson RJ, Benjamin DR, Sievers EL, Senter PD, Alley SC (2010) Intracellular activation of SGN-35, a potent anti-CD30 antibody-drug conjugate. Clin Cancer Res 16:888–897
9. Singh AP, Sharma S, Shah DK (2015) Quantitative characterization of in vitro bystander effect of antibody-drug conjugates. J Pharmacokinet Pharmacodyn 27:215–225
10. Szot C, Saha S, Zhang XM et al (2018) Tumor stroma-targeted antibody-drug conjugate triggers localized anticancer drug release. J Clin Invest 128:2927–2943
11. Tada H, Shiho O, Kuroshima K et al (1986) An improved colorimetric assay for interleukin 2. J Immunol Methods 93:157–165
12. Denizot F, Lang R (1986) Rapid colorimetric assay for cell growth and survival. Modifications to the tetrazolium dye procedure giving improved sensitivity and reliability. J Immunol Methods 89:271–277
13. Septisetyani EP, Ningrum RA, Romadhani Y, Wisnuwardhani PH, Santoso A (2014) Optimization of sodium dodecyl sulphate as a formazan solvent and comparison of MTT assay with WST-1 assay in MCF-7 cells. Indonesian J Pharm 25:245–254

Chapter 24

LC/MS Methods for Studying Lysosomal ADC Catabolism

Andrew J. Bessire and Chakrapani Subramanyam

Abstract

A critical component of antibody-drug conjugate (ADC) development is identification or verification of the active released entity upon cellular uptake and exposure to lysosomal enzymes. Coupled with LC/MS, commercial human lysosomal preparations can be used as an in vitro tool to explore the release characteristics of new ADCs, and gain information on potential metabolic or chemical liabilities of new payload structures. A general method for approaching this is described for cathepsin B-cleavable as well as non-cleavable ADCs, and opportunities for tailoring the method to specific cases are indicated.

Key words Lysosomal processing, Lysosomal enzymes, Released species, Released payload, Catabolism

1 Introduction

Antibody-drug conjugates (ADCs) are generally comprised of three major components: an antibody for the selective targeting of tumor cell surface antigens, a cytotoxic payload, and a linker unit which connects these two moieties. In some ADCs the linker is omitted, and the cytotoxin is directly conjugated to residues on the antibody, typically cysteine or lysine. In general, the mechanism of payload delivery to the tumor cell involves binding of the antibody to cell surface proteins, followed by internalization of the ADC by endocytosis, and subsequent trafficking to the endosomes and lysosomes [1, 2]. Most ADCs are designed to release the cytotoxic payload in these compartments. This may occur through antibody catabolism, or by cleavage of a linker which has been designed to take advantage of proteolytic enzymes or the slightly acidic and reducing environment found in these compartments [3–7]. For example, the cleavable linker valine-citrulline *p*-aminobenzyl carbamate (vc-PABC) is a substrate for the intracellular cysteine protease cathepsin B [8]. ADCs containing this linker, or linkers with certain other dipeptide combinations, typically release the free payload without any modification. Non-cleavable-linker ADCs, however, do not

L. Nathan Tumey (ed.), *Antibody-Drug Conjugates: Methods and Protocols*, Methods in Molecular Biology, vol. 2078, https://doi.org/10.1007/978-1-4939-9929-3_24, © Springer Science+Business Media, LLC, part of Springer Nature 2020

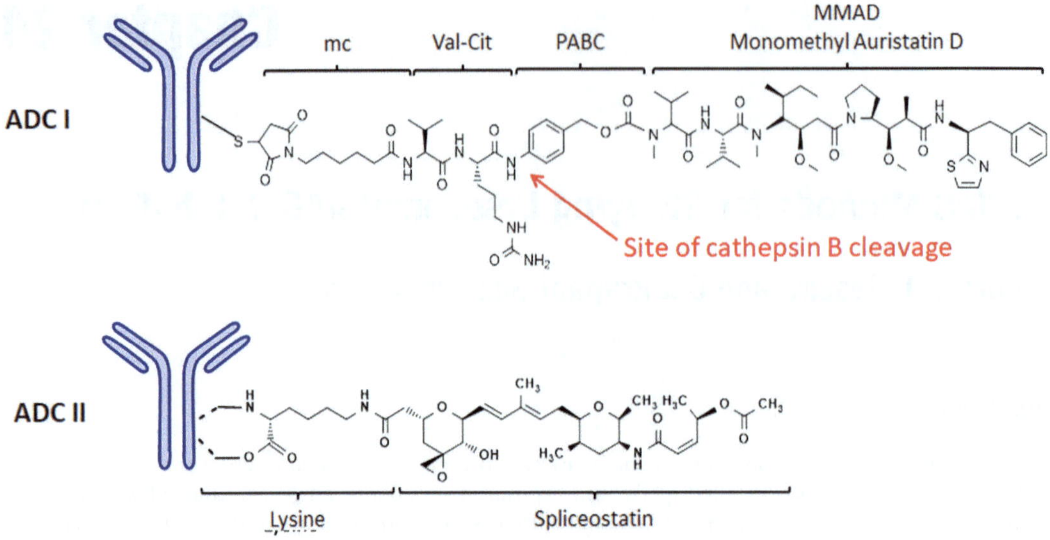

Fig. 1 Structures of ADCs I and II. ADC I contains the cleavable-linker maleimide-caproyl valine-citrulline *p*-amino benzyl carbamate (mc-vc-PABC) with the cytotoxic payload monomethyl auristatin D (MMAD). ADC II is non-cleavable, with the cytotoxic spliceostatin payload conjugated through lysine residues on the antibody. The primary released species is the lysine-spliceostatin moiety

contain a specific chemical or enzymatic trigger for payload release, but instead rely on antibody catabolism by lysosomal enzymes for production of an active small-molecule moiety [9, 10]. In this type of ADC, the active product may contain the cytotoxic molecule as a unit with the linker and one or more amino acids from the site of conjugation to the antibody. Figure 1 shows a representative ADC containing a cleavable linker (ADC I), in which vc-PABC connects the cytotoxic payload monomethyl auristatin D (MMAD) to cysteine residues on the antibody through a maleimide-caproyl moiety.

The dipeptide linker valine-citrulline-PABC is a substrate for cathepsin B, which upon cleavage results in the release of CO_2 and the *p*-aminobenzyl moiety, freeing MMAD inside of the tumor cell. ADC II is a representative non-cleavable ADC, in which the spliceostatin payload is conjugated directly to lysine residues on the antibody. Upon adequate exposure to lysosomal enzymes (other than cathepsin B), antibody catabolism occurs, ultimately releasing the lysine-bonded spliceostatin as the cytotoxic component.

Because of the variety of mechanisms that may be employed to release a cytotoxic molecule into the cell via an ADC, one step in the development of an ADC therapy should include a determination of the identity of the released species [11]. The LC/MS method(s) used to investigate this needs to be appropriate for detection and measurement of anticipated products, but general enough to discover any unanticipated species as well. Thus, every advantage should be employed during the development of the method to ensure optimal chromatography and MS, UV, etc., detection parameters. Any available standards, such as the free payload, linker-payload, or amino acid-capped linker-payload, as appropriate, should be used to inform this process.

The usual strategies of metabolite identification by LC/MS used in small-molecule research [12, 13] also apply to ADC released-species analysis. Incubations should be conducted such that dosed samples can be compared with matrix (non-dosed) controls. Also, because a number of peptides may be released as a result of lysosomal degradation of the antibody, incubations of the naked (nonconjugated) mAb are also advantageous. With these samples in hand, LC/MS data should be collected in a comparative manner to facilitate interrogation either manually or with the aid of software.

A general analytical approach to the analysis of the released species from an ADC will be described below, based upon success with several different types of payloads [14]. However, for best results, the LC/MS method should be tailored to the specific ADC being investigated.

2 Materials

All aqueous solutions should be prepared with ultrapure water (18 MΩ-cm at 25 °C). All solvents should be HPLC grade, and other reagents should be analytical grade.

2.1 Enzymatic Incubations

1. Sodium acetate buffer: 50 mM sodium acetate, pH 5.0. Add approximately 100 mL of water to a 1 L graduated cylinder or beaker. Weigh out 4.101 g of sodium acetate and add it to the vessel. Fill with water to approximately 900 mL, then mix well. Adjust the pH to 5.0 with sulfuric acid, then dilute to 1 L with water (*see* **Note 1**). Store the solution at room temperature.
2. Final incubation buffer: 2 mM tris-carboxyethyl phosphine·HCl (TCEP) in 50 mM sodium acetate, pH 5.0. Weigh 5.72 mg of TCEP·HCl and dissolve in 10 mL of 50 mM sodium acetate, pH 5.0. This solution should be freshly prepared before the experiment (*see* **Note 2**).
3. Lysosomal enzymes: Human lysosomal enzymes, Sekisui Xenotech product H0610.L, 2.5 mg/mL (*see* **Note 3**). Store this product at −80 °C until needed. Thaw the lysosomal enzymes on ice immediately prior to use. Afterwards, the unused portion of the vial can be re-frozen and thawed multiple times.

2.2 LC/MS Analysis

1. Mass spectrometer capable of data-dependent MS/MS analysis, with data processing software (*see* **Note 4**).

2. HPLC column: Halo C18, 3.0 × 100 mm, 2.7 micrometer particle size (or a comparable column, *see* **Note 5**).
3. Mobile phase: 0.1% formic acid in water (solvent "A"); acetonitrile (solvent "B").

3 Methods

3.1 Incubation Methods

1. Have a water bath heated to 37 °C at the ready.
2. Prepare labeled Eppendorf tubes containing 250 μL cold acetonitrile to quench timepoint samples from all incubations (*see* **Note 6**). For non-cleavable linker ADCs, plan to collect samples at time 0, 1, 4, and 18 h, at minimum. Cleavable linker ADCs may only require 2–6 h to go to completion, depending on incubation conditions and the location of the linker-payload (*see* **Note 7**). Buffer control incubations containing the ADC but lacking enzymes, and matrix controls containing enzymes but lacking the ADC should also be prepared and sampled in the same way.
3. Prepare all incubation mixtures on ice. The final volume should be 250 μL, made up primarily of incubation buffer (2 mM TCEP in 50 mM sodium acetate, pH 5.0; *see* **Note 8**). Dilute the lysosomal enzymes in buffer such that the final concentration (after the ADC solution is added in **step 4**) will be 0.125 mg/mL. The final ADC concentration in the incubation mixtures should be 1–5 μM, but this will be added in the next step.
4. At "Time 0 h", start the reactions by addition of the ADC to all non-control incubations. Mix the solution with the pipet, then remove a 50 μL aliquot and quench it immediately in the appropriate quench tube prepared in **step 2**. Collect "Time 0 h" samples from matrix and buffer control incubations at this time. As each tube is sampled, place it in the 37 °C water bath.
5. Remove additional aliquots at the predetermined timepoints and quench in ACN as above (*see* **Note 9**).
6. Store quenched timepoint samples in a freezer until needed for analysis.

3.2 Sample Processing

1. Remove samples from the freezer to thaw.
2. Mix the samples thoroughly after they are completely thawed, then centrifuge for 3 min at 13,000 × *g* to pellet the precipitated protein.
3. Transfer the supernatant to a suitable tube for the evaporation of solvent. Evaporate the solvent under vacuum or a stream of N_2; temperatures of 37 °C will accelerate this process (*see* **Note 10**).

4. Reconstitute the residues in 50 μL of the starting mobile phase used for analysis. Be certain that the sample is mixed well, then analyze it as soon as possible.

3.3 LC/MS Analysis

1. Equilibrate the HPLC column with the mobile phase at starting conditions. For reversed-phase applications, which typically work well for the analysis of ADC released species, a gradient of acetonitrile (solvent "B") in 0.1% formic acid (solvent "A") can be utilized as follows: 0–1 min, 5% B; 1–14 min, increase to 70% B; 14.1 min, ramp to 95% B; hold at 95% B until 16 min; 16.1 min, decrease to 5% B; re-equilibrate the column at 5% B until 19 min.
2. Perform calibration of mass spectrometer per manufacturer's instructions. A typical method will use positive-mode electrospray ionization for generation of ions. The method should be set to collect a range of full-scan data from perhaps 100–1500 *m/z*, with data-dependent MS/MS spectra collected in tandem. Be certain to enable the acquisition of MS/MS data from doubly charged ions, as these may well be observed for heavier ADC payloads.
3. The collected full-scan MS data should be interrogated for the presence of expected products. The collisionally induced dissociation (CID) spectra of these should be correlated with the structure to a degree sufficient to give confidence in the identification. Unknown products may be identified using a combination of techniques including mass defect filtering (for high-resolution instruments), precursor-ion scanning, isotope-ratio methods, etc. (*see* **Notes 11** and **12**, and refs. 12, 13). The details of these techniques are beyond the scope of this chapter.

4 Notes

1. Alternatively, commercial 3 M sodium acetate, pH 5.2 can be used and diluted down to 50 mM. Note that the pH may be less than 5.0 after dilution, so allow for adjustment of the pH before bringing up to the final volume.
2. Either 2 mM TCEP or 2 mM DTT in 50 mM sodium acetate, pH 5.0 will work for ADCs with cathepsin B-cleavable linkers or for ADCs with payloads directly conjugated to amino acids of the antibody. Some ADCs (for example, those with linker-payloads containing disulfide bonds) may be adversely affected by the reducing agent. In these cases, it may not be feasible to utilize this technique. The stability of the ADC to the buffer should be carefully evaluated by use of the buffer control (i.e., those lacking enzyme) incubations.

3. Human liver S9 fraction (20 mg/mL protein, diluted to 1 mg/mL in the final incubation mixture) can also be used as a source of lysosomal enzymes, but it contains many other extraneous materials which will make the analysis of the data more complicated due to the additional LC/MS background peaks. For cathepsin B cleavable ADCs, purified human cathepsin B is commercially available, and can be used at 1–5 U/mL. Cathepsin B may not work for non-cleavable ADCs, and even for some ADCs containing a cleavable linker, the site of conjugation may hinder or prevent the enzyme from fully releasing the payload.
4. A high-resolution mass spectrometer such as a Thermo Orbitrap or a QToF instrument provides the greatest utility for identification or verification of ADC released species. High-resolution MS provides the greatest confidence in the conclusions from these studies by enabling the use of advanced techniques, such as mass defect filtering. However, if a high-resolution mass spectrometer is not available, it is possible to utilize instruments such as an AB Sciex Q-trap or any triple quadrupole instrument, although with a greater burden on the analyst for data interpretation, and perhaps reduced confidence in the completeness of the results. The capability for MS/MS data collection is critical for this work, however. Additionally, an in-line UV detector may also be beneficial.
5. A large variety of HPLC columns is available, and many of these will likely work well. Method development should be started using a column that is already on hand, and this need not be changed if adequate retention and peak shape are observed with standards or incubations of test ADCs yielding known products.
6. For very labile ADCs, such as some cathepsin B-cleavable ADCs, cold acetonitrile may not stop the reaction quickly, and thus the released product may be observed in the "Time 0 h" sample. If this poses a problem, it may be addressed by the addition of protease inhibitors such as CA074 [15] to the quench solution, and/or a reduction in the amount of lysosomal enzyme used. The exact conditions will need to be determined experimentally if it is important to have a true "Time 0 h" sample, for example, if a kinetic time-course of payload release were being measured.
7. The sampling times and details of sample analysis can be tailored to the overall research goals. For example, if a series of cleavable linker ADCs are being compared by analysis of relative release rates, then a shorter incubation time (2–6 h) may be used. If the released entity is already known, then a simpler quantitative MS method can be used which employs Multiple Reaction Monitoring (MRM), for example, and shorter

chromatography. In the authors' experience, non-cleavable linker ADCs will require overnight incubation times and a more comprehensive method of analysis [14].

8. An acidic incubation pH is very important. ADC solutions may be slightly alkaline, so if there is any doubt about the final pH of the incubation (due to the use of a relatively large volume of a dilute ADC solution, for example), then the pH of the incubation mixture should be checked. The enzyme activity will be reduced as the pH of the incubation approaches neutral conditions.

9. For quantitative methods in which the released payload is well known, the chromatography can be developed in such a way that the starting mobile phase contains a high percentage of ACN, which may obviate the need to evaporate the solvent from quenched samples, as described subsequently in "Sample Processing." This does not lend itself to the analysis of unknown released species, since it may be difficult to achieve adequate chromatographic resolution for thorough data analysis.

10. **Steps 2** through **4** may be problematic for payloads containing chemically labile groups, such as epoxides. In these cases, heat should be avoided, and the minimum time should be used for evaporation of solvent. In extreme cases, an HPLC column suitable for the analysis of proteins can be used in the LC/MS method in order to avoid the necessity of precipitating proteins. For this approach, the timepoint samples from **steps 2** to **4** under Incubation Methods should not be quenched in acetonitrile, but rather should be quickly frozen upon collection. When thawed, the samples should be thoroughly centrifuged, and the supernatant analyzed as quickly as possible using the protein HPLC column. This has the advantage of minimizing unintended alteration of the analytes during sample processing, but adds the complication of additional protein (mAb) peaks in the MS and UV data set, which can be a major interference in the analysis. Additionally, the lysosomal enzymes may still be active upon sample thawing, so a true "Time 0 h" sample may be difficult to achieve.

11. To illustrate, Fig. 2 shows chromatograms following the incubation of ADC II with lysosomal enzymes for 18 h. The major peaks originating from the ADC are clearly observable by comparison of the 18-h ADC sample with the 18-h Matrix Blank sample, which contained lysosomal enzymes but not the ADC. Many of the observable peaks in the ADC incubation are peptides resulting from degradation of the mAb, and these do not contain the spliceostatin payload [16]. One of the more abundant is the peptide ALPAPIE, with *m/z* 710.409^{+}, which

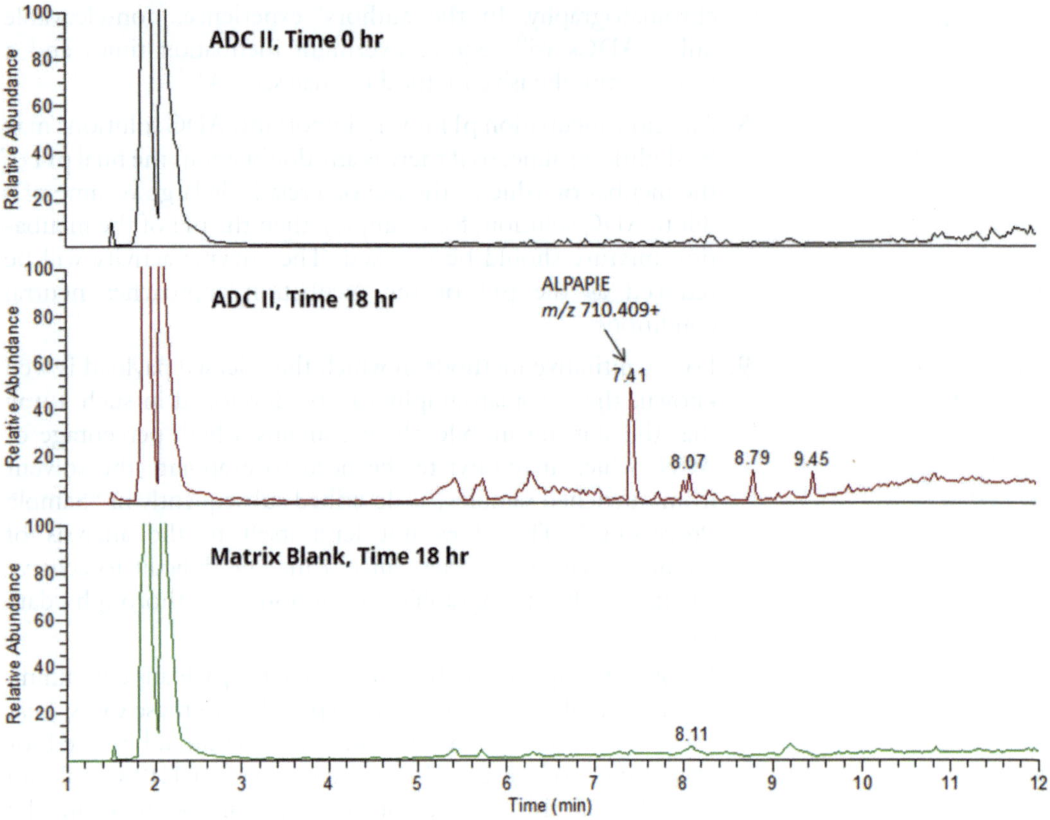

Fig. 2 Chromatograms of non-cleavable ADC II containing the cytotoxic spliceostatin payload conjugated through lysine residues on the antibody. ADC-related peaks can clearly be observed by comparison of the 18-h ADC sample to the 18-h matrix blank sample

is observed at 7.41 min. A combination of approaches can be used to identify peaks which contain the payload moiety, as described in refs. 12, 13. For example, by taking advantage of the propensity of the spliceostatin payload to lose acetic acid under CID conditions in the mass spectrometer, the constant neutral loss (NL) technique was employed to discover payload-related peaks which contain the acetate ester. Figure 3 shows a comparison of the full-scan MS data from ADC II in the upper pane, and in the lower pane a subset of the data which shows peaks from the CID spectra which have undergone a 60.02 Da loss, which is due to fragmentation of the acetate ester bond, leading to the loss of acetic acid. The spliceostatin-containing peaks are nicely visualized by this method. Note that any products for which the ester has already been hydrolyzed will be "invisible" to this particular line of interrogation.

12. Because of the expectation of free MMAD being released from ADC I due to the cleavable linker, methods were developed using standards of MMAD. In our incubation of ADC I, no

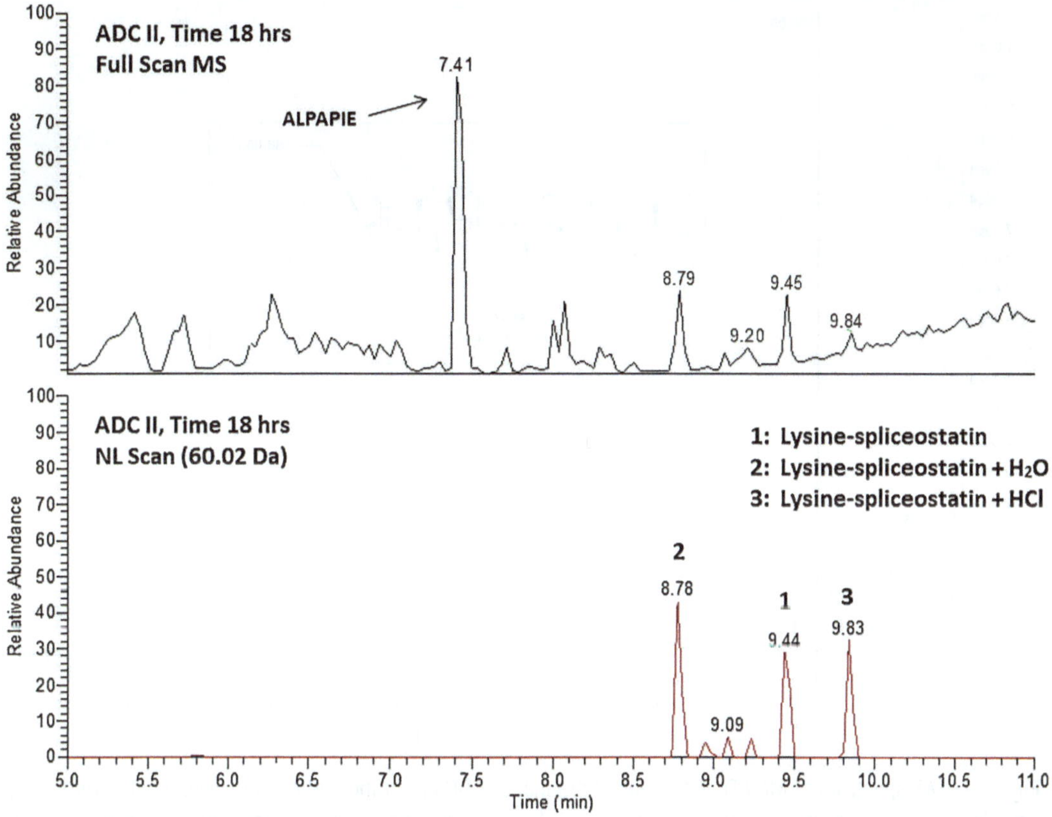

Fig. 3 Chromatograms of non-cleavable ADC II after 18 h of incubation with lysosomal enzymes. The upper pane shows the full-scan MS data, while the lower pane shows only peaks which have lost 60.02 Da in the MS/MS spectra due to the facile loss of acetic acid from the spliceostatin payload. Peaks labeled 2 and 3 are hydrolysis products most likely resulting from epoxide ring opening

other payload containing products were observed after 18 h. For purposes of illustration, however, Fig. 4 shows the CID fragmentation pattern of MMAD, in which a strong fragment ion is observed at *m/z* 188.053. This fragmentation lends itself to the precursor-ion scanning technique, in which sample components which lose *m/z* 188.053 upon CID can be identified and the masses of the parent related back to the ADC. This technique is a good way to find unexpected payload-related components, with the caveat that it will only show species in which this ion is not modified or already lost through chemical or metabolic processes. An instrument capable of all-ions fragmentation, SWATH, or a comparable method can be used for this, or, if high-resolution instruments are not available, hybrid instruments such as a quadrupole-ion trap or a triple quadrupole can be used.

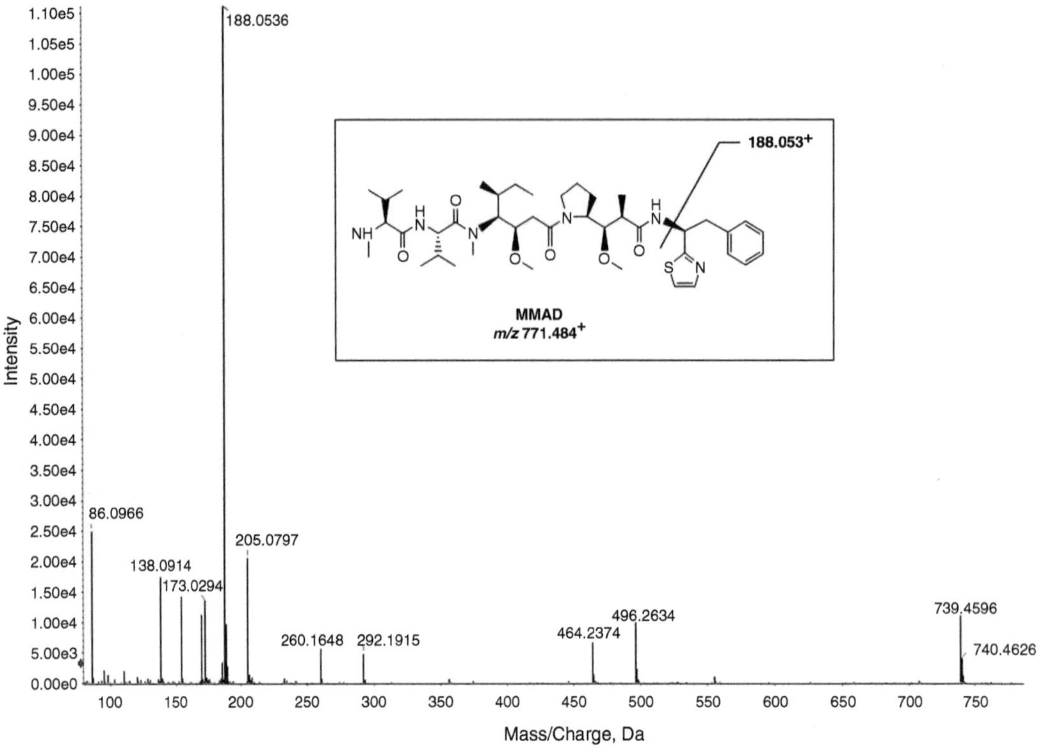

Fig. 4 MS/MS spectrum of MMAD, the released product of ADC I after incubation with lysosomal enzymes. An abundant fragment ion is observed at *m/z* 188.053 Da. This provides a convenient way to observe products which contain the auristatin payload by use of the precursor-ion scanning technique, provided that this moiety is not lost or modified chemically or through metabolism

References

1. Aboud-Pirak E, Sergent T, Otte-Slachmuylder-C, Abarca J, Trouet A, Schneider YJ (1988) Binding and endocytosis of a monoclonal antibody to a high molecular weight human milk fat globule membrane-associated antigen by cultured MCF-7 breast carcinoma cells. Cancer Res 48:3188–3196
2. Sutherland MS, Sanderson RJ, Gordon KA et al (2006) Lysosomal trafficking and cysteine protease metabolism confer target-specific cytotoxicity by peptide-linked anti-CD30-auristatin conjugates. J Biol Chem 281:10540–10547
3. Omelyanenko V, Gentry C, Kopeckova P, Kopecek J (1998) HPMA copolymer-anticancer drug-OV-TL16 antibody conjugates. II. Processing in epithelial ovarian carcinoma cells in vitro. Int J Cancer 75:600–608
4. Hamann PR, Hinman LM, Beyer CF et al (2002) An anti-CD33 antibody-calicheamicin conjugate for treatment of acute myeloid leukemia. Choice of linker. Bioconjug Chem 13:40–46
5. Doronina SO, Toki BE, Torgov MY, Mendelsohn BA et al (2003) Development of potent monoclonal antibody auristatin conjugates for cancer therapy. Nat Biotechnol 21:778–784
6. Willner D, Trail PA, Hofstead SJ et al (1993) (6-Maleimidocaproyl)hydrazone of doxorubicin--a new derivative for the preparation of immunoconjugates of doxorubicin. Bioconjug Chem 4:521–527
7. Braslawsky GR, Kadow K, Knipe J, McGoff K et al (1991) Adriamycin(hydrazone)-antibody conjugates require internalization and intracellular acid hydrolysis for antitumor activity. Cancer Immunol Immunother 33:367–374
8. Dubowchik GM, Firestone RA, Padilla L et al (2002) Cathepsin B-labile dipeptide linkers for lysosomal release of doxorubicin from internalizing immunoconjugates: model studies of enzymatic drug release and antigen-specific

in vitro anticancer activity. Bioconjug Chem 13:855–869

9. Doronina SO, Mendelsohn BA, Bovee TD, Cerveny CG et al (2006) Enhanced activity of monomethylauristatin F through monoclonal antibody delivery: effects of linker technology on efficacy and toxicity. Bioconjug Chem 17:114–124
10. Erickson HK, Park PU, Widdison WC, Kovtun YV et al (2006) Antibody-maytansinoid conjugates are activated in targeted cancer cells by lysosomal degradation and linker-dependent intracellular processing. Cancer Res 66:4426–4433
11. Kraynov E, Kamath AV, Walles M et al (2015) Current approaches for ADME characterization of antibody-drug conjugates: an industry white paper. Drug Metab Dispos 44:617–623
12. Zhu M, Zhang H, Humphreys WG (2011) Drug metabolite profiling and identification by high-resolution mass spectrometry. J Biol Chem 286:25419–25425
13. Ma S, Chowdhury SK (2011) Analytical strategies for assessment of human metabolites in preclinical safety testing. Anal Chem 83:5028–5036
14. Bessire AJ, Ballard TE, Charati M, Cohen J et al (2016) Determination of antibody-drug conjugate released payload species using directed in vitro assays and mass spectrometric interrogation. Bioconjug Chem 27:1645–1654
15. Murata M, Miyashita S, Yokoo C et al (1991) Novel epoxysuccinyl peptides. Selective inhibitors of cathepsin B, in vitro. FEBS Lett 280:307–310
16. Puthenveetil S, Loganzo F, He H et al (2016) Natural product splicing inhibitors: a new class of antibody-drug conjugate (ADC) payloads. Bioconjug Chem 27:1880–1888

Chapter 25

Assessing ADC Plasma Stability by LC-MS Methods

Cong Wei

Abstract

Plasma stability of ADCs can have a profound impact on ADC efficacy and safety. LC-MS methods enable the detection and characterization of ADC to evaluate its stability in plasma. Here we describe a procedure and LC-MS method for assessing ADC plasma stability.

Key words Antibody–drug conjugate (ADC), Immunoaffinity capture, LC-MS, Drug-to-antibody ratio (DAR), Anti-human Fc Ab, Biotinylation

1 Introduction

Antibody–drug conjugates (ADCs) have emerged as an important class of targeted therapeutics for treating cancer. It is important for the ADC to remain stable while in circulation in order to achieve targeted delivery of tumor-fighting payloads and minimize adverse effects on normal cells. LC-MS, involving high-performance liquid chromatography coupled with mass spectrometry, has made a tremendous impact in multiple fields including the characterization and quantification of ADC in biological matrices. Previous methods describe the evaluation of plasma stability by LC-MS for aliquots taken up to 96 h [1]. The drug-to-antibody ratio (DAR) of each incubated sample was demonstrated by LC-MS intact protein analysis; however, the sensitivity could be a challenge at the later time-point samples. Here we describe a procedure and LC-MS method to determine DAR on the reduced ADCs following the immunoaffinity capture (Fig. 1). We have achieved sufficient sensitivity for DAR determination of conventional cysteine-conjugated ADCs up to 144 h incubation (Figs. 2 and 3). A similar procedure has been used to determine both in vitro and in vivo ADC plasma stability for both conventional conjugated ADC and site-specific conjugated ADC [2, 3].

There are also other LC-MS methods for monitoring ADC plasma stability besides determination of DAR profiles. One is to

L. Nathan Tumey (ed.), *Antibody-Drug Conjugates: Methods and Protocols*, Methods in Molecular Biology, vol. 2078, https://doi.org/10.1007/978-1-4939-9929-3_25,

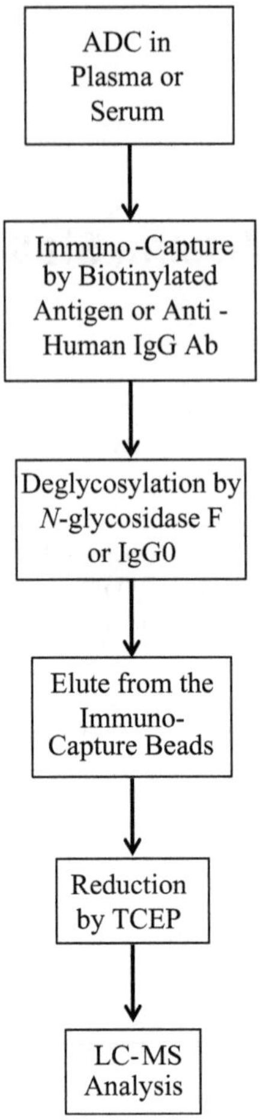

Fig. 1 Schematic illustration of sample preparation workflows for DAR analysis on reduced or fragmented ADC

quantify the total conjugated payload using cathepsin cleavage following the immunoaffinity capture of ADC [3]. This method may provide better sensitivity and allows a quantitative evaluation than the DAR determination for ADC plasma stability assessment. Furthermore, in the supernatant after the immunoaffinity capture of ADC, use of an anti-payload antibody or an anti-albumin antibody can capture the migrated payloads forming adducts with albumin in the plasma samples for stability assessment [3]. Quantification of the migrated payloads using cathepsin B cleavage following the capture of payload-albumin adducts can provide a quantitative assessment on the payload migration level of ADC stability. On the other hand, quantification of free payload (unconjugated payload) using a simple step of acetonitrile crash in the plasma incubation samples can give a quantitative estimate on the level of free released payload for ADC plasma stability assessment [2, 3].

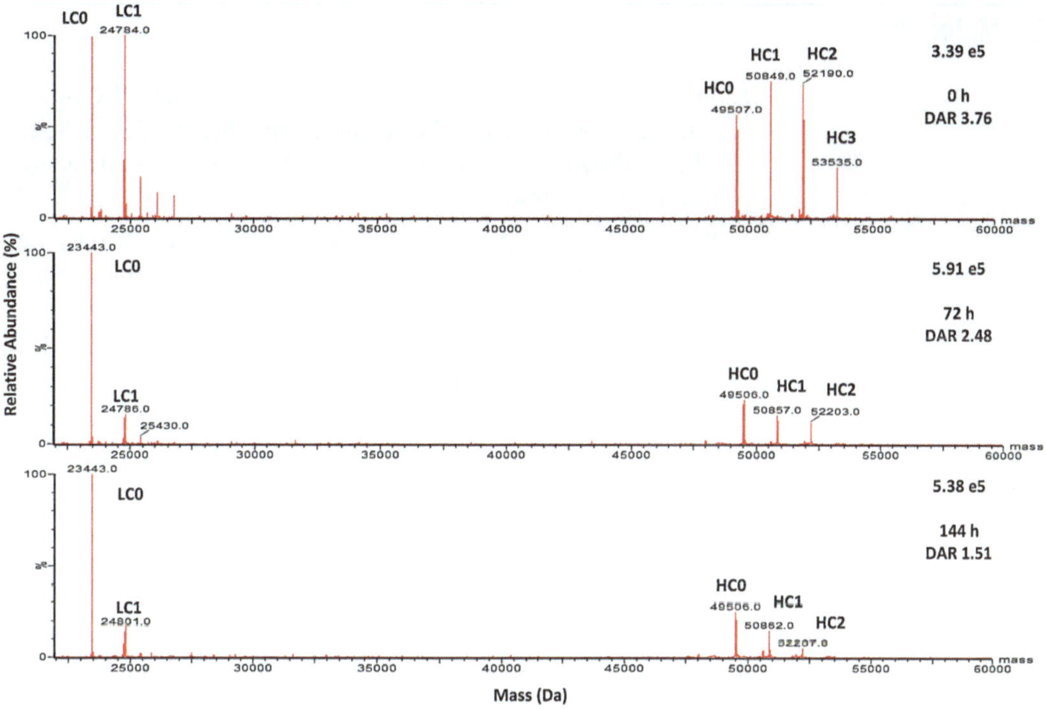

Fig. 2 Representative mass spectra of conventional cysteine-conjugated ADC for DAR determination from plasma incubation at 0, 72, and 144 h. LC0 and LC1 are the intensity (AUC) of the signal for the light chain with 0 and 1 payload, respectively; HC0, HC1, and HC2 are the intensity (AUC) of the signal for the heavy chain with 0, 1, and 2 payloads, respectively. The average DAR values are calculated using the intensity of each peak. For example, the average DAR value at 72 h for this sample was calculated as 2.48

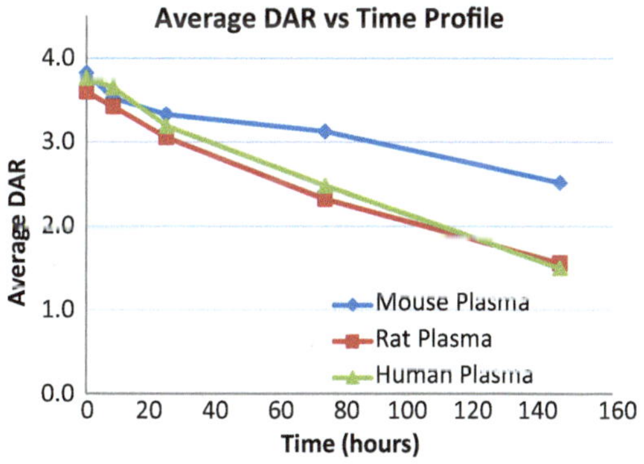

Fig. 3 Average DAR profiles of a conventional cysteine-conjugated ADC Trastuzumab-maleimido-caproyl-valine-citruline-p-amino-benzyloxy-carbonyl-payload from the in vitro plasma incubation

2 Materials

1. High-performance liquid chromatography (HPLC)-grade water and acetonitrile (ACN) are from Thermo Fisher Scientific (Waltham, MA). All other reagents and solvents are analytical or HPLC grade.
2. Water used in the procedure is HPLC-grade water or ultrapure water (prepared by purifying deionized water, to attain a sensitivity of 18 MΩ-cm at 25 °C).
3. Dulbecco's Phosphate Buffered Saline (PBS) is obtained from Lonza (Walkersville, MD).
4. Fresh mouse, rat, monkey, and human plasma containing sodium heparin are purchased from BioIVT Inc. (Westbury, NY).
5. Biotin-SP-conjugated AffiniPure goat anti-human IgG1 Fcγ fragment-specific antibody (minimal cross-reaction to bovine, horse, and mouse serum proteins) is purchased from Jackson ImmunoResearch Laboratories Inc. (West Grove, PA).
6. Biotinylated goat anti-human IgG1 antibody (minimal cross-reaction to monkey serum proteins) is purchased from Bethyl Laboratories Inc. (Montgomery, TX).
7. IgG0 for deglycosylation is obtained from Genovis Inc. (Cambridge, MA).
8. Tris(2-carboxyethyl)phosphine (TCEP) is purchased from Sigma-Aldrich Chemical Co. (St. Louis, MO).
9. BEH300 C4, 1.7 μm, 0.3 × 100 mm iKey column is from Waters Corporation (Milford, MA).

3 Methods

3.1 Incubation of ADC with Plasma

1. Dilute ADC of interest (~1.5 mg/mL) into mouse, rat, monkey, or human plasma to yield a final solution of 50 μg/mL ADC in plasma (*see* **Notes 1** and **2**). Prepare samples in triplicate with each species of plasma.
2. Incubate the samples at 37 °C under 5% CO_2.
3. Aliquots (50 μL) were taken at four time points (0, 8, 24, 48, 72, and 144 h). Samples are frozen at −80 °C until analysis.
4. All matrix samples are thawed on wet ice.

3.2 Deglycosylation of ADC for DAR Analysis

1. Aliquot 25 μL of plasma/serum samples into 96-well Eppendof protein LoBind plate (*see* **Note 1**).
2. Reconstitute IgG0 into water to prepare 20 U/μL of IgG0 as a stock solution.

3. Add 2.0 μL of IgG0 (20 U/μL) to 48 μL PBS, add 50 μL of this buffer to each tube.
4. Vortex for 5 min at room temperature.
5. Incubate at 37 °C for 1.5 h.

3.3 Immunoaffinity Capture and Reduction for ADC DAR Analysis

1. Add to samples 5 μL of capture antibody [biotinylated anti-human Fcγ fragment specific (1.0 mg/mL) for mouse and rat plasma, biotinylated goat anti-human IgG1 antibody (1.0 mg/mL) for cyno monkey plasma, and biotinylated-antigen or biotinylated anti-idiotype mAb for human plasma].
2. Incubate at 37 °C for 1 h.
3. Incubate for another 1 h at room temperature under gentle shaking.
4. Wash the Dynabead MyOne Streptavidin T1 beads twice with PBS containing 0.05% Tween-20, and then wash the beads twice with PBS.
5. Resuspend the beads in PBS.
6. Add 40 μL of washed beads to each ADC sample.
7. Incubate at room temperature for 40 min under shaking (*see* **Note 3**).
8. Use a magnetic plate to pull down the beads.
9. Wash the samples with 200 μL PBS containing 0.05% Tween-20. Repeat three times (*see* **Note 4**).
10. Wash the samples with 200 μL PBS for two times.
11. Wash the samples with 200 μL water for two times.
12. Elute the bound ADC with 55 μL of 2% of formic acid (FA) in water (v/v) by gently shaking for 15 min.
13. Use a magnetic plate to pull down the beads. Transfer 50 μL aliquot of each sample into a new plate.
14. Add 5 μL of 200 mM TCEP (final conc. 20 mM) to reduce the ADC to light and heavy chain.
15. Gently shake the plate at room temperature for 20 min.

3.4 LC-MS Method for ADC DAR Analysis

1. Set up the mobile phase A as 0.1% FA in water (v/v) and the mobile phase B as 0.1% FA in acetonitrile (v/v) in the HPLC system.
2. Set the LC column temperature at 85 °C.
3. Inject each sample (5 μL) into Xevo G2 Q-TOF mass spectrometer (Waters, Manchester, UK) coupled with nanoAcquity UPLC (Waters) using BEH300 C4, 1.7 μm, 0.3 × 100 mm iKey column, and carry out the intact protein analysis.

4. Perform the chromatographic separation at a flow rate of 0.3 μL/min using a linear gradient of mobile phase B from 5% to 90% over 7 min.
5. Conduct the data acquisition with MassLynx software, and use the mass acquisition range from 700 Da to 2400 Da.
6. Perform the data analysis including deconvolution using Biopharmalynx software (Waters). The following equation was used for average DAR calculation for conventional conjugated ADC:

$$\text{Average DAR} = \left(\frac{LC_1}{(LC_0 + LC_1)} \times 2\right) + \left(\frac{HC_1}{(HC_0 + HC_1 + HC_2 + HC_3)} \times 2\right) + \left(\frac{HC_2}{(HC_0 + HC_1 + HC_2 + HC_3)} \times 4\right) + \left(\frac{HC_3}{(HC_0 + HC_1 + HC_2 + HC_3)} \times 6\right)$$

where LC_0 and LC_1 are the intensity (AUC) of the signal for the light chain with 0 and 1 payload, respectively; HC_0, HC_1, and HC_2 are the intensity (AUC) of the signal for the heavy chain with 0, 1 and 2 payloads, respectively.

4 Notes

1. When the sensitivity is a challenge for DAR determination, it is suggested to increase the ADC incubation concentration (e.g. 200 μg/mL) and/or aliquot higher volume (e.g. 100 μL) for sample preparation.
2. Centrifuging the plasma at 1000 × *g* for 5 min prior to the incubation is recommended in order to remove insoluble proteins.
3. Incubate at room temperature for 40 min with shaking, and make sure the beads are fully suspended.
4. Try to minimize the total wash time to less than 40 min (~5 min/wash), so as to reduce dissociation of payload. Typically, 1 min shake to resuspend the beads, 3.5 min for beads to settle down on magnet, and 1 min to remove wash buffer.

References

1. Shen BQ, Xu K, Liu L et al (2012) Conjugation site modulates the in vivo stability and therapeutic activity of antibody-drug conjugates. Nat Biotechnol 30(2):184–189
2. Grafmuller L, Wei C, Ramanathan R et al (2016) Unconjugated payload quantification and DAR characterization of antibody-drug conjugates using high-resolution MS. Bioanalysis 8 (16):1663–1678
3. Wei C, Zhang G, Clark T et al (2016) Where did the linker-payload go? A quantitative investigation on the destination of the released linker-payload from an antibody-drug conjugate with a Maleimide linker in plasma. Anal Chem 88 (9):4979–4986

Chapter 26

Determination of ADC Concentration by Ligand-Binding Assays

Hsuan-Ping Chang and Dhaval K. Shah

Abstract

Total antibody, conjugated antibody or antibody-conjugated drug, and free drug are key analytes required to establish exposure–response relationships for ADCs. Therefore, bioanalytical strategies for ADCs include ligand-binding assays (LBA) and LC–MS/MS methods. Here we describe detailed methodology to develop a solid-phase-based enzyme-linked immunosorbent assay (ELISA), which is the most widely used LBA to quantify large-molecule components of ADC in biological matrices such as plasma, serum, tumor, or tissue homogenates. The approach presented here is designed to quantify total antibody concentrations in ADC containing samples, and can be easily adapted to quantify conjugated antibody concentrations.

Key words Antibody–drug conjugate (ADC), Biodistribution, Ligand-binding assay (LBA), Pharmacokinetics (PK), ELISA, Sandwich ELISA

1 Introduction

A ligand-binding assay (LBA) can be defined as an assay in which the key step is an equilibrium reaction between the ligand (analyte) and the binding molecule (e.g. a protein or antibody) that is directed against the ligand of interest. The end point of this reaction typically reflects the concentration of the analytes present in the sample. LBA can assume a variety of forms and include various reagents. For example, the ligand-binding molecules can be antibodies, antibody fragments, receptors, transport proteins, or even oligonucleotides. Techniques to detect and quantify the reaction end point can include radioactivity, fluorescence, luminescence, chemiluminescence, and UV/visible spectrometry. The LBA format can also take the form of a competitive or noncompetitive assay, with solution- or solid-phase configurations. This flexibility in the methodology allows LBAs to be developed for a variety of purposes, and these assays generally provide high sensitivity and high throughput. In fact, most of the pharmacokinetics (PK)

L. Nathan Tumey (ed.), *Antibody-Drug Conjugates: Methods and Protocols*, Methods in Molecular Biology, vol. 2078,
https://doi.org/10.1007/978-1-4939-9929-3_26,

determinations and immunogenicity assessments for biotherapeutics are performed using LBA. Out of all the LBA formats, solid-phase-based enzyme-linked immunosorbent assay (ELISA), which utilizes a nonradioactive reaction end point, is the most widely used format for the assessment of biotherapeutics PK [1, 2].

Measurement of ADC PK in the biological samples presents a unique challenge due to its complex molecular structure. Typically, three different analytes including total antibody, antibody-conjugated drug or conjugated antibody, and free drug are measured to correlate with the efficacy or toxicity of ADCs. Consequently, the bioanalysis strategy for ADCs usually require large-molecule LBA methods and small-molecule LC-MS/MS methods [3, 4]. Based on the binding properties of the analyte and the assay reagents, LBA methods can be used to quantify total antibody concentration (i.e. antibody with or without drug attached) or conjugated antibody concentrations (i.e. antibody with one or more drugs attached) [4, 5]. Using capture and detection reagents that bind to the antibody component of the ADC enables quantification of total antibody. This approach has been applied in several ADC studies, including anti-CD33-Calicheamicin ADC [6]; T-DM1 [7], and mAb-MMAE conjugates [8–13]. On the other hand, applying a capture or detection reagent that binds to the conjugated drug component of the ADC enables quantification of conjugated-antibody [4]. Many studies have utilized anti-drug-specific antibody as a capture antibody to quantify conjugated antibody [5, 7, 14–17], whereas some studies have used anti-drug antibody as a detection reagent [5, 11, 18–21].

In this chapter, we describe a sandwich ELISA method to quantify total antibody concentrations in biological matrices such as plasma, serum, tumor, or tissue homogenates. This sandwich ELISA method can be easily adapted to quantification of conjugated antibody concentrations. However, it should be noted that conjugated antibody ELISA is very sensitive to the choice of the anti-drug antibody, and therefore the key aspect in such assay development is to identify an anti-drug antibody that is minimally influenced by the drug load (i.e. Drug:Antibody Ratio or DAR) [5]. Figure 1a, b show a representative sandwich ELISA arrangement to quantify total-antibody and conjugated-antibody concentrations, respectively. A detailed diagram describing the sandwich ELISA procedure employed by us to quantify total-antibody concentrations is presented in Fig. 2.

2 Materials

Prepare all solutions using ultrapure water (prepared by reverse osmosis to attain a specific resistance of 18 MΩ at 22 °C). All

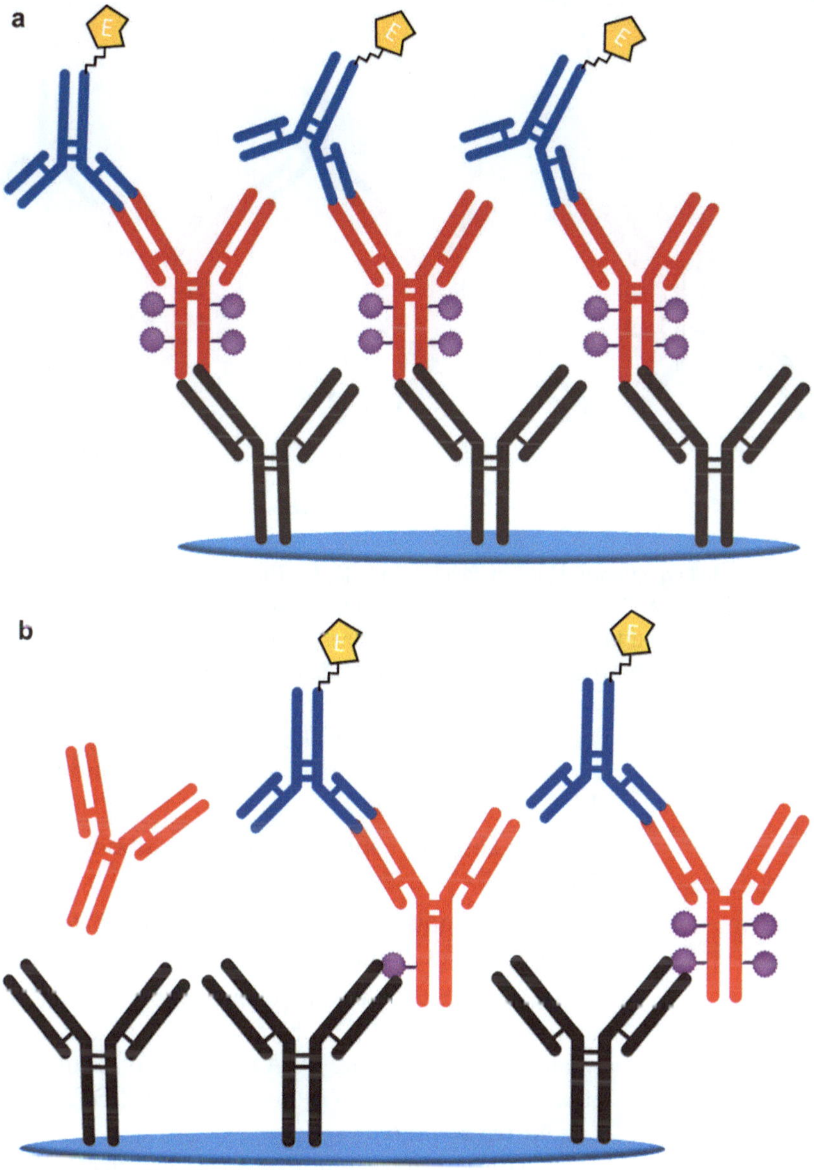

Fig. 1 Representative sandwich ELISA arrangements to measure ADC components. (**a**) Total-antibody ELISA; (**b**) Conjugated-antibody ELISA

reagents should be stored at 4 °C (unless indicated) and warmed up to room temperature before use.

1. ELISA microplates: 96- or 384-well, polystyrene-based hydrophilic passive binding surface (*see* **Note 1**).
2. Blocking buffer: 1× PBS or 1× TBS containing 1% bovine serum albumin (*see* **Note 2**).
3. Wash buffer: for PBS-based wash buffer use 0.05% v/v Tween 20 in 1× PBS, for tris-based wash buffer dissolve 6.06 g tris

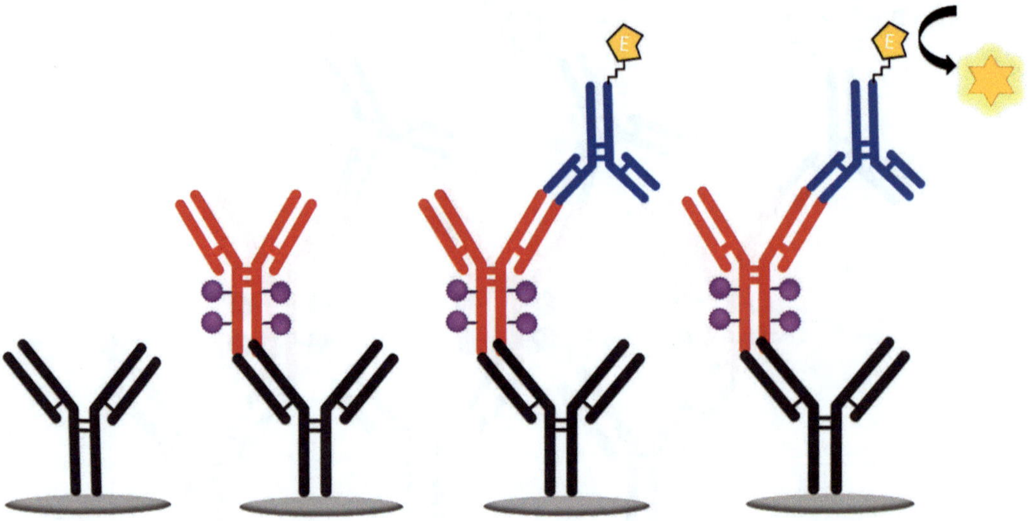

Fig. 2 A schematic detailing different steps of sandwich ELISA. (1) The plate is coated with primary antibody; (2) sample is added and the ADC is allowed to bind to the primary antibody; (3) enzyme-conjugated secondary antibody is added and allowed to bind to the sample; (4) finally, the substrate is added and converted to a colored product by the enzyme, which is read by an appropriate detector

base, 8.2 g NaCl, and 6.0 mL 6 M HCL in 1 L distilled water (adjust the pH between 7.2 and 7.8, and conductivity between 14,000 and 16,000).

4. Primary antibody: anti-human IgG antibody (Fc-specific) (*see* **Note 3**).
5. Secondary antibody: Alkaline phosphatase (AP) conjugated anti-human IgG antibody (Fab specific) (*see* **Note 4**).
6. Substrate: PNPP (*p*-nitrophenyl phosphate disodium salt), diethanolamine (DEA) substrate buffer (5×, 5.1 M diethanolamine, pH 9.8). Dilute DEA from 5× to 1× using dH_2O, and dissolve each mg of PNPP in 1 mL of 1× DEA (*see* **Notes 5** and **6**).
7. Microplate reader: equipped with absorbance, fluorescence, luminescence, or other read modes, along with programmable kinetic endpoint measurement via multiple-wavelength linear scan or area scan.
8. ADC standard: ADC stock solution, which should be made with the same batch of ADC that is in the analytes (*see* **Notes 7–9**). In this example, for quantification of trastuzumab-vc-MMAE in plasma or tissue homogenates, ADC standard curve ranging from 1000 ng/mL to 0.98 ng/mL was generated. An 11-point standard curve generated using two-fold serial dilutions from ADC stock solution is recommended. Prepare at least 120 μL volume for each standard concentration.

3 Methods

All procedures are carried out at room temperature, unless otherwise indicated.

1. Prepare primary antibody-coated 384-well ELISA microplates as following. Add 60 μL of anti-human IgG-F(ab′)2 fragment cross-adsorbed antibody (5 μg/mL, diluted in 20 mM Na_2HPO_4) per each well of the 384-well plate. Cover the plates with 384-well plate lids or plastic film sheets. Incubate the plates at 4 °C overnight or at room temperature for 2 h (*see* **Note 10**).
2. At the end of incubation, remove the excess primary antibody solution, and wash the plate with washing buffer followed by deionized water for a total of three times. Block the remaining reactive sites by adding 90 μL of blocking buffer (1% BSA prepared in PBS or TBS) per well. Cover the plate and incubate for 1 h at room temperature on a horizontal orbital microplate shaker (e.g. 0.125″ orbit, set at 500 ± 50 rpm) (*see* **Notes 11** and **12**).
3. Add samples and standards to the plate. For analyzing our representative ADC trastuzumab-vc-MMAE, we add 30 μL of sample per well (*see* **Note 13**). Seal the plate with plastic film and incubate at room temperature for 2 h on a horizontal orbital microplate shaker.
4. Wash the plate with washing buffer followed by deionized water for three times, and add the secondary antibody (30 μL per well). In this example, cross-adsorbed alkaline phosphatase (AP) conjugated $F(ab')_2$ fragment of human IgG antibody (0.5 mg/mL), diluted 1:2500 in washing buffer, is added to the plate. Seal the plate with plastic film and incubate at room temperature for 1 h on a horizontal orbital microplate shaker.
5. Wash the plate with washing buffer followed by deionized water for three times. To detect the AP conjugated antibody, add 30 μL of PNPP substrate (1 mg/mL diluted in 1× DEA) per well (*see* **Notes 14** and **15**).
6. Read the change in absorbance using kinetic mode at 405 nm for 40 min, using microplate reader (*see* **Note 16**). Total antibody concentrations are calculated by interpolation from a four parametric standard curve. Figure 3 shows a representative standard curve, along with a fitted curve, generated using a total antibody ELISA developed for ADCs.

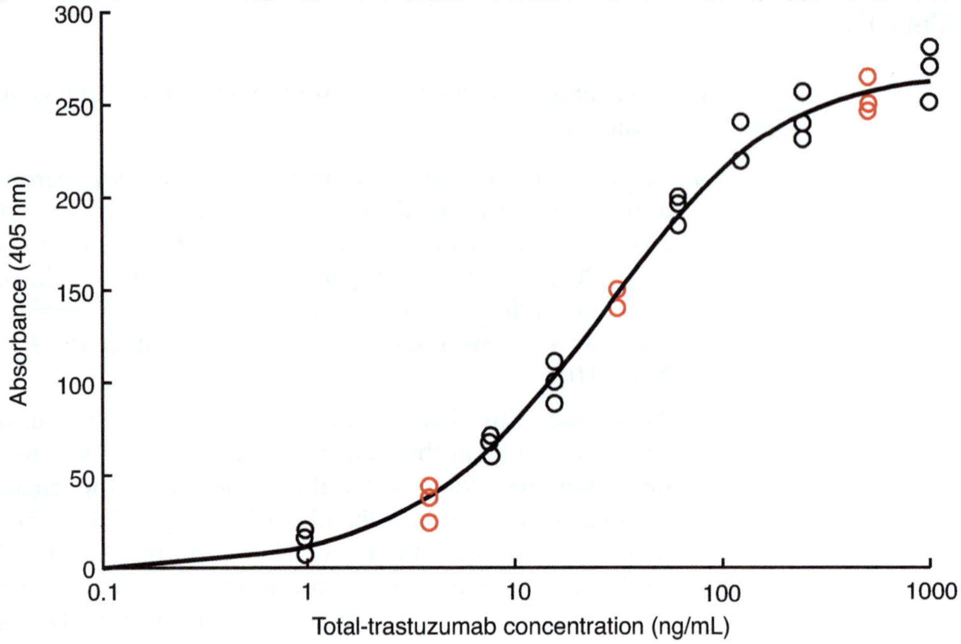

Fig. 3 Representative standard curve from an ELISA performed to quantify total antibody concentrations in ADC containing tissue matrix. Solid line represents curve fitting using a 4-parameter equation. Open circles are measured signals at each ADC concentrations

4 Notes

1. The polystyrene-based hydrophilic passive binding surface of microplate binds to high amounts of IgG. The choice of 96- or 384-well depends on the amount and the number of the samples. The working volume for 96-well and 384-well are 40–280 μL and 10–130 μL, respectively. In this example, we have used 384-well microplate.
2. Commercial product such as package powder dissolved in 1 L of distilled or deionized water, or 10× PBS or 10× TBS further diluted into 1× solution can be used. Please store the blocking solution at 4 °C.
3. It is important to evaluate the nonspecific cross-reactivity of antibodies. For rodent studies, choose antibodies with minimum reactivity to mouse and rat. Usually the cross-reactivity is less between the goat anti-human IgG antibody and the goat anti-mouse IgG antibody. Both monoclonal and polyclonal antibodies can be used as the capture and detection antibodies in sandwich ELISA. Monoclonal antibodies provide monospecificity toward a single epitope, which allows fine detection and quantitation of small differences in antigen. Often a polyclonal antibody is used as the capture antibody to catch as much

antigen as possible, and a monoclonal is used as the detecting antibody to provide improved specificity. Polyclonal antibodies are generally less expensive (about fivefold) to produce than monoclonal antibodies, and thus the selection of these molecules should be based on cost and specificity criteria.

4. Alkaline phosphatase (AP) and horseradish peroxidase (HRP) are commonly used enzymes conjugated to secondary antibodies.

5. PNPP diluted in DEA buffer is widely used to detect AP. The reaction produces a water-soluble yellow product that absorbs light at 405 nm. Commonly used substrates for HRP include OPD (*o*-phenylenediamine dihydrochloride), TMB (3,3′,5,5-′-tetramethylbenzidine), and ABTS (2,2′-Azinobis [3-ethylbenzothiazoline-6-sulfonic acid]-diammonium salt). OPD, TMS, and ABTS turn in to amber, blue, and green colors after the reaction with HRP.

6. DEA is effective at concentrations from 10 mM to 1 M.

7. ADC concentration is determined by comparing the sample response to that of a standard whose concentration is known. Samples and standards should be processed in the same manner by mixing them with same matrix or reagent. In addition, samples and standards should be prepared in the same plate and the absorbances should be measured in the same run. Dilution factor should be pre-optimized in order to let the sample concentrations lie within the standard curve range. Dilution factor should be kept consistent between sample and standard.

8. Based on our experience, for quantifying total antibody in ADC samples the standard curve should be made using ADC stock solution (e.g. trastuzumab-vc-MMAE) and not antibody (e.g. trastuzumab) stock solution. For example, same batch of trastuzumab-vc-MMAE stock solution, but not pure trastuzumab, should be used to establish the standard curve for trastuzumab-vc-MMAE quantification. We have compared two standards curves generated by either trastuzumab-vc-MMAE or trastuzumab stock solutions. The signals for ADC standard curves are lower than trastuzumab standard curve. As such, one can erroneously report lower concentrations of total antibody in the ADC sample if the standard curve generated using pure antibody.

9. Prepare standard curve by making serial dilutions of the ADC stock to obtain a desired range of concentrations. Here, trastuzumab-vc-MMAE is used as a standard, and the optimal range of standard curve is around 1–500 ng/mL for plasma, tumor, and most of the tissue samples. When conducting serial dilutions, make two- or three-fold dilutions and avoid large

single-step dilutions. If the dilution is more than 500-fold, use multiple steps. Avoid dilutions that require pipetting a small volume (<5 μL). Mix each dilution well, but avoid creating bubbles or foaming. Always include a negative control (i.e. matrix without analyte).

10. We recommend to centrifuge the microplate at 800 rpm for 30 s after adding the primary antibody.
11. We also recommend to centrifuge the microplate at 800 rpm for 30 s after adding the blocking buffer.
12. Washing buffer volume should be higher than the coating buffer volume added to each well. In this example, we use 3 cycles of washing. Do not let the plate dry between wash steps. After finishing the wash, you can turn the plate upside-down and tap the plate gently on paper towels to remove residual buffer.
13. After adding samples, we do not recommend to centrifuge the microplate. Centrifugation may cause precipitation of components in the matrix, especially for tissue samples, resulting in heterogeneous distribution of samples in the wells.
14. PNPP solution should be prepared fresh just before the use. Protect it from light. Discard unused reagent.
15. Before washing the microplate, we recommend to run plate dimension optimization for the plate reader. This enables the plate reader to determine the exact positioning of the plate being used. During this time, the position of each corner well of the plate is measured.
16. Since in this example the kinetic mode of reading is used, the plate should be read immediately (i.e. in less than 5 min) after adding the substrate solution.

References

1. Gorovits B et al (2013) Bioanalysis of antibody-drug conjugates: American Association of Pharmaceutical Scientists antibody-drug conjugate working group position paper. Bioanalysis 5(9):997–1006
2. Khan MN, Findlay JWA (2009) Ligand-binding assays development, validation, and implementation in the drug development arena. Hoboken, NJ Wiley
3. Khot A, Sharma S, Shah DK (2015) Integration of bioanalytical measurements using PK-PD modeling and simulation: implications for antibody-drug conjugate development. Bioanalysis 7(13):1633–1648
4. Kaur S et al (2013) Bioanalytical assay strategies for the development of antibody-drug conjugate biotherapeutics. Bioanalysis 5 (2):201–226
5. Stephan JP, Kozak KR, Wong WL (2011) Challenges in developing bioanalytical assays for characterization of antibody-drug conjugates. Bioanalysis 3(6):677–700
6. Dowell JA et al (2001) Pharmacokinetics of gemtuzumab ozogamicin, an antibody-targeted chemotherapy agent for the treatment of patients with acute myeloid leukemia in first relapse. J Clin Pharmacol 41(11):1206–1214
7. Lewis Phillips GD et al (2008) Targeting HER2-positive breast cancer with trastuzumab-DM1, an antibody-cytotoxic drug conjugate. Cancer Res 68 (22):9280–9290

8. Pollack VA et al (2007) Treatment parameters modulating regression of human melanoma xenografts by an antibody-drug conjugate (CR011-vcMMAE) targeting GPNMB. Cancer Chemother Pharmacol 60(3):423–435
9. Hwu P et al (2009) A phase I/II study of CR011-vcMMAE, an antibody-drug conjugate (ADC) targeting glycoprotein NMB (GPNMB) in patients (pts) with advanced melanoma. J Clin Oncol 27(15S):9032–9032
10. Sznol M et al (2009) Pharmacokinetics (PK) of CR011-vcMMAE, an antibody-drug conjugate (ADC), in a phase (Ph) I study of patients (pts) with advanced melanoma. J Clin Oncol 27(15S):9063–9063
11. Junutula JR et al (2008) Site-specific conjugation of a cytotoxic drug to an antibody improves the therapeutic index. Nat Biotechnol 26(8):925–932
12. Singh AP, Shah DK (2017) Measurement and mathematical characterization of cell-level pharmacokinetics of antibody-drug conjugates: a case study with Trastuzumab-vc-MMAE. Drug Metab Dispos 45 (11):1120–1132
13. Singh AP et al (2019) A cell-level systems PK-PD model to characterize in vivo efficacy of ADCs. Pharmaceutics 11(2):pii: E98
14. Stephan JP et al (2008) Anti-CD22-MCC-DM1 and MC-MMAF conjugates: impact of assay format on pharmacokinetic parameters determination. Bioconjug Chem 19 (8):1673–1683
15. Xie H et al (2004) Pharmacokinetics and biodistribution of the antitumor immunoconjugate, cantuzumab mertansine (huC242-DM1), and its two components in mice. J Pharmacol Exp Ther 308(3):1073–1082
16. Kovtun YV et al (2006) Antibody-drug conjugates designed to eradicate tumors with homogeneous and heterogeneous expression of the target antigen. Cancer Res 66(6):3214–3221
17. Advani A et al (2010) Safety, pharmacokinetics, and preliminary clinical activity of inotuzumab ozogamicin, a novel immunoconjugate for the treatment of B-cell non-Hodgkin's lymphoma: results of a phase I study. J Clin Oncol 28 (12):2085–2093
18. DiJoseph JF et al (2004) Antibody-targeted chemotherapy with CMC-544: a CD22-targeted immunoconjugate of calicheamicin for the treatment of B-lymphoid malignancies. Blood 103(5):1807–1814
19. Alley SC et al (2008) Contribution of linker stability to the activities of anticancer immunoconjugates. Bioconjug Chem 19(3):759–765
20. Tolcher AW et al (2003) Cantuzumab mertansine, a maytansinoid immunoconjugate directed to the CanAg antigen: a phase I, pharmacokinetic, and biologic correlative study. J Clin Oncol 21(2):211–222
21. Sanderson RJ et al (2005) In vivo drug-linker stability of an anti-CD30 dipeptide-linked auristatin immunoconjugate. Clin Cancer Res 11 (2 Pt 1):843–852

Index

L. Nathan Tumey (ed.), *Antibody-Drug Conjugates: Methods and Protocols*, Methods in Molecular Biology, vol. 2078, https://doi.org/10.1007/978-1-4939-9929-3, © Springer Science+Business Media, LLC, part of Springer Nature 2020

MIX
Papier aus verantwortungsvollen Quellen
Paper from responsible sources
FSC® C105338

If you have any concerns about our products,
you can contact us on
ProductSafety@springernature.com

In case Publisher is established outside the EU,
the EU authorized representative is:
Springer Nature Customer Service Center GmbH
Europaplatz 3, 69115 Heidelberg, Germany

Printed by Libri Plureos GmbH
in Hamburg, Germany